Breaking Negative Eating Patterns and Remembering Your True Self

This book is a practical self-help manual that provides step-by-step guidance on applying a whole-self approach for eating disorders and eating difficulties grounded in Schema Therapy.

Structured in two parts, the book addresses how to overcome the thinking, emotional, and behavioural patterns that drive eating difficulties, using powerful experiential strategies for change. It helps readers understand the factors that drive and maintain their eating and body image patterns and offers effective techniques for overcoming them. Readers will learn to reconnect with their true self that lies beneath these protective patterns, discovering new ways to meet their deepest needs. Templates and worksheets provide useful resources that support recovery.

The first of its kind, this book supports those suffering from eating disorders and serves as a reference and adjunct to face-to-face therapy for therapists and clinicians.

Susan Simpson, DClinPsy, is Australian Clinical Psychologist and Schema Therapist who has lived and worked in Scotland for over 25 years. She is both a clinician and researcher, specialising in whole-person trauma-informed approaches to eating disorders, and is co-author of clinician guides *Schema Therapy for Eating Disorders* and the *Cambridge Guide to Schema Therapy*.

"Eating disorders can be very difficult to overcome. Even if one is able to access psychotherapy, there are days and often weeks between appointments. This is where this self-help book comes into its own providing an innovative array of practical tools to assist with the journey towards recovery. It is easy to read and understand and provides essential clinical skills to deal with the significant challenges that confront those with an eating disorder. With this book by your side, you will not feel alone. It is a wonderful resource to have."

Emeritus Professor Stephen Touyz, *University of Sydney, Australia*

"*Breaking Negative Thinking Patterns and Remembering Your True Self* distils theory and knowledge of schema therapy and related modalities with the author's clinical wisdom. The result is an engaging, compassionate and practical resource which is well placed to enhance in-person therapy and/or provide guidance towards recovery for people experiencing eating disorders."

Professor Phillipa Hay, *Western Sydney University, Australia*

"The true self is calling. It's time to come home.' This is Susan Simpson's message to anyone struggling with an eating disorder. This is in the spirit of influential figures like Kierkegaard, Nietzsche, Jung and Winnicott who pointed to the centrality of finding and living from one's authentic self. With rich clinical examples and approachable everyday metaphors and exercises, this wonderful book shows that this is no abstract idea, but a project that can be intelligently and compassionately embarked on in very practical ways. Her lucid synthesis of current scientific research with clinical insights from the increasingly influential schema therapy approach, Simpson shows how deadening psychological patterns that result in mere surviving, rather than energized thriving, can be understood and steadily and radically transformed. I will be recommending this book widely and not only to clients with eating disorders."

Kalsched, D. (2013). Trauma and the soul: A psycho-spiritual approach to human development and its interruption. Routledge.

Professor David Edwards, *Rhodes University, South Africa*

"Grounded in decades of clinical practice, this deeply wise and wonderfully practical book draws on key strands of contemporary psychotherapy to guide readers on a clear and flexible path to integration and recovery. Highly recommended for individuals experiencing eating or other mental health difficulties, as well as carers, clinicians, and all who want to better understand the beautiful messiness of being human."

Dr. Beth Shelton, *Counselling Psychologist and Eating Disorder Sector leader*

Breaking Negative Eating Patterns and Remembering Your True Self

A Self-Help and Support Book

Susan Simpson

Routledge
Taylor & Francis Group
LONDON AND NEW YORK

Designed cover image: Natalya Matyushina

Illustrations by Dominika Sambor

First published 2027
by Routledge
4 Park Square, Milton Park, Abingdon, Oxon OX14 4RN

and by Routledge
605 Third Avenue, New York, NY 10158

Routledge is an imprint of the Taylor & Francis Group, an informa business

British Library Cataloguing-in-Publication Data
A catalogue record for this book is available from the British Library

ISBN: 978-1-032-41022-7 (hbk)
ISBN: 978-1-032-41021-0 (pbk)
ISBN: 978-1-003-35587-8 (ebk)

DOI: 10.4324/9781003355878

Typeset in Galliard
by Apex CoVantage, LLC

Access the Support Material: www.routledge.com/9781032410227

To Craig, Finn, and Rory—thank you for your unconditional love, and for always being true to who you are.

Contents

Figures

Tables

Characters

Character 1 Sophie	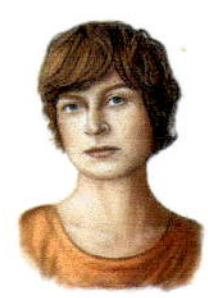	26
Character 2 Tony	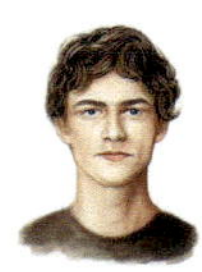	53
Character 3 Samantha	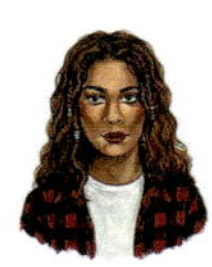	25
Character 4 Harriet	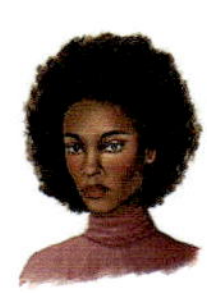	11
Character 5 Melissa	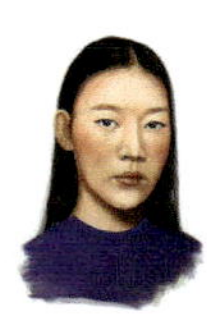	9

Acknowledgements

A huge thank you to **Kaja Dwulat** for her incredible support, creativity, honesty, and feedback throughout this book-writing journey and to **Dominika Sambor** for her wonderful artistic contributions. I am also deeply grateful to **Hannah Slater** for her brave, generous insights and to **Corinne Reid, Andrea Papitsch-Clark, Jacqui Finnigan, and Emma Mawdsley** for their thoughtful feedback on the manuscript. Finally, I wish to thank the many people with eating disorders who have helped me understand their inner world.

Introduction

Introduction: How to Use This Book

> *There's a disconnect between that clever, clever brain and human heart, love, and compassion. Only when head and heart work in harmony can we attain our true human potential.*
>
> —Jane Goodall (1).

This book is an invitation to remember yourself—reconnecting with parts of you that became buried when survival became more urgent than authenticity.

Beneath the eating difficulties, beneath the coping strategies that once helped you manage overwhelming feelings, there's a calmer, wiser part of you still waiting—the part that knows how to feel joy, trust your instincts, and be genuinely yourself. That part has been waiting for conditions that make it safe enough to emerge. Together, we'll create those conditions.

What You've Been Looking For

Do you recognise yourself in any of these?

- Constant battles with food—overeating, undereating, or swinging between both
- Guilt after "unhealthy" foods or missed exercise
- A life shaped by pleasing others or chasing approval
- Therapies that focused on food but not on you

If so, this book was written with you in mind. Eating difficulties make sense when we understand the context in which they began—they are often an understandable response rather than a sign that something is wrong with you. They often signal that essential emotional needs—safety, acceptance, belonging, freedom—have not yet been met.

You may have tried approaches that addressed eating patterns but didn't quite reach what was underneath. Perhaps you sensed that treatment helped

DOI: 10.4324/9781003355878-1

on the surface, but didn't fully get to what was really going on. You're not alone. Many people describe feeling like they're living behind a mask, going through the motions of life without truly inhabiting their own experience. They sense that their eating difficulties are just the surface of something much deeper—a disconnection that developed as a way of surviving when being real felt too risky.

This book offers a different path. Instead of fighting your symptoms, we'll come to understand them as expressions of your intelligence and adaptability. Instead of focusing solely on food, we'll explore what it means to reconnect—with yourself, with others, and with the world around you.

A Different Kind of Recovery

Eating patterns often emerge as ingenious attempts to meet emotional needs when direct expression felt unsafe. Restriction may have brought a sense of control amid chaos; bingeing may have offered comfort when no one else could. These patterns reflect creative ways of coping—ways that once supported survival, and can, over time, begin to limit the life you long for.

The same intelligence that built those patterns can also guide you towards new, life-giving ways to meet your needs.

What Makes This Approach Different

Rooted in Schema Therapy[1] and body-based approaches, this model looks beyond symptoms to the whole person. You'll learn to:

- **Reclaim lost parts of yourself**—your playfulness, creativity, and capacity for joy
- **Understand your adaptations** as intelligent responses to real pain
- **Integrate thinking and feeling** so your inner world works in harmony
- **Nourish yourself** with genuine emotional "vitamins": safety, connection, mastery, freedom, and healthy boundaries
- **Heal the split** between your clever brain and compassionate heart that allows for authentic living

This isn't about changing into someone else. It's about finding your way back to the person you've always been beneath the layers of protection.

Your Journey Back Home

Recovery is less about changing eating behaviours and more about coming home to yourself—rediscovering passions, trusting your instincts, and forming relationships where you can be real instead of performing. The path is rarely linear; it includes setbacks and small moments of recognition. Real healing is messy, human, and deeply personal.

This looks different for different people. For some, it means reconnecting with interests that got lost along the way; for others, learning to trust their own perceptions and feelings after years of self-doubt. The path is rarely linear. Real healing unfolds through setbacks, breakthroughs, small moments of recognition, and gradual shifts in how you relate to yourself and the world.

How This Book Works

This book can accompany your therapy journey or serve as a standalone resource, depending on your needs and circumstances. If you're currently working with a therapist, the concepts and exercises here can deepen and support that work. If you're exploring on your own, the framework provides a comprehensive map for understanding and transformation.

Everything you need to do the work is here in these pages. Where we couldn't go into depth—because this is already a lot to hold—you'll find optional online appendices and supporting materials if you want to explore particular topics more fully or revisit tools in more detail.

A note about medical safety: If you're experiencing physical complications from restrictive eating, bingeing, purging, or other eating behaviours, it's important to work with medical and/or dietetic professionals to ensure your safety. The psychological healing described in this book requires adequate physical nourishment to support your brain and body's capacity for change and integration.

The chapters build upon each other, moving from understanding how your patterns developed to meeting the different parts of yourself to practical work on integration and change. Take your time with each section—this isn't material to rush through but wisdom to absorb gradually.

What Lies Ahead

In the pages that follow, you'll discover that beneath the eating difficulties lies someone with unique gifts, perspectives, and ways of connecting with the world. You'll learn that your struggles reflect your system's remarkable capacity to adapt and survive under challenging circumstances.

The journey back to yourself begins with understanding how your adaptations developed, continues through reclaiming the parts of you that went into hiding, and leads to a life where all aspects of yourself can contribute to your flourishing.

As Jane Goodall[2] reminds us, it's only when head and heart work together that we reach our true potential. That integration—between thinking and feeling, between independence and connection, between all the different parts of who you are—is both the path and the destination of the work ahead.

Most importantly, you'll find that what has been hidden is not lost. The part of you that knows how to feel, connect, and create has been waiting for the conditions to emerge. This book will help you build those conditions—step by step, gently and persistently—until your life begins to feel like your own again.

It's time to come home.

A Note on Language

Throughout this book, I often use the pronouns "she" and "her" when introducing clients and examples. This helps keep the writing simple and coherent. However, eating difficulties affect people of all genders. If you identify as male, nonbinary, or with any other gender, please know that these stories and tools are for you. Feel welcome to substitute the language that best reflects who you are.

You belong here.

Notes

1 Tippett, K. & Goodall, J. (Autumn, 2020). The Shadow of Humanity and the Spirit of Animals A conversation. Orion Magazine. Jane Goodall is a pioneering primatologist and anthropologist whose decades of research revolutionised our understanding of the emotional lives of animals. Her work bridged the gap between scientific observation and compassionate connection, demonstrating that true understanding requires both rigorous thinking and open-hearted empathy.

2 Schema Therapy, developed by Dr. Jeffrey Young, helps people recognise the early patterns that shape how they relate to themselves and others and works with their different modes—or parts of self—to repair emotional injuries and meet core needs. For further details on Schema Therapy for Eating Difficulties, see Appendix 1.

1 Understanding Your Eating Difficulties

A Novel Whole-Self Approach

A Moment of Recognition

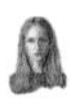 Emma stands before her bathroom mirror, toothbrush in hand. She's done this a thousand times, yet something feels off. The eyes staring back seem both hers and not hers—like meeting an old friend she somehow lost.

For three years, Emma's world has revolved around rules about food and exercise. They once offered control, safety, and even identity. The strategies that once saved her now feel like a life raft she never stepped off—keeping her afloat, yet far from the shore of her own life. If Emma's story feels familiar, you're not alone. Many people sense this disconnection—not just from their bodies but from their being. The person you were meant to become feels buried beneath coping patterns that once made life safer. This chapter begins the process of understanding that disconnection and tracing the path back towards yourself.

Nature Always Finds a Way—How You've Adapted

When a plant grows in the shadows, it twists toward the light. Its shape tells the story of how it survived. The same is true for you. Your eating behaviours are signs of creative intelligence responding to scarcity—scarcity of safety, acceptance, or freedom to be yourself.

Your Adaptations

Perhaps showing emotion was not welcome, so food became a safer language for distress. Perhaps connection felt risky, so control over eating became your reliable companion. Each behaviour arose for a reason: to meet needs that felt otherwise unreachable.

These evolved as workarounds. But what kept you safe yesterday may now block the sunlight you need today.

Reflection: Instead of asking "What's wrong with me?" try "What have my eating patterns been protecting me from—or trying to give me?"

DOI: 10.4324/9781003355878-2

When Changing Behaviours Isn't Enough: The Missing Piece

Many treatments focus on thoughts and behaviours alone. They can be useful, even life-saving, but they often overlook the purpose behind the patterns. Change lasts only when we meet the need the behaviour once met.

The goal is to gently expand beyond coping by creating conditions where your real needs—connection, safety, expression—can be met directly. To understand these adaptations more clearly, we'll explore how your inner world is organised—the crew that keeps your ship sailing.

Your Inner Sailing Ship—Meeting Your Crew

Imagine your inner world as a sailing ship navigating unpredictable seas. Each part of you is a crew member with a role: some steer, some patch sails, some keep lookout. When the weather is calm and the crew communicate well, the voyage feels purposeful. But when storms come, the crew may lose connection and forget they're on the same team.

At the heart of the ship lives your *Inner Child*—the sensitive, curious, feeling part who senses wind and tide, who knows what brings joy or danger. She represents your emotional truth and capacity for wonder.

The *Wise Captain*, your inner leader, combines heart and reason—listening to the child's intuition whilst charting a steady course. When these two work together, you steer with both courage and compassion.

But when our environments discourage emotion or independence, the captain never fully develops, and the child retreats below deck. Survival-focused crew take command—efficient and analytical but mostly rigid and disconnected from feelings.

Emma's story shows how this happens: growing up where emotional expression felt unsafe, she learned to control herself through self-denial. Food restriction became both discipline and a distress call. The result? A clever mind steering without the heart's compass.

Recognising this inner split is the first step towards healing. The goal isn't to fire the survival crew—it's to reunite them under wiser leadership. To do that, we first need to understand what keeps the crew—and you—alive and thriving. Beneath all our strategies lies a simple reality: the human system depends on emotional nourishment as much as the body depends on food. But what happens when these real nutrients are scarce or inconsistent? Our systems find substitutes.

Emotional Vitamins—What Your System Actually Needs

Plants grow in response to the soil, light, and care available to them. Human beings are no different. When a tree struggles to grow, we don't ask, "What's wrong with you?"—we look at the conditions it has been growing in. This way of seeing invites understanding rather than shame. When our bodies lack nutritional nourishment, they weaken. When our emotional nourishment runs low, something similar happens to our inner world: we lose colour, curiosity, and connection.

These invisible nutrients—*Emotional Vitamins* (2)—are the psychological equivalents of sunlight, water, and soil. They allow us to feel safe, alive and capable of growth. When they're scarce, we adapt in creative but costly ways.

Two Pillars of Emotional Health

Human thriving rests on two fundamental groups of vitamins: *Connection* and *Autonomy*. Think of them as the two legs you stand on (3). When they're balanced, you feel grounded; when one is weak, you limp through life.

Connection Vitamins—Belonging, Safety, and Warmth

These nourish the heart side of being human.

Vitamin:

- **Safety and Stability**: The experience of having a *safe harbour*—someone emotionally available, predictable, accepting. As children, this often comes from caregivers who were mostly present and responsive, allowing us to feel protected even when we made mistakes. When this need is unmet, we grow up scanning for danger or fearing rejection; closeness can feel either desperately needed or too risky to trust. Stability allows us to be vulnerable without fear of losing connection.
- **Connection and Belonging**: The felt sense that you matter to others and have a secure place in their hearts. This grows when you are seen, listened to, valued, and cherished, simply for being who you are—not for what you achieve or how you appear. In early life, it's nurtured through attuned relationships that communicate, "You are wanted here." When this vitamin runs low, we may search endlessly for approval, mould ourselves to fit in, or withdraw to avoid more rejection. Genuine belonging allows your whole system to settle, so you can simply be.
- **Play and Spontaneity**: The freedom to explore, laugh, and create, without performance or fear of judgement. In childhood, it shows up when adults delight in your joy rather than manage it—when curiosity and silliness are welcomed, not shamed. Play restores vitality; it teaches flexibility and helps emotions flow. When this need is unmet, life becomes overly serious or constrained, and pleasure can feel unsafe or undeserved. Reclaiming play is how the heart remembers it's alive.

When these vitamins flow freely, the world feels safe enough to reach out, risk closeness, and enjoy being alive.

Autonomy Vitamins—Identity, Freedom, and Mastery

These feed your sense of self—your ability to act, choose, and create.

Vitamin:

- ***M*astery**: The sense of being capable and effective in the world. It begins when caregivers encourage effort rather than perfection—celebrating curiosity, persistence, and small triumphs. This vitamin grows through ***small doses of challenge followed by support***—the experience of "I can try, and it's safe to fail." When it's missing, effort feels humiliating, mistakes feel catastrophic, and achievement becomes the only route to self-worth. True mastery restores confidence through the joy of learning and creating, rather than control.
- ***F*reedom to Express Needs and Emotions**: The permission to have your own thoughts, feelings, and preferences—and to voice them without fear of rejection or punishment. In early life, this need is met when adults listen and respect your individuality, even when they disagree. When it's unmet, you may silence your opinions, over-adapt to others, or rebel against control. Reclaiming this freedom means rediscovering your own voice and trusting that it deserves to be heard.
- ***L*imits and Boundaries**: The experience of structure that protects rather than confines. Healthy limits teach that both your needs and others' needs matter. In childhood, this comes from caregivers who set consistent rules with warmth, modelling mutual respect. When limits are **too harsh or controlling**, children may grow fearful of losing freedom and push back in protest; when too loose, life can feel chaotic and unsafe. Balanced boundaries allow connection **without suffocation**.

When these are present, you can stand on your own feet and stay connected to others—firm roots and flexible branches.

The Delicate Balance

Connection without autonomy can feel smothering; autonomy without connection can feel lonely. True wellbeing comes when both sets of vitamins circulate together—when you can say, "I belong here, and I am still myself."

Yet many environments struggle to provide this balance. Some families and educational settings offer closeness but little space for individuality; others prize achievement whilst overlooking tenderness. Many cultures hold self-control and independence in high regard, while emotional openness is sometimes less visible or supported.

When our emotional vitamins are out of balance for too long, our system finds ways to adapt.

Melissa's Story: The Cost of Scarcity

 Melissa grew up in a family full of care but short on boundaries. Everyone sacrificed for everyone else. Love meant depletion. She learned that to need was to be a burden. To protect others, she shrank her appetite for food, comfort, and attention.

Restrictive eating became her moral compass: *If I take nothing, I can't hurt anyone.* Her body obeyed; emotionally she starved. The split between thinking and feeling widened, leaving her outwardly capable yet inwardly empty.

Your Emotional Provisions Check-In

Imagine six barrels in the hold of your inner ship—each one representing an emotional vitamin. How full were they in your early life, and how full are they now? (There's nothing to get right—just notice what you find.)

Ask yourself:

- Which barrels feel full?
- Which run low when stress hits?
- How do I try to refill them—through people, through achievements, through food, through control?

Notice patterns rather than judging them. Every adaptation tells a story about what your system needed and how it survived. As you start receiving these emotional nutrients again—through balanced, stable relationships, genuine self-expression, and nourishing routines—your mind and body begin to move in the same direction.

See Appendix 2 for the Provisions Barrels Worksheet.

When Real Vitamins Are Scarce—The Creative Solutions Begin

When the genuine sources of nourishment—safety, belonging, freedom—become scarce or unpredictable, the human system gets creative in how it copes.

Like a plant stretching toward artificial light, you found ways to keep living. These makeshift substitutes may have looked like control, discipline, or comfort sometimes even shaping your relationship with food and your body. They kept you going. But over time, what once helped you survive may have gradually taken charge of the whole garden.

The Birth of Creative Substitutes

Eating patterns often arise as substitute sources of the vitamins we couldn't safely receive. They provide genuine, if temporary, relief—structure instead of chaos, detached comfort instead of connection, mastery where a sense of choice and agency was hard to access. Each pattern carries its own logic:

Connection Vitamin Substitutes

- **Safety and Stability** → Rigid rules and routines bring order when relationships feel unpredictable.
- **Connection and Belonging** → Restriction of food or self-deprivation may create a sense of purity or worthiness; bingeing can offer the warmth of comfort that was missing; rituals around food might generate a sense of predictability and certainty when other aspects of life feel out of control.
- **Play and Spontaneity** → Eating rituals or secret indulgence in food can become the only moments where pleasure feels permitted.

Autonomy Vitamin Substitutes

- **Freedom to Express** → Skipping meals or eating in secret may speak what words cannot: *I need space. I can say what I feel and need. I can decide on my own destiny.*
- **Mastery** → Counting, controlling, and perfecting food or exercise offers tangible achievement when emotional mastery feels impossible.
- **Limits and Boundaries** → Food rules create firm edges when life's boundaries are either too harsh or too loose.

Each behaviour reflects intelligence at work—your system protecting itself in the only way it knew how.

Samantha's Story: Comfort in Disguise

 Samantha grew up in a family where being "tough" was a point of pride. When loneliness or sadness crept in, her dad's cheerful "Toughen up, sunshine!" made it clear that tears weren't an option. Food became the comfort she could reach for instead. Bingeing became her secret shelter, a reliable way to feel cared for when her nervous system needed warmth in a household that prized stoicism.

The Hook of Temporary Relief

These patterns work—for a while. They bring calm, focus, even a sense of identity. That's why letting go can feel impossible: each behaviour once offered something essential. But just as a plant can't thrive forever under fluorescent light, we can't flourish on substitutes alone. They sustain life but dim vitality.

Over time, these creative solutions begin to reinforce the very split that caused the problem: the clever brain stays in charge whilst the feeling heart waits below deck.

Reframing the Story

Instead of seeing your eating patterns as enemies to conquer, try viewing them as letters from your past self—each one saying, "I did what I could with what I had." Your task now isn't to tear those letters up, but to read them with compassion and decide what their messages mean for the person you're becoming.

Next, we'll explore what happens when the ship loses its captain—the Wise Self—and how survival mode takes the helm. Understanding this leadership vacuum sets the stage for re-establishing balance and genuine nourishment.

The Lost Inner Captain and Survival-Mode Leadership

When genuine emotional nourishment is scarce, the part of you designed to steer your life—the Inner Captain—doesn't fully get to grow into their role. They are still there, but without enough guidance and attunement early on, a stable sense of self and direction doesn't fully take shape.

In their place, a quick-thinking emergency crew takes the wheel. These inner Protectors know how to keep the ship afloat during storms, but they're not trained for long voyages. They operate on short-term safety, scanning constantly for danger, tightening every rope. In the process, they keep the vessel moving—but only in circles.

How the Captain Gets Lost

Your Inner Captain—the Wise Self—develops through consistent experiences of being understood, guided, and supported. When those "training conditions" are missing, leadership defaults to whoever shouts the loudest: the parts that promise control or protection. These parts are brilliant crisis managers. They keep emotions contained, relationships smooth, and danger at bay. Yet they do so by narrowing your range of feeling and choice. The cost of safety is freedom.

When the Crew Runs the Ship

Once survival modes are in charge, every decision becomes about avoidance:

- Avoid rejection.
- Avoid abandonment.
- Avoid failure.
- Avoid need.

The crew mistakes emotional shutdown for safety. Over time, life becomes a series of calculated manoeuvres rather than an authentic journey. You might recognise this as the constant inner tension between parts of you—one urging control, another craving release. Both are trying to protect you, but neither can steer the whole vessel alone.

Harriet's Story: Safety through Disappearing

As a child, 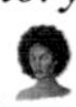 Harriet learned that strong feelings invited punishment or ridicule. When trauma struck later, she had no safe harbour to turn to. Her system decided that the best way to survive was to disappear.

Food restriction became her muted protest and her protection at once: *If I become small enough, no one can hurt me.* Her emergency crew worked tirelessly—monitoring calories, chasing perfection, silencing the pain below deck. It succeeded in keeping her functioning but at the cost of vitality, spontaneity, and connection.

Recognising the Pattern

If you've been living in survival leadership for years, it can feel almost normal—like running on high alert is just "how you are." But that state isn't your natural rhythm; it's how your system learned to cope.

Reclaiming your Inner Captain means holding appreciation for the crew and the roles they've played, while gradually restoring leadership so that wisdom, empathy, and direction come from a place of steadiness rather than fear.

The First Step Back to the Helm

The process begins with simple awareness:

Who's steering right now?

When you notice the inner voices that drive perfection, avoidance, or control, pause before reacting. Gently reassure this side of you: "It's okay. I know you're trying to keep me safe." This small act of recognition begins to build trust in your inner system. It shows each part that you're willing to listen and understand—that you see it has its own story and a good reason for being there.

There's no expectation of change at this stage, no need to fix or force anything. These are *tiny first steps*—moments of compassionate contact with yourself. Awareness itself is the beginning of transformation.

In the next section, we'll explore how to move from mere survival to genuine thriving—learning to draw on real nourishment instead of substitutes and allowing the captain and crew to work together as a united team. Awareness of who's at the helm opens the doorway to a new phase—one where leadership begins to return to wisdom rather than fear.

From Surviving to Thriving—Accessing Real Vitamins

Our brains and bodies are built for change. Even when patterns have been in place for decades, due to neuroplasticity and our brains' lifelong capacity to learn and grow, the human system can rewire and grow new connections. What once kept you safe doesn't have to define you forever. The same creativity that built your coping patterns can now build your recovery.

Healing begins when we stop trying to fight the old adaptations and start listening to what they've been trying to achieve. Recovery is about gradually creating conditions where you can get your emotional needs met in healthier, more direct ways. When those needs are nourished, the pull of eating-based coping naturally lessens.

Recovery involves acknowledging what's been lost—time consumed by eating difficulties, relationships strained, experiences missed, nourishing emotional vitamins that you deserved but didn't receive. This grief is a normal part of healing. We'll explore this more deeply as you progress.

Developing Your Wise Self

Developing this new way of living means strengthening your Wise Self—the inner leader capable of guiding every part of you with steadiness and compassion. She doesn't silence your protective parts but listens to their fears, thanks them for their work, and shows them new ways to feel safe. This process builds an internal sense of *earned security*: the lived experience that you can have needs, express emotion, and stay connected without catastrophe following.

As this sense of safety grows, the old split between self-protection and vitality begins to mend. You may notice that moments of joy, hunger, sadness, and creativity start to feel less threatening. Instead of oscillating between control and collapse, you begin to experience a more grounded rhythm—an inner state where self-awareness and spontaneity coexist.

Real Vitamins versus Substitutes

Accessing "real vitamins" means learning to recognise the difference between temporary substitutes and genuine nourishment.

Substitute forms of mastery and achievement might look like relentless attempts to control eating weight or shape, whereas real mastery feels like engagement, curiosity, and pride in small steps of progress. Substitute belonging might come from external approval, whilst real belonging arises when you can be known as you truly are.

As these genuine sources of nourishment accumulate, recovery stops being about restriction or control strategies—it becomes about *participation*: being fully alive in your own experience. The more you strengthen this authentic way of meeting needs, the less you'll rely on food to carry emotional messages.

Integration, Not Elimination

The goal is to bring your different parts into balance, rather than trying to get rid of them. Every coping strategy contains fragments of wisdom about what mattered to you—safety, order, love, freedom. Rather than erasing them, recovery is about expanding your repertoire.

Eating-based coping may once have been your only route to relief; now it can become one of many options, gradually replaced by choices that sustain rather than deplete you.

When these inner parts begin working together under the guidance of your Wise Self, life stops revolving around survival. It starts expanding towards meaning, purpose, and genuine connection. The work ahead is not to perfect yourself, but to remember how to live as a whole, responsive, and fully human being.

Your Whole-Self Recovery Journey

True recovery is about helping every part of you to find its rightful place in the system. The patterns that once helped you survive still hold valuable information about your needs, fears, and strengths. Healing means allowing these parts to collaborate rather than compete, creating an inner environment where integration can finally occur.

When your inner world works together—when protective parts trust that they no longer need to run the show, and your Wise Self can guide from a place of steadiness—you begin to experience what we might call *joined-up living*. Life starts to feel more in sync. The part that plans and the part that feels, the part that protects and the part that longs for connection, can finally communicate. Decisions start to feel both grounded and real.

What Whole-Self Recovery Looks Like

This is what whole-self recovery looks like: more aligned, less about being perfect. You start to respond rather than react, to express needs directly rather than through food or control, and to build relationships that include rather than erase your authenticity. The focus shifts from managing symptoms to cultivating aliveness.

The path ahead isn't linear. It winds, circles, and doubles back, because growth is rarely tidy. Progress may appear in small moments—choosing rest instead of overworking, expressing emotion rather than suppressing it, noticing hunger as information rather than a threat. Each small act of reconnection is a sign that your internal leadership is growing stronger.

The Journey Ahead

The chapters that follow will guide you step by step through this process. You'll learn how to recognise the social and cultural influences that shaped your adaptations, meet and understand the parts of yourself that carry old roles, rebuild connection with your Wise Self, and experiment with new ways of meeting needs in everyday life. Along the way, you'll develop relationships—both inner and outer—that support your ongoing growth.

Ultimately, this work is about *reclaiming sovereignty*—being able to guide your life in a way that feels true to you. It's not about control or self-denial but a steady confident way of living in line with your own values and needs. When your Wise Self leads with compassion, the energy once spent on maintaining defences becomes available for creativity, intimacy, and joy.

Permission for Imperfect Recovery

You also have permission for imperfect recovery. Healing is not a final destination or a flawless state—it's a practice of staying in relationship with yourself, even when you wobble. Integration means allowing contradictions to coexist: strength and vulnerability, independence and belonging, effort and rest. It's the capacity to live as a whole, complex human being rather than a project to be managed.

As you move forward, remember that what has been hidden is not lost. The part of you that knows how to feel, connect, and create has been waiting for the conditions to emerge. This book will help you build those conditions—step by step, gently and persistently—until your life begins to feel like your own again. This journey isn't about returning to who you were before the eating disorder or to the pain that shaped that time. It's to reconnect with the parts of you that became lost or silenced, and learning to live, breathe, and relate from them again.

Gentle Experiments to Try

You've now been introduced to a way of understanding eating difficulties that goes far beyond food. This is not a quick fix but a process of remembering—of reuniting with the parts of you that have been waiting for safety, expression, and care. As you move forward, it can help to begin noticing, in simple everyday ways, how your system communicates and what it's asking for.

Think of these short reflections as gentle experiments—ways of listening to yourself with curiosity instead of criticism.

1. The Daydream Experiment

For the next week, give yourself permission to engage in a gentle *daydream fantasy.* Each morning, as you move through your usual rituals—showering, brushing your teeth, getting dressed—let your imagination wander.

Visualise this simple magic: you put down this book, step out of the room, and as you close the door behind you, your eating difficulties dissolve—completely gone, as if they never existed.

Now take a slow breath and allow the picture to unfold naturally. Without forcing or analysing, notice:

- What is different in your life now that food, weight, and control no longer take centre stage?
- What do you notice first—inside you or around you?
- What would you **do more** of?
- What would you **do less** of?
- What would you **start doing** that you've held back from?
- What would you **stop doing** that no longer feels necessary?
- What might begin to fill the space that the eating difficulties once occupied?

Then, turn your curiosity toward any edges or unease that arise:

- Is there anything about this imagined freedom that feels *unsettling* or *frightening*?
- Do new problems or worries appear—either for you or for people around you—when the old problem disappears?
- What, if anything, still feels missing or incomplete even in this fantasy of recovery?
- What hopes surface? What fears?

Spend a few minutes writing down whatever you discover each day. There are no right or wrong answers—just gentle noticing.

Rather than being about wishful thinking, this is a way for your *Wise Self* (Inner Captain) to glimpse what true freedom might feel like and to begin understanding both the desires *and* the fears tied up with change. Every image or feeling that surfaces—pleasant or uneasy—offers valuable information about what healing will ask of you and what it might give back in return.

Come back to this exercise as you move through recovery, observing how your mind and body respond at different points along the way.

2. Emotional Nourishment Scan

At different points in your day, pause and ask: *What kind of nourishment do I most need right now?* Is it comfort, rest, laughter, company, honesty, solitude, or movement? There's no right answer. The goal is simply to start recognising when you reach for food, control, or avoidance as a substitute for another kind of sustenance. Each moment of awareness is a step towards real nourishment.

3. Gratitude for Adaptation

Before you sleep, take a moment to thank your system for its creativity. Even the most painful behaviours began as attempts to care for yourself in some way. Gratitude here is about acknowledging your resilience and the ways you've tried to get through. This simple shift from blame to understanding can begin to dissolve shame and open space for healing.

Journalling Prompt Reflections: Understanding Your Eating Difficulties

Set aside 10 minutes with your journal:

- What idea in this chapter created a sense of recognition—that "yes, this is me" feeling?
- Which emotional vitamins felt most scarce in your early life?
- What creative solutions did your system develop when those vitamins were missing?
- If your eating patterns could speak, what might they be trying to tell you?

Each of these reflections helps you strengthen the relationship between awareness and compassion—the foundation of whole-self recovery. Over time, this gentle curiosity becomes your compass, guiding you towards genuine nourishment and away from old habits of self-criticism or control.

In the next chapter, we'll look more closely at how your eating patterns formed in context—exploring the social, cultural, and relational forces that shape the ways we learn to meet our needs. Our inner worlds never exist in isolation. The way you've learned to think, feel, and cope has been shaped not only by your own experiences but also by the cultural, relational, and biological environments you grew up in. The emotional vitamins available to you were filtered through family histories, social expectations, and unspoken cultural rules about whose needs matter and which emotions are welcome.

Understanding these influences is the next step towards living as the person you were always meant to be: grounded, free, fully alive.

2 When Eating Difficulties Emerge

How Temperament, Culture, and Connection Intertwine

In a world shaped by performance and protection, it is genuine presence that truly nourishes us.

Emma's Question

Emma sits in her therapist's office, hands curled around a mug she's barely tasted. "Why me?" she asks at last. "Why did I end up with an eating disorder when my sister didn't? We grew up in the same house."

It's a question that echoes through many therapy rooms. Emma's sister seems effortlessly confident—comfortable in her body, sure of her place in the world. Emma, meanwhile, has spent years counting, measuring, and apologising for existing. Her life has been ruled by invisible arithmetic: calories, grades, approval.

There is no single answer to her question, only an intertwining story—a story of temperament, culture, and early relationships that shaped how her system learned to stay safe.

Eating patterns rarely appear out of nowhere. As we explored in Chapter 1, they develop as creative responses to environments that felt unpredictable or overwhelming. They emerge when parts of us decide that controlling food, shape, or appearance might offer the safety and acceptance that ordinary human connection couldn't provide.

This chapter explores those three intertwining strands:

1. *The temperament you were born with*
2. *The cultural messages that shaped what was valued or shamed*
3. *The quality of connection that taught you how to translate emotion into relationships*

When these strands braid together under stress, eating difficulties can arise as intelligent—if costly—attempts to meet needs and stay safe.

Discovering the Mindsets That Drive Eating Difficulties

From your first breath, your brain began forming mindsets: shortcuts for predicting what will happen next and how to stay safe. Mindsets tell you whether

DOI: 10.4324/9781003355878-3

the world welcomes or rejects your needs, whether feelings lead to comfort or criticism, and whether you are welcomed as you are or feel you must adapt yourself to stay connected.

When these internal blueprints are tinged with shame, fear, or guilt, they begin to narrow your range of being. Parts of you step forward with strategies:

- *If I can control my body, I'll finally be enough.*
- *If I don't need anything or anyone, no one can leave me.*
- *If I keep others happy, I'll stay safe.*

Each strategy began as protection. Over time, though, the protection became the prison.

Understanding how these patterns formed is about compassionately tracing the logic of your system—so that what once felt like something was wrong with you begins to make sense.

Part 1: Your Natural Temperament

Your Temperament Blueprint

You were born with a particular nervous system style—a temperament as real as eye colour or height. Temperament is a bit like a washing label—it shapes how deeply you feel, how quickly you recover, and how sensitive you are to the world inside and around you.

The Three E's of Temperament

Each of us arrives in the world with a unique nervous system pattern—a biological rhythm that influences how we feel, think, and act. Temperament traits are like *coordinates* to understand your internal weather patterns and how your system responds to uncertainty. Research has identified three core dimensions that appear especially relevant for people who struggle with eating and body image difficulties:

Environmental Sensitivity (ES): how deeply you process and respond to the world around and within you.

Emotionality (EN): how strongly and how often you experience emotions, particularly distressing ones.

Effortful Control (EC): your capacity to pause, focus, and choose a response rather than react automatically.

Each of these traits exists on a spectrum—no two people are alike—and each contains both *vulnerability* and *strength*. With the right support they can grow into empathy, creativity, and wisdom. In less supportive environments, they can feel overwhelming, or show up as perfectionism, or emotional withdrawal.

ES: The Orchid–Tulip–Dandelion Spectrum

ES describes how finely tuned your radar is to sensory, emotional, and social cues. This idea has been described by researchers Boyce and Ellis using a simple botanical metaphor (4). Some people are like *dandelions*—steady and adaptable, thriving almost anywhere. Others are *tulips*, flourishing in many conditions but wilting under sustained stress. And then there are *orchids*, exquisitely responsive to their environment: they may struggle under harsh conditions but bloom magnificently when nurtured.

If you recognise yourself as an orchid, you probably:

- Notice tiny shifts in other people's tone, posture, or mood.
- Feel easily overstimulated by noise, clutter, or conflict.
- Absorb others' feelings as if they were your own.
- Feel moved by beauty, art, or nature in ways that can be overwhelming.

Research (5) shows that sensitivity itself is *not* the problem—it's the fit between temperament and environment that determines whether this trait becomes a gift or a vulnerability. When a sensitive child grows up surrounded by emotional warmth, gentle structure, and caregivers who help name and regulate feelings, this trait matures into empathy, creativity, and intuition.

But when the environment is overstimulating, emotionally chaotic, or lacking in close, attuned relationships, the same sensitivity can become exhausting. Without external soothing, the nervous system struggles to self-regulate. Many sensitive children spend long periods alone or in emotionally barren settings, learning to dampen their internal volume through overcontrol, pulling back from connection, or self-soothing. Eating-based coping often becomes a way to dampen sensory and emotional overload when the world feels too much.

Recovery isn't about toughening up but rather building an environment—inside and outside—that helps your sensitivity feel safe. What allows an orchid to flourish is the right balance of warmth, light, and consistency.

EN: Feeling Deeply

EN refers to how readily negative, difficult emotions arise and how intensely they are felt.

High EN is a natural variation in how the nervous system processes emotion. Problems can arise when a child with high EN grows up in environments where emotions are dismissed, ridiculed, or feared—where *connection vitamins* such as acceptance and emotional attunement are in short supply (6).

In those settings, a child learns that strong feelings are dangerous or unwelcome. Without modelling or co-regulation, emotion becomes dysregulated—too big to manage alone. Many people with eating difficulties learned early that the only safe ways to manage these internal storms were through *overcontrol* (suppressing and perfecting) or *undercontrol* (acting out or numbing).

When met with attunement, however, EN transforms into depth, compassion, and authenticity. It gives you the capacity to feel joy and sorrow in full colour. The aim isn't to shrink your feelings but to build environments—and relationships—that can hold them safely.

EC: The Capacity to Pause and Choose

EC is the part of temperament that helps you manage impulses, stay focused, and follow through on what matters to you. It's the ability to pause, take a breath, and consider options before reacting—to guide your behaviour rather than be driven by every feeling, urge, or spike of uncertainty.

People vary naturally in this trait:

- **High EC** means you're organised, reliable, and good at thinking things through before acting. You can plan ahead, resist temptations, and keep sight of long-term goals.
- **Low EC** means you may act quickly on impulse, emotion, or the discomfort of not knowing what will happen next. You might start things enthusiastically but struggle to finish or find it hard to slow down when feelings run high.

Like other temperament traits, EC is shaped partly by genes and partly by early experience.

When children grow up with calm, consistent adults who help them settle when upset and think through what to do next, this ability tends to strengthen. When that guidance is missing—for example, if early years are unpredictable or there is a lack of stability—the trait can stay less developed, leaving emotions and impulses harder to manage.

High EC brings persistence and focus, but if pushed too far it can harden into perfectionism. Lower EC brings spontaneity and creativity, but without enough steadiness it can slip into chaos.

With understanding and practice, EC can always be strengthened. It's like a muscle: supported gently, it grows flexible and strong enough to help you steer your life with balance.

One additional trait I wanted to add in here is *Novelty-Seeking*. This trait is more common in some people with eating disorders, especially those with bulimia nervosa.

Novelty-Seeking—Chasing the Spark

Some people are born with a temperament that craves novelty, adventure, stimulation, and change. They get bored quickly, light up with new ideas, and come alive with movement, play, or adventure.

When Novelty-Seeking has safe outlets for creativity, exploration, and self-expression, it fuels vitality and growth. But when those outlets are unavailable—or when caregivers fear, shame, or suppress spontaneity—the same drive has to go somewhere. Without attuned guidance, Novelty-Seeking can be channelled into risky or self-soothing behaviours: binge eating, purging, compulsive exercise, substance use, or other impulsive coping patterns. This is particularly common in binge–purge–type eating difficulties, where the system reaches for intense, fast relief.

The issue isn't the trait itself but the lack of healthy pathways for curiosity, play, and exploration. Creating safe ways to express that energy—through art, movement, humour, connection, or adventure—allows this trait to become a source of aliveness rather than chaos.

Melissa's Story: The Gift and the Weight of Sensitivity

From an early age,  Melissa could read the room like a script. If her mother sighed at the end of a long day, Melissa would tidy the kitchen before being asked. If her father's voice sharpened, she would quiet her laughter. No one told her to do these things; her body simply knew.

Her sensitivity, which could have become artistry or intuition, turned instead into vigilance. By adolescence, she was scanning constantly—others' moods, teachers' approval, the smallest shift in her waistband.

When she began restricting food, it brought a sense of relief. Hunger muted the noise of her internal world. Numbers were cleaner than emotions. Her family saw a conscientious, health-minded teenager; they didn't see the child trying to quiet a nervous system overloaded by empathy.

In therapy years later, Melissa could finally name both sides of her sensitivity: the beauty of perceiving so much and the exhaustion of feeling responsible for it all.

Her work was not to become tougher but to build environments—and relationships—that honoured her nature instead of overwhelming it.

Temperament as Both Vulnerability and Gift

Your temperament is not fixed and does not determine your future. All temperament traits hold potential. Sensitivity can become artistry, empathy, and wisdom. Emotional intensity can fuel passion, creativity, and love. EC can support perseverance and purpose.

The key here is *fit*. When environments match temperament, strengths flourish. Recent research shows that when there is a mismatch between a child's temperament and the type of environment and caregiving they receive, this can increase vulnerability to developing problems such as eating disorders (6). Eating-based coping strategies become a way of filling the gap.

As child psychiatrist and researcher David Rettew (7) describes it, temperament is like the internal weather system that we're born with: we can't change whether we're sunny, windy, or storm-prone—but we can learn how to forecast and prepare.

For further details on temperament, see Appendix 3.

Reflection

- Do you recognise yourself more as an Orchid, Tulip, or Dandelion?
- Which situations leave you overstimulated, and which bring you alive?
- How has your temperament been misunderstood—as "too sensitive," "too intense," or "too driven"?
- What environments or relationships have allowed your natural temperament to feel safe?

> **Note on Neurodivergence**: Many of the temperament traits we've explored—high ES, intense EN, and differences in EC—are also common features of neurodivergent conditions such as autism and ADHD. Research shows significantly higher rates of eating disorders amongst neurodivergent individuals. Neurodivergent brains process sensory information, emotions, and social situations differently, creating both remarkable gifts and unique vulnerabilities. An autistic person might develop restrictive eating patterns as a way of managing sensory sensitivities around food textures or eating environments. Someone with ADHD might turn to binge eating as a way of managing intense emotions or seeking dopamine stimulation their brain needs. Neurodivergent traits, like temperament traits, are simply different ways of experiencing the world that can become strengths when properly understood and supported.

Part 2: Cultural Mindsets That Drive Eating and Body Image Disturbances

Your temperament is just the starting point. How it develops depends enormously on the cultural waters you've been swimming in—the unspoken hierarchies about who holds power, whose emotions matter, who deserves nourishment, and what makes a body "acceptable."

These cultural mindsets work through seduction. They promise that if you just sail toward their island—thin enough, controlled enough, productive enough, selfless enough—you'll finally arrive at safety, worth, and belonging. But these islands are mirages. The closer you sail, the further they recede. Meanwhile, the real island—*the island of self*, where your authentic needs, values, and voice reside—drifts further behind you.

Let's explore how these cultural currents shape eating difficulties.

Cultural Subjugation: When Hierarchies Define Your Worth

We don't develop eating disorders in a vacuum. We live in cultures built on hierarchies—systems that rank people, emotions, bodies, and needs along scales of "better than" and "less than." These hierarchies maintain themselves through a cunning paradox: they convince you that becoming *smaller, quieter,* and *more controlled* will make you *more valuable.*

But "valuable" in this system never means "powerful" or "free." It means "acceptable within the hierarchy." The smaller you become—the less space you take, the fewer needs you express, the more you fit the cultural ideal—the less power you actually hold to advocate for yourself, ask for what you need, or challenge the system itself.

This is how ***subjugation*** *maintains itself: by making the diminished condition feel like achievement.*

These hierarchies show up in multiple, overlapping forms:

Patriarchal hierarchies teach that traditionally masculine traits (strength, stoicism, independence, competition) hold higher status than traditionally feminine ones (emotional attunement, vulnerability, interdependence, collaboration). Your worth becomes something you must *earn* through performance and control rather than something you possess simply by being human.

Racist hierarchies enforce Eurocentric beauty standards and colourism, teaching that certain skin tones, features, and body types are inherently more valuable than others.

Ableist hierarchies equate productivity with worth, treating bodies and minds that don't conform to narrow definitions of "normal" or "functional" as less deserving of care, rest, or accommodation.

Heteronormative hierarchies police gender expression and sexuality, punishing anyone who colours outside rigid lines of how bodies "should" look and behave.

All use the same mechanism: *create standards you can never quite meet and then convince you that trying harder is the solution* rather than questioning the standards themselves.

Within these hierarchies, your body becomes a *commodity to be evaluated and improved* rather than a home to be inhabited with care. Vulnerability becomes weakness. Emotional needs become inconvenient problems to manage or eliminate. And you learn to *compete rather than connect,* to rank yourself constantly against others—and against the impossible ideal.

Emotion Hierarchies: When Feelings Become the Enemy

Cultural hierarchies influence both how people are valued and *which parts of human experience are welcomed or sidelined.*

Many modern cultures have developed a hierarchy of emotions that elevates logic and rationality above intuition and emotional intelligence. So called "negative" emotions—sadness, fear, anger, shame—sit at the bottom of this hierarchy, treated as problems to solve rather than information to understand, inconveniences to manage rather than meaningful signals.

This emotion hierarchy serves subjugation perfectly: *if you can't feel or name what's happening inside you, you can't recognise when your needs are being ignored or your boundaries are being violated.* Disconnection from emotion keeps hierarchical systems stable.

Within this hierarchy, stoicism and "mental toughness" are praised whilst emotional expression is dismissed as dramatic, *too much*, or self-indulgent. For highly sensitive people, this cultural message is particularly damaging. Their natural gift for feeling deeply becomes reframed as a sign of defectiveness that needs to be overcome. They learn to apologise for their sensitivity rather than recognise it as a capacity.

Our culture rewards the analytical, controlling, productivity-focused parts of us whilst treating embodied wisdom—rest, pleasure, intuition, and emotional attunement—as suspicious or lazy. We're encouraged to operate from the neck up, valuing cognitive control over bodily knowing. This creates a particular vulnerability for eating difficulties, which often develop precisely in the gap between what your body knows it needs and what your thinking mind believes is acceptable.

 **Samantha's family** exemplified this emotion hierarchy. Her parents were high achievers who genuinely believed they were teaching her resilience through their emphasis on pushing through difficulties without complaint. Her father's favourite response to her emotional struggles was "Toughen up, sunshine!" whilst her mother consistently suggested exercise as the solution to every feeling.

When Samantha felt sad about a friendship ending, the message wasn't "Tell me about your sadness so I can understand and comfort you." Instead, it was "Go for a run and you'll feel better."

Over time, Samantha learned that her emotions were inconvenient for others and evidence of her own weakness—that she sat lower in the hierarchy of "acceptable" people. Her binge–restrict cycle became her way of managing this impossible situation—bingeing when the pain of suppressing her emotions became unbearable and then restricting to punish herself for having feelings in the first place.

Scarcity Hierarchies: When "Not Enough" Becomes Your Identity

The scarcity mindset creates hierarchies of deservingness: who deserves nourishment, care, and resources. Under scarcity thinking, there isn't enough to go around, so we must carefully ration our needs and constantly prove our worthiness.

This mindset operates on the belief that taking your share means depriving others, that having needs makes you selfish, and that anything beyond survival requirements is excessive or wasteful. It teaches you that to be valuable within the hierarchy, you must need *less* than everyone else.

Under scarcity hierarchies, we become hypervigilant about not being "too much"—not taking up too much space, not needing too much attention. We learn to shrink ourselves to avoid depleting others' limited supply of patience, energy, or care.

Sophie's story illustrates how a scarcity mindset gets passed down through generations. Her parents had grown up during times when resources were genuinely limited, when survival required making do with less.

They unconsciously carried this scarcity forward into their parenting, living frugally even when they could afford more, always choosing the cheapest option regardless of quality, treating any form of pleasure or indulgence with suspicion. Their love was genuine but expressed through sacrifice—they went without so Sophie could have what she needed.

But Sophie's sensitive system picked up on the subtext: *My needs deplete others. My wants are greedy. Taking care of myself means taking away from people I love.*

Her restriction became her solution to this impossible equation. Through it, she could demonstrate that she needed absolutely nothing, that she could survive on less than anyone else, that she would never be a burden. This scarcity mindset created a painful cycle: rigid restriction proving she needed nothing, followed by binges when deprivation became unbearable, followed by harsher punishment.

These hierarchies—patriarchal, emotional, scarcity-based—create the conditions for confusion about your worth. They teach you that you're not inherently valuable, that love and belonging must be earned, that your needs are burdensome, and that taking up space requires justification.

And then, as if on cue, two seductive solutions appear on the horizon—two mirage islands promising rescue from the hierarchy's impossible demands.

The Two False Solutions: Seductive Islands That Keep You Lost

When cultural hierarchies leave you feeling not enough, two solutions seem to shimmer on the horizon: *Perfectionism* promises you can *earn* your way to worth through achievement and control. *Consumerism* promises you can *purchase* your way to worth through acquiring the right body, lifestyle, or products.

Both are mirages. Both promise to lift you up the hierarchy whilst actually keeping you locked in its logic. You're still accepting that worth must be earned or purchased rather than inherent. You're still measuring yourself against external standards. You're still sailing away from the island of self.

Perfectionism: The Achievement Island

Perfectionism promises: "If you can just be perfect enough—controlled enough, disciplined enough, achieve highly enough—you'll finally deserve love and escape judgement."

This island assures worth through *doing, controlling,* and *earning.* It tells you that the hierarchy isn't the problem—you simply haven't worked hard enough yet to climb it. If you can just get straight As, maintain the perfect weight, never make mistakes, always stay composed, always put others first, never burden anyone with your needs—*then* you'll finally be safe.

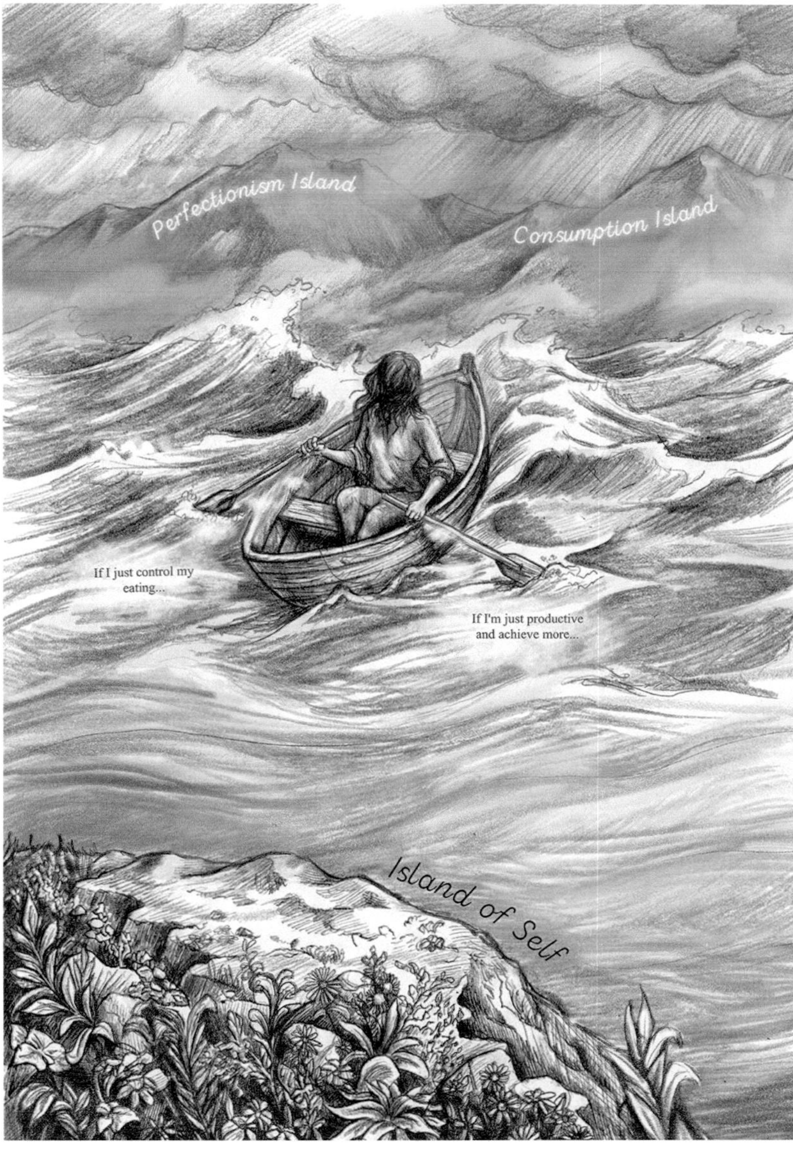
Perfectionism Island
Consumption Island
If I just control my eating...
If I'm just productive and achieve more...
Island of Self

Figure 2.1 Girl rowing to "Island of Self"

But perfectionism constantly moves the goalposts. No matter what you achieve, it finds new flaws to focus on, higher standards to meet, and new territories to conquer. There is always something more to prove. This is how the island maintains its mirage quality—it stays perpetually just out of reach.

Within eating difficulties, perfectionism shows up as:

- All-or-nothing thinking about food, exercise, and body
- Rigid rules that must never be broken

- Self-punishment when you "fail" to meet impossible standards
- The belief that control over your body will finally grant you the acceptance and safety you've been seeking
- Using restriction, overexercise, or other compensatory behaviours to demonstrate your discipline and worthiness

Faye's Story: Perfectionism as Proof of Worth

 **Faye's story** illustrates how perfectionism becomes the solution to hierarchical pressure. Growing up in a family that valued achievement and having "everything together," she learned that approval came through meeting high standards. Her parents weren't intentionally harsh—they genuinely believed they were motivating her to reach her potential.

But Faye's sensitive temperament translated their expectations into internal tyranny. Every B+ became evidence of laziness. Every emotional outburst became proof of weakness. Every extra kilogram felt like a personal failing.

Her binge–restrict cycle became the perfect expression of this perfectionist trap—dieting with rigid perfection until the deprivation became unbearable, then bingeing in a moment of "failure," followed by punishing herself through more restriction. She was simultaneously trying to climb the hierarchy through perfect control and being crushed by its impossible standards.

The perfectionism promised: *Be controlled enough and you'll finally be valuable.* But the smaller and more controlled she became, the less power she actually held to advocate for herself or challenge the standards crushing her.

Consumerism: The External Rescue Island

If perfectionism promises worth through *doing*, consumerism promises worth through *having*. This mindset tells us: "If you can just buy, consume, or acquire the right things—the right diet, body, lifestyle, achievements—you'll finally be valuable."

Consumerism masquerades as the solution to all the previous hierarchies. It promises that the answer to patriarchal competition, emotional emptiness, and scarcity thinking lies in consuming the right products, services, or experiences—that you can *purchase* your way up the hierarchy or out of your pain.

This mindset teaches you to look outside yourself for solutions to internal problems, particularly your deep loneliness and disconnection. It's perhaps the most seductive of the mirage islands because it comes wrapped in self-care language, wellness promises, and empowerment marketing.

Diet Culture as Consumerism's Perfect Tool

Diet culture is perhaps the clearest example of consumerism targeting eating disorder vulnerability. It sells the promise that the right diet, exercise programme, supplement plan, or body modification will solve not just your physical "problems" but your emotional ones too.

The message is clear: *Thinness will finally grant you the acceptance and power the other hierarchies deny you. The right body will make you lovable. The perfect diet will give you control. The disciplined lifestyle will prove your worth.*

But like all mirage islands, diet culture promises keep receding. There's always a new diet to try, a new body goal to achieve, and a new product that will *finally* be the answer. You're encouraged to consume your way to thinness through meal replacements and diet programmes, then consume your way to "health" through supplements and cleanses, and then consume your way to "wellness" through organic everything and expensive fitness memberships.

The consumption extends beyond just buying products:

- Consuming achievement (collecting qualifications, accolades, promotions to prove worth)
- Consuming approval (constantly seeking validation from others)
- Consuming busyness (staying productive to avoid feeling)
- Consuming control (using perfectionist rigidity as consumerism of another kind)

The common thread: the answer to your internal struggles lies somewhere *outside yourself*—on one of those distant islands rather than in returning to the island of self.

The Trap Both Islands Share

Whether you're chasing the Perfectionism Island through rigid control and achievement or the Consumerism Island through diet culture and external solutions, you're still accepting the hierarchy's basic premise: *that your worth is conditional, that you must earn or purchase belonging, that the problem is you rather than the system.*

Both solutions keep you:

- Measuring yourself against external standards
- Competing with others (and yourself) rather than connecting
- Looking outside yourself for validation
- Believing you must change to be acceptable
- Sailing further from the island of self

Recovery means recognising these islands for what they are—mirages that promise rescue whilst keeping you lost. It means turning your boat around and sailing back toward the island of self, where your inherent worth has been waiting all along.

Reflection: Recognising Cultural Messages in Your Story

- Which mindsets feel most familiar from your family, community, or peer groups?

- How do your eating patterns help you comply with these cultural expectations?
- What messages did you absorb about emotions, needs, and your body?

Internal Othering: How Cultural Hierarchies Live Inside Us

These cultural hierarchies don't just create divisions between people—they teach us to create divisions *within ourselves*. We learn to "other" our own hungry body, our emotional needs, and our "weak" or "messy" parts—to reject and view these parts as "not-me" (8).

The false solutions of perfectionism and consumerism intensify this internal othering. They give us tools to attack ourselves with: "This part of me that needs, that feels, that wants—that's the shameful part that's preventing me from reaching the Perfectionism Island. That's the undisciplined part that requires the Consumerism Island's products to fix."

Recovery means returning to the island of self—reclaiming your right to need, to feel, to take up space, to exist outside these imposed hierarchies. It means recognising that the problem was never you; it was always the system that convinced you to sail away from your own worth in pursuit of conditional acceptance that was always designed to recede.

Part 3: Early Relationship Mindsets

The Family Recipe

These cultural hierarchies form the water all families swim in. But it's within our earliest, most intimate relationships where we either receive or miss the specific emotional vitamins our particular temperament needs to stay afloat. The broader cultural currents shape what's valued or shamed, but family relationships determine whether you learn to navigate those currents with an internal life raft—or whether you're left swimming alone.

The "Family Recipe" Metaphor: Think of your family's approach to love and care as a *recipe* that's been passed down through generations.

Imagine that your great-great-great-grandparents had a family recipe for chocolate cake, which had been passed down through the generations to them. During their lifetime, they may have endured a war or famine, followed by great hardship when food was scarce, and it was impossible to buy the usual ingredients. Your ancestors continued to bake their cake according to the family recipe, but as one of the ingredients—baking soda—was unavailable, they skipped that part of the recipe.

As time passed, generation after generation became accustomed to making do with the flat cake. The cake still turned out tasty, full of many other rich ingredients, but no matter what they tried, it was flat. The familiar recipe was passed on without that missing ingredient, with no one questioning it. Some tried to compensate by adding a thick layer of cream. Of course, in reality, no-one was at fault—it was simply an ingredient that had become lost between generations.

All of us have ancestors who were impacted by the traumas of war, famines, migration, slavery, pressures of long working hours in difficult conditions, and feeding large families. When basic survival is a struggle and trauma is commonplace, some of the key emotional vitamins that lead to resilience and well-being can go by the wayside.

Research on epigenetics—how trauma affects our biology across generations—suggests that trauma and chronic stress can influence how the genes of following generations express themselves (9)—though this doesn't mean trauma is "hardwired" or unchangeable. Patterns of sensitivity, tension, and emotional reactivity and vulnerability to eating difficulties can be passed on, but they can also be interrupted and healed.

When Love Doesn't Translate: The Gap between Intention and Impact

Most parents love their children deeply and want to provide the best care possible. But various factors can interfere with their ability to provide the specific emotional vitamins each child needs:

Mismatched Temperaments: A highly sensitive child born to parents who are naturally less emotionally reactive might not receive the level of emotional attunement they need.

Intergenerational Trauma: Parents who experienced their own childhood trauma, neglect, or emotional deprivation often struggle to provide emotional vitamins they never received themselves.

Cultural Pressures: The toxic cultural mindsets we explored earlier don't just affect individuals—they shape entire family systems.

Life Circumstances: Even well-intentioned parents can struggle to provide consistent emotional attunement when they're dealing with mental health challenges, financial stress, work demands, physical illness, or other overwhelming circumstances.

Early Separation or Loss: Extended separations due to hospitalisation, work demands, family breakdown, or other circumstances can disrupt the attachment process even when they're unavoidable.

Care That Is Attuned to Specific Emotions and Needs

When emotional vitamins are delivered in a consistent and attuned way—the right needs met at the right times—we learn to correctly interpret our body sensations and connect them to specific emotional or physical needs. We learn to tell the difference between feeling hungry and lonely; cold and sad; physically full and angry; tired and overwhelmed.

However, if these needs are not met in an attuned way, this can lead to confusion over the meaning of inner signals. For example, when babies and children do not feel consistently and sufficiently soothed, they can respond by learning not to cry at all, even when they need something, by disconnecting and numbing their body sensations.

This is not about whether we are loved—but about how our needs have been responded to, influenced by factors often out of our control. To a large extent, this is influenced by the interaction of the child's temperament alongside the strengths and limitations of the caregiving available.

Melissa's Family Recipe

Melissa's grandparents lived through times when resources were genuinely scarce, when families had to focus on basic survival rather than emotional connection. Love got translated into providing, protecting, and ensuring children had the material necessities for success.

This recipe worked well in some ways—Melissa received excellent practical care, educational support, and material security. But crucial ingredients her temperament needed had dropped out over the generations: emotional validation, permission to have preferences that differed from her parents', and the experience of being loved simply for who she was rather than for how well she met expectations.

Her parents weren't withholding these ingredients intentionally—they were following the only recipe they knew, trying to give their daughter the best version of love they had received and understood.

When the Three Strands Intertwine: How Schema Mindsets Form

By now, you've seen how each strand—temperament, culture, and early relationships—shapes who we become. When these strands fit together well, a child's needs for safety, love, and freedom are met naturally. But when they pull in different directions, the developing system adjusts, and *schema mindsets* take root.

A schema mindset is like a pair of tinted glasses or an old script we keep following—the brain's way of predicting what will happen next and reducing uncertainty, even when those predictions are painful. Once formed, these mindsets work in the background to shape perception and behaviour: we notice what confirms them, overlook what challenges them, and often find ourselves drawn to people or situations that replay the same story.

Imagine a sensitive child growing up in a culture that prizes self-control over emotional honesty, in a family that shows love through doing rather than through attunement. To stay connected, that child learns to manage feelings instead of expressing them. Years later, this becomes a familiar rule for living: "If I stay in control, I'll be safe; if I show too much, I'll lose love." What looks like a problem in adulthood began as a solution in childhood—an attempt to hold onto safety and belonging, the only way the child knew how.

Common Schema Mindsets in Eating Disorders

The following mindsets often emerge where particular emotional vitamins (listed in Chapter 1) were scarce:

Abandonment: When love and presence felt unpredictable, the child learned that support can vanish without warning. *Others won't be there for me when I need them. I'm all alone.*

Emotional Deprivation: When others were kind but emotionally unreachable, the child internalised: *People care, but they don't really see or understand me. Others see my needs as a burden.*

Defectiveness/Shame: When criticism, comparison, or subtle disapproval coloured early relationships, the child concluded: *Something inside me is fundamentally wrong or unlovable.*

Mistrust: When the world felt unsafe or unpredictable, trust in others—and sometimes in one's own body—fractured. *I can't trust others. I can't trust myself.*

Social Isolation: When differences led to exclusion or misunderstanding, the child concluded: *I don't belong. I'm fundamentally different.*

Subjugation: When harmony and compliance were prized above individuality, the child learned: *Voicing my needs brings conflict or guilt. I must allow others to take control, hide my anger and mould myself to others' expectations.*

Enmeshment: When emotional boundaries were blurred—when a parent or loved one's mood dictated everyone else's—the child learned: *I don't know where I end and others begin. To stay close, I must give up being separate.*

Unrelenting Standards/Perfectionism: When achievement and self-control were equated with worth, the child internalised: *I must strive to be good enough and reach the standards expected of me. I must do more, be more, prove more.*

Emotional Inhibition: When emotional expression was discouraged—punished, minimised, dismissed, or silently disapproved of—the child learned: *My feelings cause problems. If I stay controlled and contained, I'll be acceptable. It's safer to be composed than to be real.*

Negativity/Pessimism: When early experiences were marked by chronic criticism, anxiety, or a focus on what could go wrong, the child learned: *Something bad is always around the corner. If I stay vigilant and expect disappointment, I won't be caught off guard. Hope is risky; caution keeps me safe.*

Each of these mindsets tells a story of adaptation: a way of managing the tension between a sensitive inner world and an imperfect outer one.

Take the *Emotional Deprivation* schema mindset. It often develops when a child's caregivers are physically present but emotionally distant—perhaps loving in principle but unable to tune into the child's inner world. The child learns early that strong emotions are unwelcome or ignored. They might receive practical help—meals cooked, lifts to school—but not the warmth of being comforted when sad or celebrated when joyful.

Over time, the child's nervous system adapts by expecting *less*. They learn not to ask, not to hope, not to depend. When others later try to offer care, it may feel foreign or unsafe. A small voice inside says, "No one will really be there for me," and relationships start to echo that expectation. They might choose emotionally unavailable partners or push away those who try to get close, recreating the loneliness they fear most.

From the outside, this can look like independence or emotional control. Inside, it's often a deep, unacknowledged hunger to be met and understood. Recognising this pattern invites understanding rather than blame. It helps us see how a sensitive nervous system learned to survive in a world that couldn't always meet its emotional needs.

For a comprehensive list of schema mindsets relevant to eating disorders, see Appendix 4.

The Meeting Point of the Three Strands

The schema mindsets form precisely where the three strands meet.

- **Temperament** determines how strongly we feel and how deeply we process experiences.
- **Culture** shapes which feelings and needs are deemed acceptable.
- Through repeated interactions, **Early Relationships** teaches us whether our inner experiences will be met or misunderstood.

When these interact in supportive ways, the child develops flexible, self-compassionate schemas—beliefs like "I'm lovable even when imperfect" or "I can need others and still be independent."

When they collide, rigidity and self-blame fill the gap.

Sophie embodies this fusion. Shaped by scarcity culture and a self-sacrificing family, she absorbed the message that needing less was the highest form of goodness. Her restriction became an act of loyalty to those who had survived on little—a silent continuation of an ancestral story.

Faye illustrates the perfectionist dimension. Her sensitive, detail-oriented temperament made her an excellent student, yet it also heightened her sensitivity to subtle disappointment. She grew up in a culture that equated success with virtue and in a family that expressed love through achievement. When she faltered, she felt defective; when she succeeded, she felt temporarily safe.

Each person's pattern made sense in context. Their eating difficulties were creative responses to complex histories.

When you recognise how emotional vitamins were missing—when you see clearly what should have been different—grief naturally arises. This is healthy. It means you're finally acknowledging the truth of your experience rather than minimising or explaining it away. Your Lost Child has been holding this grief; as your Wise Self emerges, she can finally express it.

The Hidden Wisdom in Your Story

When you begin to see your eating patterns through this lens, they start to make sense. Each behaviour reflects an unmet need and an intelligent attempt to meet it indirectly.

Restriction can signify the need for boundaries. Bingeing can express a hunger for comfort. Overexercise might translate the wish to feel competent in a world that feels overwhelming.

The aim of recovery is not to silence these signals but to decode them—to understand what each part of you has been trying to communicate. Once you know the message, you can meet the need directly.

Breaking the Cycle

When you provide yourself with the emotional vitamins that were missing, the old schema mindsets begin to loosen. You no longer need to rely on the same protective strategies because your system senses that real nourishment is available.

Safety is rebuilt through consistency, curiosity, and compassion—qualities that gradually rewire old expectations.

Generational cycles shift when we provide ourselves with missing emotional vitamins. The scarcity that once bred self-denial gives way to generosity; the perfectionism that once sustained belonging yields to authenticity. By understanding your story in context, you become both the beneficiary and the healer of your lineage.

Gentle Experiments to Try

Life Story Time Line Exercise: Use the worksheet in Appendix 5 to map your life story from birth to now, noticing both the nourishing and difficult moments that shaped your relationship with yourself, your body, and others. *Focus on the events themselves and any patterns or beliefs (schema mindsets) you notice forming—you'll learn about the specific "parts" (modes) that developed in response in the next chapter.* The aim is to see your story more clearly, so that you can begin to reshape it with compassion.

Journalling Prompt Reflections: When Eating Difficulties Emerge

- Which schema mindsets felt most familiar? When did you first learn these patterns?
- How do they make sense when viewed through your temperament, culture, and relationship history?

- How did your temperament (ES, EN, EC, NS) interact with your environment?
- What cultural messages about bodies, emotions, or worth did you absorb?
- Looking at your life story timeline, what connections do you notice between difficult periods and your eating patterns?

Looking Ahead: Meeting Your Inner Crew

Understanding Schema Mindsets and Modes

Before we go further, let's clarify two important concepts you'll see throughout this book. These terms are distinct, and understanding the difference helps you make sense of your inner world.

Schema Mindsets are lasting core beliefs about yourself, others, and the world—conclusions you drew from early experiences. They act like old predictive maps that colour what you expect from yourself, others, and the world. Once formed, they operate quietly in the background, shaping your perceptions without you always realising it.

Examples of schema mindsets:

- "I'm defective." (Defectiveness schema)
- "Others will abandon me." (Abandonment schema)
- "I must be perfect to be acceptable." (Unrelenting Standards schema)
- "My needs make me a burden." (Subjugation schema)

Schemas are also the nervous system's way of reducing uncertainty. Recovery means gently revising these old "certainties" while building a new source of safety through the steady bond between your Wise Self and your Inner Child.

Modes are moment-to-moment emotional states and coping strategies—the different parts of you that show up in response to triggers. They're like crew members on your inner ship, each with specific roles and strategies.

Examples of modes:

- Lost Child (feeling state—holds emotions and vulnerability)
- Overcontroller (coping strategy—uses control and rules for safety)
- Inner Critic (attacking state—uses shame as protection)
- Wise Self (healthy leadership—provides grounded guidance)

Think of It This Way: Schemas create the conditions; modes are how you navigate them.

Your schemas tell you the world is dangerous (core belief formed in childhood). Your modes are the feeling states and strategies you developed to stay safe in that world (parts that activate in the present moment).

When your Abandonment schema gets triggered (someone cancels plans), your Overcontroller mode might activate (restrict food to regain sense of control), and your Lost Child Mode surfaces (feels rejected and alone).

When your subjugation schema gets triggered (someone expects you to accommodate their needs), your People Pleaser Mode might activate (agree even when it hurts you), and your Impulsive Child Mode surfaces later (rebels through binge eating). The subjugation schema—suppressing your authentic needs and desires to avoid conflict or abandonment—shows up powerfully in eating patterns. In Chapter 8, you'll discover how both binge urges (rebellion against suppression) and struggles with recovery discomfort (exhaustion from prolonged subjugation) often stem from this same root pattern of self-silencing.

Throughout this book:

- When I talk about *schemas/schema mindsets*, I'm referring to those underlying beliefs formed long ago.
- When I talk about *modes*, I'm referring to the parts of you that are active right now, in this moment.

This distinction matters because recovery involves both understanding where your beliefs came from (schema mindsets) and learning to work with the parts that show up daily (modes).

The next chapter turns from the external to the internal world—from how your patterns developed to how they now live inside you. You'll meet the different modes or parts of yourself—the crew members of your inner ship—each of whom developed to help you navigate these emotional seas. You'll learn how to recognise them, understand their motives, and begin leading them with compassion and clarity.

The journey ahead means coming into a relationship with your own story—listening to what it still asks of you and responding with care. Each time you choose awareness over avoidance or compassion over criticism, you loosen the old knots that shaped you. In doing so, you begin to model a different way of being, one that gradually shifts the emotional inheritance passed forward to those who follow.

3 Meeting Your Inner Crew

Listen, oh beautiful soul. Every day a new feast comes running into your life. Always a new experience. Your body is like a guest house, receiving company from the hidden world. Some are positive, some are tragic, and still others who are frantic. All mirroring your needs. All showing you ways to expand. All challenging your beliefs. Whoever that comes from these unseen lands, receive it without regret. Welcome all that come to you, with no judgment. Remember, every visitor, here a short time, meant only for your growth.
The wound is the place where the Light enters you.

—*Your Body is a Guest House*, Rumi. (Translated and interpreted by Shahram Shiva)[1]

In Chapter 2, you discovered the schema mindsets—those lasting core beliefs formed in childhood when emotional vitamins were scarce. You learned how temperament, culture, and early relationships intertwine to create these internal blueprints about yourself, others, and the world. But these are only part of the story. They're the conclusions you drew long ago.

What's happening right now, in this present moment, involves something more dynamic—the different parts of you that activate in response to those old beliefs. These are your "modes": the moment-to-moment emotional states and coping strategies that show up when life triggers those schema mindsets.

Think of it this way: your Defectiveness schema mindset is the old belief "I'm fundamentally flawed." Your Lost Child Mode is the part of you feeling that shame right now. Your Inner Critic mode is the voice attacking you for feeling it. Your Overcontroller mode is the strategy of trying to fix it through perfection and control.

This chapter introduces you to these different parts—your inner crew. You'll discover how they developed, why they operate the way they do, and how they've been trying to help you navigate a world that once felt overwhelming. Understanding these modes is essential because recovery isn't about changing your beliefs through logic alone—it's about learning to work with the parts of yourself that are active in each moment.

Let's meet them.

DOI: 10.4324/9781003355878-4

Part 1: Understanding Your Inner World

The Mirror

 Emma stands before her bathroom mirror, brushing her teeth. Same routine, same face, same reflection she's seen thousands of times. But this morning, she pauses to really look.

The woman staring back looks familiar—same eyes, same mouth, same cheekbones. Yet Emma has the strangest sensation that she's looking at a stranger. Or maybe several strangers, layered one on top of the other like a badly edited photograph.

There's the Emma who smiled at colleagues yesterday, the one who spent two hours calculating tomorrow's food intake, the one who wanted to cry when her sister called but couldn't remember why. Which one is real?

Behind those familiar eyes, she senses someone younger. Someone who once knew exactly what she wanted, what she felt, what she needed. Someone who got lost somewhere along the way. If you've ever had this feeling—that the person you show the world isn't quite the person you actually are—you're not alone. And you're not confused. You're just meeting your inner crew for the first time.

The Truth about Who You Are

We grow up believing we're one person with one mind, one personality, and one consistent "self" that shows up the same way all the time. But if you've lived with eating difficulties, you already know this isn't true.

You know what it's like to desperately want to eat normally while another part of you is already calculating how to compensate. You know the experience of feeling two ways about the same thing—wanting connection but pushing people away, craving freedom but clinging to rules, longing for rest but unable to stop moving. This is not a sign that something's wrong with you—just evidence that you're human.

All of us—every single person—are made up of different parts. Think of them as different sides of your personality, different aspects of who you are that developed at different times for different reasons. Some parts are visible to others, operating where everyone can see them. Others stay hidden, working behind the scenes in ways you might not even notice.

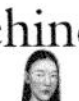 **Melissa** sits in her kitchen, frozen. She needs to buy yoghurt. Simple enough. But one voice in her head is calculating fat content, comparing prices, insisting she find the cheapest option even if it's past its expiration date. Another voice is getting angry: *Why can't I just buy what I want? Why does everything have to be so hard?*

She stands there, unable to move, pulled in opposite directions by parts of herself she didn't know existed until right now.

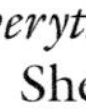 Faye knows the pattern too well. When her "diet" is going well, she feels on top of the world—in control, achieving something, hopeful that this

time will be different. But, eventually, the emptiness creeps in. The boredom. The numbness. And she knows what's coming: that familiar urge to binge building like a wave she can't outrun. "It's like I'm swept away," she says. "Like a runaway train with no brakes."

Both women are operating without an inner leader. Both are being steered by parts of themselves that once served a purpose but haven't updated with the times. And both are exhausted from the constant internal conflict.

The first step is beginning to understand these different parts. To see why they developed and how they might work together instead of against each other.

That's what this chapter is about.

Your Inner Crew: An Overview

Think of your internal crew as having four main groups:

Inner Child Modes carry your emotions and vulnerability. Our Inner Child Modes are the key to connection and closeness—both within ourselves and with others. They are the parts of us that know and feel the truth of our experience, even when other parts use eating patterns to obscure this from ourselves. The Lost Child holds feelings you might not even know you have—loneliness, shame, longing, and joy. Other child parts include your Feisty Child (the part that pushes back when boundaries are crossed), your Impulsive Child (the freedom-seeking part that can't stand restriction), and your Contented Child (the playful, authentic you that emerges when you feel safe).

Protector Modes are the survival strategies you unconsciously developed when life felt overwhelming. They include your People Pleaser, your Overcontroller, your Detached Protector, and your Helpless mode. As we explored in Chapter 1, these parts emerged as creative responses to missing emotional vitamins and difficult circumstances. They're the parts visible to others—the roles you play to navigate the world.

The Inner Critic operates a bit like your Protector Modes—though it certainly doesn't feel protective. This part learned to keep you safe through harsh self-attack, absorbing cultural messages, family standards, and schema-based conclusions. It uses shame and guilt as protective mechanisms, genuinely believing these harsh methods will keep you safe from rejection and inadequacy. We'll explore this complex protective part in detail below.

The Wise Self[2] is your inner leader—the part of you that can coordinate all these different voices, understand what each one needs, and guide your internal world with both strength and compassion.

When emotional vitamins are available consistently, inner child parts flourish and your Wise Self naturally develops. But when certain needs go unmet,

Protector Modes take over, and your Lost Child gets pushed out of awareness where her feelings can't threaten your survival.

Now let's explore what happens when this crew loses coordination.

Understanding Schema Mindsets, Raw Spots, and Your Crew's Response

Picture your internal world when Protector Modes are running the show. Some parts work frantically while others are locked away, banging on walls, trying to be heard. No one's coordinating. Everyone's working at cross-purposes.

Your mind gets preoccupied with food rules, calorie calculations, body checking, or planning binges—anything to avoid what's underneath. The loneliness. The sadness. The emptiness. Your Lost Child is trying to get your attention, but your Protector Modes have sealed her away.

Remember the schema mindsets from Chapter 2? Each one developed when specific emotional vitamins were missing. When those mindsets get triggered in the present moment—by a comment, a situation, a memory—they activate what we call *emotional raw spots* in your Child Modes.

The *schema mindset* is the old conclusion ("I'm too much," "I'm not enough," "I'm unlovable") and includes an "emotional raw spot"—the feeling that lives in your body when that mindset gets activated—the shame, the loneliness, the panic, the emptiness.

The Pattern

When someone criticises you, your Defectiveness mindset might trigger. Immediately, your Lost Child feels that familiar raw spot—the bodily sensation of shame, of being fundamentally flawed. Before you can even identify what you're feeling, your Protector Modes jump in: your Overcontroller tightens food rules to regain control, your Detached Protector goes numb, your Critic attacks you for being "too sensitive."

The eating-related behaviours are your Protector Modes' attempts to manage the pain of those raw spots—to prevent them from being touched or to numb them quickly when they surface.

This creates a predictable chain: Trigger → Schema Mindset Activated → Raw Spot Felt → Critic Attacks → Protector Modes Deploy → Eating Behaviour Follows.

Transforming the Pattern

In recovery, instead of letting Protector Modes immediately cover over the raw spot with eating behaviours, you learn to pause. You notice: "Ah, something just triggered me. I can feel that familiar ache in my chest, that tightness in my throat."

In that pause, your Wise Self can reach your Lost Child before the Protector Modes do. This is where healing happens—not in avoiding triggers but in meeting them differently.

When your Wise Self can say, "I see you're hurting. That person's comment touched that old wound. Let me stay here with you"—the raw spot begins to heal. Your Lost Child learns: I don't have to manage this alone. Someone is here. I'm not too much.

Over time, as your Wise Self consistently meets those missing emotional vitamins—offering the connection, validation, or boundaries that were scarce in childhood—the raw spots become less tender. The schema mindsets lose their grip. And the Protector Modes can finally relax, knowing your Lost Child is being cared for.

Recovery is about transforming triggers from emergencies into portals—opportunities for your Wise Self to practice meeting the needs your Lost Child has carried all along.

As Jane Goodall reminds us, "Only when head and heart work together can we reach our true potential." Your Lost Child holds the heart—feelings, needs, and authentic desires. Your Wise Self holds integrated wisdom—both thinking and feeling working in harmony. Your Protector Modes split these apart, letting your clever brain run the show whilst your feeling heart stays locked below deck. Recovery means bringing them back together.

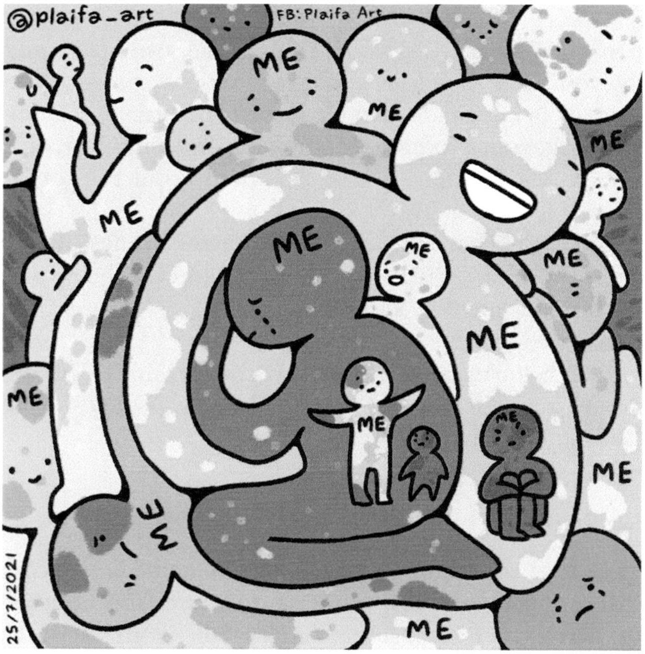

Figure 3.1 Plaifa Art (Plaifa Jungjaroennorasuk)

Part 2: Meeting Your Inner Crew

Now that you understand how your inner world becomes fragmented, let's meet each crew member individually. We'll start with your Child Modes—the parts that hold your emotional truth.

Meeting Your Child Modes

The Lost Child

There's a part of you that's been waiting.

She might be eight years old or five or twelve. She remembers things you've tried to forget. She feels things you've learned to numb. She needs things you've trained yourself not to want.

She's your Lost Child—the vulnerable, feeling part of you that holds your capacity for connection, creativity, and authentic emotion. In spite of the pervasive denial of vulnerability across our society, this side represents our common humanity, the vulnerability at the core of who we all are. Vulnerability is the "gold thread" of authenticity that runs through us all.

For many people with eating difficulties, this part has been hidden so long that they don't remember she exists. The Lost Child lives within your body and alerts you to your physical and emotional needs. She holds the hunger for emotional vitamins that were scarce—she knows what you needed then and still need now.

The Golden Buddha: Finding Your True Worth

There's a story of a Thai statue that beautifully illustrates the "gold" of the Child within. In the 1950s, a well-known statue of the Buddha in Bangkok began to show cracks due to drought and heat. Some monks came to inspect it and shone their torches into the widest cracks. To their astonishment, they caught a glimpse of gleaming gold under the layers of dull clay.

It was revealed that this was a statue made of pure gold that had been covered in clay 600 years earlier to protect it from invading soldiers. While all of the monks were killed by the soldiers, the golden Buddha had survived with the layers of clay covering its true value.

Just as this statue was covered for its own protection, so the inherent worth of our Child Modes becomes covered by Protector Modes—the parts whose role is to keep the Child hidden, presenting to the world what our culture expects or demands of us.

When we experience troubled times in early life that lead to loneliness, shame, guilt, humiliation and poor self-image, this creates emotional wounds—raw spots that remain active in our nervous systems and are reactivated within relationships in our adult lives. When triggered, we can find ourselves feeling overwhelmed and reacting in ways that feel out of proportion to the situation.

How She Shows Up in Your Life

Melissa's Lost Child carries the weight of never being quite good enough. She feels rejected, unwanted, inferior—desperate for someone to see past the performance, to value her for something other than achievement or appearance. She feels ashamed of normal emotions and needs, as if wanting comfort or connection makes her fundamentally flawed. She's been trying to communicate the only way she knows how: through body sensations, through eating urges, and through the inexplicable feeling that something is desperately wrong even when everything looks fine from the outside.

Faye's Lost Child remembers the day her dog died—not just the event, but the ache that followed, the grief that had nowhere to go because no one in her family knew how to help her hold it. She remembers the cakes her mum offered, the well-meaning attempt to "cheer her up," and how she learned in that moment: sadness gets replaced, not felt. Emptiness gets filled, not acknowledged. Her Lost Child carries years of feeling different, somehow on the outer—not through anything anyone said, but through absence. Through always being slightly invisible. She still feels this emptiness—a hollow ache that means she's alone even in the company of others, a sense that she'll never quite belong.

In restrictive eating patterns, low weight can become a language. Sometimes it says, "I'm vulnerable. I need help. Please see me." At other times it functions as armour—"I'm untouchable, I don't need anything, I can manage alone." For some, it's a way to disappear altogether, to feel safe through invisibility. Each message carries the same longing underneath: to be seen, understood, and safe in connection.

In binge patterns, the behaviour says: I'm so hungry—not for food but for connection, comfort, freedom, expression. It's a pressure valve releasing what can't be contained anymore.

Recognising Your Lost Child[3]

Your Lost Child (10) is your emotional self—the part of you that's been waiting to belong, be seen, and understood. The vulnerable part of you that is at the heart of your humanity.

She might feel:

- Like a lonely child valued only by "proving" herself through achievement or appearance or by meeting others' needs
- Longing for nourishment, protection, and someone to finally see her
- Anxious, sad, empty, guilty, and ashamed of existing
- Inferior, undeserving, and powerless

Due to missing emotional vitamins in childhood (connection, validation, empathy, nurturance), she believes she is a burden and undeserving of love. She feels guilty and ashamed of normal emotions and needs. She feels different and inferior. She feels unattractive and ashamed at both an emotional and a bodily level.

This mode is often hidden, and you may not be aware of its existence. But she's there, waiting—holding the truth of your experience, the capacity for joy and sorrow, the longing to finally be seen without having to earn it.

Her Voice: "I feel sad and lonely. I'm not enough. I don't belong. No one really sees me."

The Feisty Child

There's another feeling your Inner Child carries that is often overlooked: a sense of injustice or anger. We might only sense it as a tight chest, a tension in the jaw, and a slow simmer of "something isn't right." Other times it's bigger, as feelings of fury at the unfairness of it all, at how your needs are dismissed, at how hard you've had to work just to feel acceptable. When something feels unfair, she refuses to go along quietly. And as trauma physician Gabor Maté notes, when your *emotional immune system* is ignored or overridden, the physical immune system often pays the price—long-term suppression of anger can place the body under considerable strain (11).

This is your Feisty Child—your *emotional immune system*. She holds the truth of what happened that shouldn't have and what didn't happen that should have. She speaks up the moment something feels unjust, controlling, dismissive, or misaligned with your needs—although her voice might not reach the surface as it's pushed back down by Protector Modes.

For many people with eating difficulties, she has been silenced for years. Anger felt risky—too threatening to relationships, too likely to cause rejection or conflict. So her protest turned inward: into self-attack, perfectionism, restriction, bingeing, or punishing the body.

But anger is never the enemy. It is *information*—a signal that a boundary has been crossed or a need has gone unmet. When expectations feel controlling, she pushes back. When needs are ignored, she protests.

Her voice says: "I've been ignored for too long—and I won't disappear to keep the peace."

Emma knows this feeling well, though she rarely calls it anger. It appears as tightness in her chest when her sister asks for yet another favour, as irritation when her flatmate leaves the dishes again, as the silent resentment of always accommodating everyone else. Her family "didn't do anger." They did polite; they did "no fuss." So Emma learned to say "it's fine," while her Feisty Child raged unseen—redirected into perfectionism, restriction, or self-punishment.

Faye's anger lives even deeper underground. She doesn't know who she's angry with—her parents loved her, after all—but beneath the numbness is the fury of a child who felt overlooked and emotionally dismissed. During binges, the anger gets swallowed with the food, pushed down to preserve the family story that everything was "fine." Still, her Feisty Child waits . . . hoping someone might finally acknowledge that she has been hurting for a very long time.

The Impulsive Child

Then there's the part that jumps first and thinks later. This is your Impulsive Child—the freedom fighter, the part that can't stand restriction, that needs relief now, that acts on impulse without considering consequences.

She feels like she can never get enough. Like there's a famine coming and she'd better get what she needs before it's too late. She acts to get her way, to meet her needs, to grab whatever's available before it's gone again. *Impulsive bingeing isn't about not having enough willpower.* This part breaks through when she's been deprived for too long—a frantic attempt to meet needs that have repeatedly been silenced. It is also a backlash against feeling controlled or over-restricted—a protest against losing her freedom, especially when life feels like endless obligation or self-discipline without relief.

This part can't tolerate discomfort. Can't sit with difficult feelings without distraction. Can't be alone with herself without something to numb the experience. For her, *boredom or emotional deadness can feel like an emergency*—a trapped, airless state she'll do almost anything to escape. Restriction signals deprivation, and deprivation signals crisis.

Impulsive bingeing or self-harm can function as a means of meeting needs or desires (before the next "famine") or as a backlash against demands to be "good" or tightly controlled.

Her voice: "I deserve this, I need it NOW!" or "I need my freedom now!"

Better to take what you can get while it's available.

Some people have a more prominent Impulsive Child when certain traits are present—such as high Novelty-Seeking temperament, lower Effortful Control, or neurodivergent wiring (such as ADHD). In environments that feel shaming, rigid, or overly controlling, her energy grows stronger as she fights to protect a basic need for *freedom, stimulation, and aliveness.*

Her impulsivity is her way of saying, "I'm alive, I want to feel, I want to be free." In recovery, the goal is for your Wise Self to channel her energy toward genuine needs for stimulation, play, and connection—without the chaos that once surrounded them.

The Undisciplined Child

This part of you reacts like a tired, frustrated child who's had enough of being told what to do. She gets overwhelmed quickly, hates feeling pushed, and has very little tolerance for boredom, repetition, or long-haul effort. Small tasks feel huge; recovery can feel like an endless list of "shoulds."

On the surface she can look unmotivated or avoidant—but her reaction is emotional, immediate, and rooted in *a deep aversion to feeling trapped in obligation.* Even small tasks can feel like losing her freedom for the whole day.

She's pushing back against demands that feel bossy, heavy, or unfair. What makes this tricky is that often the "authority" she's resisting isn't coming from someone else at all—it's coming from your own internalised expectations, the demanding voices you absorbed in childhood.

Her inner protest sounds like:

"I don't want to!"
"You can't make me."
"This is too much . . . I'm done."
"I'm bored, I hate this, don't make me do it."

She shuts down because no one helped her learn persistence through *small doses of struggle followed by support*—the kind of scaffolding that grows confidence. Instead, effort felt like pressure, criticism, or defeat. She may also have grown up feeling controlled, shamed, or over-directed—so even when *you* try to guide yourself kindly, it triggers that old wiring.

Her Core Experiences

- Low tolerance for boredom or repetition—"boring" feels suffocating, not just dull.
- Overwhelm and depletion ("I'm tired before I even start")
- Pushback against perceived authority ("don't control me!")
- Reacting to internalised demands, not actual external ones
- Swinging between brief effort and total shutdown

Her Message: "I'm overwhelmed, I'm bored, and I don't want to be pushed. I don't know how to keep going when things feel effortful."

Wise Self Response: "You're not being difficult—you're tired, discouraged, and reacting to old pressure. I'm not here to boss you. We'll go slowly, with choices, breaks, and small steps. I'm beside you—we'll take this one step at a time, with breaks and choices, so effort doesn't feel like losing your freedom."

With this kind of gentle pacing and emotional companionship, she gradually discovers:

"Maybe I can try . . . as long as you don't push me, and we take it slowly."

The Contented Child

Here is a child part that you might have forgotten exists. She's playful. Spontaneous. Hopeful. Calm. Creative. Fully alive in her body.

This is the part that emerges when you feel safe enough to simply be. When emotional vitamins are present, she comes out to play. She feels valued, cared for, and understood. She trusts her body's signals. She asks for what she needs without shame.

She views her body as a positive part of herself—something to enjoy, to express feelings through, to experience pleasure with.

For most people reading this book, the Contented Child has been in hiding for years. But she's not gone. She's just waiting for conditions safe enough to emerge.

In this mode, you are playful, spontaneous, hopeful, calm, creative, and embodied. You feel valued, cared for, understood, capable, energetic, confident, protected, and safe. You can interpret body signals and ask for needs to be met. You view your body as your source of vitality and use it for play, expression of feelings, and pleasurable activities.

Her voice: "I'm allowed to say what I feel and ask for what I need. I'm allowed to play and have fun! I feel alive and free!"

In Practice

As Faye was growing up, she didn't have the opportunity to learn how to make sense of her inner body sensations. There was no one in her family who could describe how they were feeling, so there was no one who could tune into her world and really understand or deeply "know" her. Food became her language for expressing what couldn't be said.

Melissa's family provided excellent practical care but struggled with emotional attunement. She grew up never quite knowing where her mother ended, and she began. When she tried to follow her own life goals that didn't quite fit with her mother's expectations, her mother would act offended, reminding Melissa of all the sacrifices she had made for her. By losing weight, her body found another language: *These are my boundaries. This is where I end, and you begin.* The hard edges of her bones substituted for the identity she couldn't claim through words. Not eating became a way of setting boundaries and substituting for missing emotional vitamins for autonomy, freedom, and a separate self/identity.

Your Lost Child has been speaking through your body all along. You just haven't had anyone to translate.

For Faye, her eating became a way of filling the "emptiness" inside, substituting for her need for missing vitamins of affection, understanding, and nurturance. For Melissa, not eating became a way of setting boundaries and substituting for missing emotional vitamins for autonomy, freedom, and a separate self/identity.

Beneath eating difficulties, there is almost always a hidden child waiting to be heard and seen. This approach is about finding this lost part of yourself and creating space for her to exist—her body sensations, feelings, and thoughts.

Understanding Emotional Fluency

Emotional fluency—our ability to be aware of and work with our emotions—depends on how tuned in we are to the "language" of the body. Your ability to read your body's signals is what researchers call *interoception.* When your interoceptive skills are strong, you become adept at interpreting signals from your body as cues for what you need—whether they be physical needs, such as hunger, thirst, and warmth, or emotional needs such as being safe, seen, and soothed.

Table 3.1 What Am I Really Feeling? When Emotions are Mistaken for Hunger or Fullness

Inner Child Feeling	*Eating Pattern Misinterpretation*	*Eating Urge or Behaviours*
Overwhelmed, confused	I'm too full	Skipping meals, vomiting, exercise
Sadness	I'm heavy	Lose weight to lighten the feeling
Loneliness, boredom, anxiety	I'm hungry	Eating to fill inner emptiness
Guilty	I'm too much, a burden	Under-/overeat to punish self
Ashamed	I'm a problem, wrong	Lose/gain weight to hide self

Relying too heavily on logic whilst neglecting the wisdom held in our bodies can stand in the way of understanding the sensations that alert us to our emotional needs. Over time, this can impact significantly our wellbeing and deprive us of our potential to develop a rich inner emotional world.

Research shows that people with eating difficulties often experience heightened sensitivity to bodily sensations—particularly in the gut, heart, and lungs—while finding it harder to make sense of what those sensations mean or whether they are emotional and physical sensations (12, 13, 14).

The Paradox of Connection

What makes connecting with your Child Modes so difficult is that you might not want to.

Many people resist this work. It might feel childish, simplistic, or embarrassing. You've worked hard to be an adult, to be independent, and to leave behind those feelings of neediness and vulnerability. The last thing you want is to revisit them.

But the paradox is that when you disconnect from your Child Modes, you also disconnect from the emotions that tell you what you truly need. Joy, playfulness, love, sadness, shame, and anger—all of these have roots in childhood experience. That experience lives in your memory, in your body, informing how you navigate relationships and life itself.

When you ignore your Child Modes, you abandon the part of yourself that holds the truth of your reality. You lose your sense of direction. You become reliant on others to tell you who you are, what you should want, and what you should feel.

This makes you extra vulnerable to abandonment—not because others will necessarily leave but because without an internal foundation, losing external validation feels like losing yourself.

The alternative is different. When you have a strong bond between your Wise Self and your Child Modes—when you commit to never abandoning yourself—then other people's coming and going doesn't shatter you. It still hurts. Relationships still matter. But your sense of self remains intact.

You can be there for yourself while also reaching out for connection with others. Not self-sufficient isolation. Not desperate dependence. Something in between: interdependence rooted in a stable internal foundation.

This is why trust is so important in this work. If you can connect with someone you trust—whether a therapist, a close friend, or eventually yourself—who will be sensitive and supportive rather than dismissive, you might find yourself more willing to explore childhood memories, desires, regrets, and disappointments. Having someone who will validate those experiences can help you expand them into deeper emotional fulfilment in your present-day life.

Reflection Point

Which of these Child Modes do you recognise in yourself? Which one feels most familiar in your daily life?

Consider a recent eating-related struggle you've had. Looking back, can you identify what your Child Modes might have been feeling underneath the surface? Was it:

- Loneliness and seeking connection?
- Anger about being controlled or overlooked?
- Overwhelmed and needing comfort?
- Shame about your need for connection?
- Guilt about taking up space?
- Something else entirely?

To what extent are you able to talk openly and authentically about your emotions with others in your life? How is this similar or different to others in your family?

Meeting Your Protector Modes[4]

The Survival Crew

Now we meet the parts that have been running your life.

These are the Protector Modes—the survival strategies that stepped up when your Lost Child's feelings became too overwhelming, when expressing your authentic self felt too dangerous, when you needed solutions, and these were the only ones available.

Each Protector Mode was developed when specific emotional vitamins were missing. Your Overcontroller might have emerged when Freedom to

Express or Healthy Limits were scarce. Your People Pleaser when Safety and Stability felt conditional. They developed for good reasons, they've been working hard, and they have good intentions. But they're also keeping you stuck.

Each Protector Mode has a specific job: keep the Lost Child's feelings contained, prevent vulnerability from surfacing, manage relationships so you don't get hurt again, and create the illusion of control when everything feels chaotic.

They live in your body in particular ways. Learning to recognise these physical signatures helps you identify which mode is operating.

In Chapter 4, we'll explore each mode's fears, fantasies, and the cycles they create. For now, let's simply meet them.

Detached Protector

Emma sits on her couch, scrolling through her phone for two hours. She couldn't tell you what she's looking at. The day stretches ahead, empty and flat. She should probably eat, shower, and respond to her friend's text from three days ago. She does none of these things.

This is Emma's Detached Protector—the part that numbs everything. Emotions get flattened. Relationships stay superficial. Life happens at a distance, as if she's watching through thick glass.

This part has many tools: restriction that creates numbness, work that fills every moment so there's no space to feel, sleep that offers escape, and exercise that exhausts into blankness.

This part learned early: needing others leads to disappointment. Showing vulnerability invites rejection. Better to disconnect and shut down, even if that means being completely isolated inside yourself.

This mode can also show up as cynicism or sarcasm, such as brushing off the concept of emotional needs and questioning whether any of it really applies to you. Or a "passive simmering" or irritation that comes with pushing needs and emotions underground.

Voice: "I don't need to feel anything. Emotions are pointless. I'm fine on my own."

Detached Self-Soother

While the Detached Protector creates general numbness, the Detached Self-Soother offers something more active—specific behaviours that promise relief and comfort, even if temporary.

Bingeing. Self-harm. Substances that take the edge off. Alcohol. Screen time that stretches into hours. Exercise that goes past pleasure into mechanical repetition. These activities manage overwhelming feelings when emotional vitamins have been triggered but are in short supply.

Sometimes, vomiting follows the binge—a way to "cancel out" the shame the binge created. One behaviour to manage feelings, another to manage the feelings about the first behaviour.

For Faye, whose family navigated difficulty through silent endurance, this mode became her most reliable companion. It promises relief without requiring vulnerability, comfort without risking rejection.

Voice: "At least this is reliable. At least this is something I can count on when everything else feels out of control."

Overcontroller

Melissa's alarm goes off at 5:45 AM. She's already awake.

By 6:00 she's logged her food for the day. By 6:15 she's on the treadmill. Her mind is already organising tomorrow: client meeting, "safe" snack, emails, the same carefully measured meal she eats every day.

This is Melissa's Overcontroller—the general who runs her life with military precision. It promises: If you just follow the rules perfectly and control everything tightly enough, you'll finally be safe.

Emma's Overcontroller emerged almost politely—much like Emma herself. It doesn't shout demands. Instead, it insists: "Just be efficient. Plan everything. If you're organised enough, controlled enough, no one will notice you need anything." It spent two hours last night calculating tomorrow's food, keeps her schedule so packed there's no space for feelings to surface, and rewrites emails until they're perfect—so neutral that no one could possibly be offended, or notice her, or ask how she's really doing.

This part tries to convert old painful feelings into their opposites—turning shame into pride, powerlessness into control, vulnerability into invincibility. It takes pride in overruling basic human needs. Feelings are viewed as weak or self-indulgent. The body exists only as transport for the head—something to manage and direct.

This mode was often learned early that feelings were unsafe. Perhaps emotional expression brought criticism or rejection. Perhaps feelings seemed dangerous because they overwhelmed a fragile parent. When a child must stay calm to keep the household stable, emotional suppression becomes protection.

The Overcontroller's problem-solving mindset brings temporary relief from confusion, translating life into simple categories—productive or unproductive, success or failure, attractive or unattractive. These rules create a sense of direction and safety, but they're a substitute for real emotional nourishment and connection.

The Overcontroller comes in different flavours—perfectionistic (must get everything exactly right), invincible (must need nothing), or suspicious (must stay hypervigilant to danger). We'll explore these variations in Chapter 4.

Voice: "Follow the rules. Control everything. Emotions are a weakness. You don't really need that."

Overcontroller's Different Flavours

Perfectionistic Flavour: For Melissa, this shows up as perfectionism. Every meal is measured precisely. Every workout is logged. Any deviation triggers panic, as if one unplanned snack will send everything spiralling. She maintains tight control to ensure that everything is done "properly" and to avoid criticism or humiliation. Satisfaction is always just out of reach—standards keep rising, and the pressure to do better never settles. The focus often shifts between restrictive eating, weight, shape, exercise, grades, or other forms of achievement. There is a strong pull toward order, symmetry, and doing things the "right" way, with mistakes quickly felt as getting it "wrong".

Invincible Flavour: 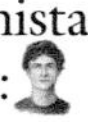 Tony's Overcontroller looks different, invincible rather than perfectionistic. His coaches taught him that missing training meant failure, so his system learned to push past pain, exhaustion, and hunger. There is a sense of power in needing nothing, in proving himself stronger than basic human limits. When injury ended swimming, restriction became a new way to express that strength. It can feel like a kind of victory over the body—rising above physical needs. Contempt for your own or others' needs. This part strives for complete invulnerability, pushing emotional needs aside. At times, exercise or eating restraint or restriction brings a sense of intensity or elevation, alongside pride, mastery, and a strong feeling of being in control. There may be momentary feelings of being 'better than' or above others.

Suspicious Flavour: Melissa's version is suspicious. If others see her vulnerability, they'll control her. If they witness her needs, they'll use them against her. Better to stay guarded, hypervigilant, one step ahead of potential betrayal. Hypervigilant to danger. Fearful that if others see your true self or vulnerability, or if you reveal you need them, they'll control or overpower you.

Melissa, whose family sacrificed everything while rarely allowing themselves anything, developed an Invincible Overcontroller that insists: "The only way to be worthy is to need nothing." Her restriction became a way of making herself smaller—a protective strategy with good intentions, even though it causes harm.

Whether perfectionist or invincible, or suspicious, the Overcontroller is organised around one core belief: control brings safety and feelings carry risk. Survival comes to depend on overriding anything soft, vulnerable, or needing.

Voice: "Stay in control. Follow the rules. Keep everything tight. Emotions aren't helpful. You don't really need that. You're stronger than your body."

Pollyanna Overcompensator

"Everything happens for a reason!" "Look on the bright side!" "I'm fine! Really, I'm great actually!" This is the Pollyanna Overcompensator—the part that learned to cope by maintaining a persistently positive attitude even when authentic feelings tell a different story.

Emma's Pollyanna mode developed when her family couldn't handle negativity. Any expression of sadness or struggle was met with "Don't be so negative!" She learned that keeping things light and upbeat was the only way to stay connected.

Now, when something genuinely difficult happens—a friend cancels plans, her eating disorder urges intensify, someone hurts her feelings—Emma immediately performs optimism: "It's totally fine! Actually, it's probably better this way!"

But underneath the performance, her Lost Child feels dismissed. The real feelings—hurt, disappointment, anger—have nowhere to go. So they get expressed through eating behaviours instead.

This mode overcompensates for underlying negativity, mistrust, and fear of being criticised or rejected. Often, the person learned early that they were responsible for buoying up depressed, emotionally fragile, or overly negative parents.

Voice: "Everything's fine! There's always a bright side. Let's not dwell on negative things."

People Pleaser

Karen sits across from her friend, nodding and smiling as she talks about relationship problems. Karen is exhausted. She had her own crisis this morning—a panic attack before work, a text from her mother laden with guilt, and a deadline she's not sure she can meet.

None of this comes up. Instead, Karen listens. Offers advice. Makes supportive sounds. When her friend finally says, "Enough about me, how are you?" Karen hears herself say: "I'm good! Just busy with work." This is Karen's People Pleaser—the part that learned to earn love through usefulness, to maintain relationships by having no inconvenient needs of her own.

This part monitors others constantly, suppresses personal preferences, and says yes when every cell screams no. It works to keep everyone happy because happiness equals safety, and conflict equals abandonment.

Karen's family showed love through sacrifice rather than emotional presence. The message was clear: your needs are a burden. Don't ask for more. So she doesn't. She helps everyone else while her own emotional reserves run dry. Then wonders why she feels so empty.

Voice: "I need to make others happy. If I'm useful and don't cause problems, maybe they'll keep me around."

Helpless Protector

"I don't know how to do this." "It's too hard." "I've tried everything and nothing works." "Can't someone else fix this for me?"

This is the Helpless Protector—the part that learned to cope by giving up personal power and waiting for rescue.

For many people, helplessness became the only reliable way to maintain a connection. If a parent needed to be needed, staying helpless kept them engaged. You might have learned that vulnerability expressed through visible struggle (illness, low weight, obvious distress) brings people closer, but vulnerability expressed through direct requests pushes people away.

This mode holds a powerful fantasy—that if you stay helpless long enough, someone will finally show up and give you what you needed all along. The perfect parent figure who will retroactively fill in all those missing emotional vitamins from childhood. The rescue you're waiting for means you don't have to grieve what you missed.

This mode also protects against facing impossible adult expectations. If you stay ill, you don't have to meet the relentless standards you've watched others struggle under—the exhaustion, the self-denial, the achievement treadmill that never stops.

The Helpless mode maintains eating disorder behaviours through seemingly legitimate reasons: "I was too busy to eat because of my studies." "I've been ill and couldn't eat." The eating disorder continues, but now it's "not my fault."

Voice: "Why won't anyone help me? Can't someone else fix this? If I get better, will you still care about me?"

For a deeper exploration of the Helpless Protector's functions, fears, and the rescue-fantasy, see Supporting Materials in Appendices.

Inner Critic: The Guard at the Hatch

When you hear harsh, attacking voices in your mind—voices using shame, guilt, and relentless criticism—you're hearing what we call the Critic.

This is the internalised voice of the cultural and schema mindsets we explored in Chapter 2. Remember those messages about bodies, worth, needs, and emotions that you absorbed from family, culture, peers, and media? Your Critic is what happened when you took those messages inside and made them your own—partly because, as a child, you naturally believed adults were right, and partly because believing "the problem is me" gave you something to work on. If you could fix yourself, maybe you'd finally be acceptable.

This internalisation was especially functional when it helped you stay connected to caregivers. If your parents couldn't tolerate your emotions or needs, learning to criticise yourself for having them helped you maintain attachment. Better to stay connected by agreeing "I'm too much" than risk abandonment by insisting "I deserve care."

The Critic's voice carries messages that are:

- **Demanding**: "You should be achieving more, doing better, being perfect."
- **Punishing**: "You're disgusting, weak, pathetic, fundamentally flawed."
- **Guilt-inducing**: "Your needs are a burden, you're too sensitive, stop being dramatic."

But the Critic isn't just old messages playing on repeat. It's also become a protective part of you—one that genuinely believes harsh self-attack will keep you safe. It learned that punishing yourself first might protect you from others' punishment. That if you deprive yourself enough, criticise yourself harshly enough, maybe you'll finally become acceptable.

For some, the Critic becomes particularly punishing, actively using deprivation, restriction, and self-harm as tools. 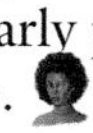 Harriet's Critic took the anger she felt at the people who dismissed her pain and turned it inward, using restriction as a way to control her own suffering rather than risk showing others how much she hurt. The punishment felt like power, until it became a prison.

In our sailing metaphor, the Critic is the guard shouting down the hatch where your Lost Child hides. It believes keeping her locked below deck—using shame and harsh criticism—is the only way to keep you safe from rejection, abandonment, and humiliation.

The Critic genuinely attempts to protect you. But its methods keep your Lost Child trapped, afraid to emerge, convinced she's fundamentally flawed.

In Chapter 6, you'll learn how your Wise Self can set boundaries with this harsh voice whilst helping it discover that protection doesn't require punishment. For now, simply begin noticing when you hear the Critic speaking—and remember, this voice isn't the truth about you. It's old messages you internalised to survive, now operating as a misguided protector.

For a more extensive list of Modes, see Appendix 6.

Finding Your Wise Self

But there's another part—the voice of quiet wisdom, easily drowned out by Protector Modes and Critic voices. Your Wise Self.

If your Critic has been loud for years, this part might feel like it's barely there. A seedling waiting to grow. But it's there—at the core of your humanity, carrying qualities like compassion, warmth, wisdom, and integrity. This is your inner leader, the captain your crew has been waiting for.

Unlike your Protector Modes, your Wise Self doesn't operate on fear—but from growth and possibility—understanding that capacities for handling life aren't fixed but can develop over time.

The Role of Your Inner Leader

A key role of the Wise Self is attuning to and caring for your Child Modes. The Wise Self is your internal witness, protector, nurturer, and coach. It doesn't judge, attempt to fix, attack, reject, pity, or abandon. It advocates—listening to your Lost Child's emotions, setting boundaries aligned with your Feisty Child's signals, encouraging play for your Contented Child, and understanding your Impulsive Child's needs.

Even if this part exists only as a small spark right now, it holds the potential to offer the care and steadiness you may have missed growing up. Your Wise Self isn't fixed—it can learn, strengthen, and grow.

Qualities Your Wise Self Develops

Your Wise Self recognises and accepts emotions and vulnerability—in yourself and others. It finds balance between feeling and thinking and manages uncertainty with more ease. It experiences body and mind as integrated rather than at war. It gives and receives nourishment without guilt. It stays present with both distress and joy without needing to escape.

When you have a strong inner leader who can tune into your Child Modes' feelings and needs, this operates as an inner compass—directing you through life based not only on rational thought but also on body wisdom: intuition, gut instincts, felt sense.

In Chapter 5, you'll learn how to remember and develop this wise presence, building the foundation for all the healing work ahead. For now, simply know: this part exists within you, waiting to be strengthened.

Connecting with Your Wise Self

Try this: Find a photograph of yourself as a child—ideally before age 12. Look at this child. Really look. Notice their expression, posture, and the look in their eyes.

What Feelings Come Up?

Can you sense vulnerability? Loneliness? Shame visible in how they hold themselves? Or pride? Joy? Some people feel warmth, a protective urge. Others feel critical, impatient, and disgusted. Some feel nothing at all.

Ask yourself:

- What feelings and thoughts emerged?
- Did I feel drawn toward this child or want to look away?
- Did I feel warmth or judgement?
- If I could speak to this child now, what would I say?

If you felt warmth, you're in touch with your Wise Self. If you felt criticism, you're identified with your Critic. But your Wise Self is still there, buried under old messages. This wise presence might feel like a warm, compassionate guide—a caring mentor within you.

Strong feelings may arise in the context of this exercise. This isn't a sign that you're doing it incorrectly or that there is anything wrong with you. Just take it step by step and feel free to return and lightly repeat when you feel able to, even if only for a minute or two.

Meeting Your Crew: A Visualisation Exercise

Before we map how your modes operate, it helps to get acquainted with them as distinct characters. Many people find that visualising or drawing their modes makes it easier to recognise when these parts are active and creates some helpful distance from being completely fused with them.

You don't need to be an artist for this exercise—stick figures work perfectly well. What matters is creating a visual representation that helps you recognise each mode when it shows up.

Getting Started

Take a piece of paper and draw a simple ship—your ship. It doesn't need to be detailed; a basic outline is enough. This is your internal world, and you're about to populate it with the crew members who've been running things.

Now, for each mode you've recognised in yourself, give them a form:

What Do They Look Like?

- How old are they? (Your Overcontroller might look like a stern adult, whilst your Lost Child might appear as your younger self at a particular age.)
- What's their posture? (Protector Modes often stand rigid or cross-armed; your Lost Child might be curled up or hiding.)
- What's their facial expression? (The Critic might be scowling; the People Pleaser might look anxious and watchful.)

Where Are They Positioned on the Ship?

- Your Overcontroller might be at the helm, white-knuckled grip on the wheel.
- Your Detached Protector might be off to the side, facing away from everyone.
- Your People Pleaser might be scanning the horizon anxiously.
- Your Lost Child is below deck—but where exactly? Huddled in a corner? Hidden behind boxes? Peeking nervously up the stairs?
- Your Critic might be standing over the hatch where your Lost Child hides.

What Are They Wearing or Carrying?

- Does your Critic carry a megaphone or a clipboard, constantly monitoring?
- Does your Overcontroller have charts, measuring tools, or a stopwatch?
- Does your People Pleaser carry a mirror to check how they're appearing to others?
- What does your Lost Child clutch for comfort—a blanket, a toy, and her knees pulled tight?

What's Their Voice Like?

- Sharp and attacking? Urgent and controlling? Flat and monotone? Pleading? Barely a whisper?

Alternative Approaches

Not everyone connects with drawing. Some people prefer to:

- Write detailed descriptions of each mode as if introducing characters in a story
- Find photos in magazines that capture each mode's essence and create a collage
- Use objects around the house to represent each mode
- Simply close your eyes and imagine the scene vividly

There's no right way to do this—choose whatever method helps you see your modes as distinct presences rather than abstract concepts.

Why This Matters

When you can visualise your modes as distinct characters occupying specific positions on your ship, you begin to see your internal world differently. Instead of being completely merged with a feeling—"I AM anxious," "I AM worthless"—you can begin to observe with some distance—"Ah, my Overcontroller has taken over the helm again. I can see her there, frantically adjusting the sails." This change in perspective is the seed of your Wise Self awakening. You're learning to be the one who can see the whole crew, rather than being hijacked by whichever member is currently loudest.

Once you've created your visual map, keep it somewhere accessible. In the exercise that follows, you'll use these crew members to map out how they interact, what triggers them, and how they've been trying to keep you safe. Having a clear image of each one makes this analytical work much more tangible; you're not working with abstract concepts but with specific characters you can now recognise.

Note: Remember, take your time with this visualisation practice. You don't need to see all your modes clearly in one sitting. Start with just one—perhaps the mode that feels most active in your life right now. Spend a few days getting to know this crew member before moving to the next. Notice: Do you like the flavour of this practice? Does it help you see yourself more clearly? Then take another step when you're ready.

Mapping Your Crew

Think of yourself with many different crew members, each with its own agenda. Some child parts feeling sad. Others running around causing disruption.

Others happy and singing. Various protector parts operating in different ways—one wanting to seal everything off, another pulling out the rule book, another monitoring everyone else.

The next step: bringing them together as a team rather than random parts working independently.

Making Your Mode Map

Step 1: Draw Your Internal World

Take paper and draw a line down the middle. One half is "hidden" (parts operating behind the scenes, out of conscious awareness). The other is "visible" (parts dominating thoughts, urges, and behaviours).

Step 2: Place Your Child Modes in the Hidden (Below Deck) Section

We can assume that right now your Child Modes might be in the "below deck" section at least some of the time. Note your Child Modes with associated words and feelings: Lost Child, Feisty Child, Impulsive Child, Contented Child. The Inner Critic might also be there, echoing schema mindsets from the past.

Step 3: Map a Recent Trigger

Now that you understand the pattern (Trigger → Schema Mindset → Raw Spot → Critic → Protector Modes → Eating Behaviour), practise tracking it with a recent situation that led to eating-related urges:

- What happened first? (The trigger)
- What schema mindset got activated? (See Chapter 2)
- What did your Child Modes feel? (The raw spot—notice the bodily sensation)
- What was your Inner Critic's message?
- Which Protector Modes stepped in?
- Which eating behaviours followed?

This tracking helps you see your unique pattern clearly. Once you can identify this chain, you have the opportunity to interrupt it—to let your Wise Self reach your Lost Child at the moment the raw spot surfaces, before the Protector Modes take over.

Step 4: Add Your Protector Modes

Most Protector Modes operate visibly, often on autopilot without your Wise Self choosing them. You likely see these as "me" rather than recognising them as parts of your larger self.

Remember: they developed with good intentions—to manage painful feelings created by missing vitamins and difficult experiences. But they also carry utopian fantasies about perfect outcomes that keep you separated from developing real resilience.

Example:  **Samantha's Map**: Two-Act Mode Cascade: When a Small Trigger Sets Off a Storm

Trigger: A friend cancels a lunch date.

Schema Mindset Activated: Emotional Deprivation ("My needs don't matter") + Defectiveness ("I'm not enough to keep her attention")

Act 1: The Sudden Drop below Deck

Below deck, a painful feeling surfaces.

Lost Child: *I feel sad. Lonely. Like I don't matter.*

Almost immediately, another voice cuts in.

Inner Critic: *Of course, she cancelled. You're the problem. You're too much. Too needy. Unlovable.*

The feelings intensify—heavy, raw.

Detached Self-Soother: *Make this stop. Eat. Numb it. Push the feelings away.*

Bingeing is a way to escape the loneliness . . . for now.

Act 2: After the Storm Breaks

When the eating stops, the relief fades. Below deck again, the *Lost Child* is left exposed.

Lost Child: *I've failed again. I'm weak. I should be ashamed.*

Inner Critic returns, louder now.

Inner Critic: *You shouldn't have lost control. What's wrong with you . . . stupid girl.*

A different protector steps forward:

Overcontroller: *Enough. You need discipline. Stop eating. Be productive. Don't feel. Get yourself back under control.*

Rules are formed. Diets planned. Feelings are shut down. The ship looks steady again above deck—but below deck, the Lost Child is still alone.

Understanding the Pattern: When something touches an old schema wound or emotional "raw spot"—the Critic's harsh voice attacks the Lost Child, whilst Protector Modes reach for familiar eating behaviours to soothe the pain.

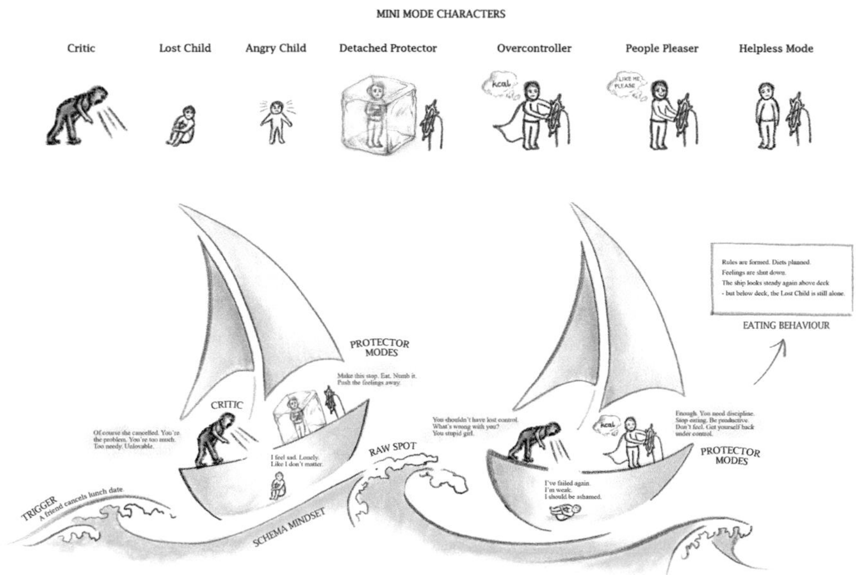

Figure 3.2 Mode Map with ship and characters

Samantha's eating behaviours are driven by her Protector Modes as an attempt to manage or shut down the emotional pain of the Child Modes. The goal in recovery is for Samantha's Wise Self to reach her Lost Child at the moment her friend cancelled—to stay with that ache in her chest and say, "You're lonely. That makes sense. Your need for connection is valid. Let's find a way to meet that need that doesn't involve your friend or food."

Reflection Point: Can you see this pattern in your experience? What happens when you restrict tightly—does pressure build? When you break rules, which Protector Modes show up afterwards?

For further guidance on making a Mode Map, see Appendix 7.

Understanding Functions

Your eating behaviours serve multiple functions, including:

Prevention (Keeping Lost Child Contained):

- Filling your mind with food/weight thoughts to avoid emotional awareness
- Creating rigid rules for control and predictability
- Using body focus as a distraction from life difficulties
- Maintaining patterns that keep you numb

Emergency Response (pushing Child Modes back down when they surface):

- Bingeing to soothe loneliness or anxiety that broke through
- Restricting to regain control when overwhelmed
- Compulsive exercise to release pent-up emotional energy such as anger
- Using substances, self-harm, and sleep to numb surface pain

The Path Forward

When you have a strong inner leader tuned into your Child Modes' needs, this operates as an internal compass. This partnership requires your Wise Self to soothe and regulate your body sensations and emotions by ensuring emotional needs get met.

This harmonisation allows a flexible, adaptable, coherent, energised, and stable self to emerge.

Inner integration means:

- Your Wise Self leads with compassion and skill.
- Your Child Modes feel heard and cared for.
- Your Protector Modes relax their vigilance and find healthier ways to contribute.
- Your Critic's influence diminishes as you recognise it as an echo needing limits.

Gentle Experiments to Try

1: Child Mode Check-Ins

Three times this week, when you notice eating-related urges, pause. Ask: "What might my Child Modes be feeling right now? What schema 'raw spot' was triggered?"

Don't try to fix anything. Just notice. Offer yourself the same compassion you'd give a friend.

2: Spot the Protector Pause

When you notice an urge to restrict food, binge, or criticise yourself, take a slow breath and ask, *Who's speaking right now?* Which Protector Mode is on deck? Then ask, *What is this part trying to protect me from?* You don't have to change anything yet—just listen. Understanding the purpose of each voice helps your Wise Self begin to guide the conversation.

Remember that the urge to criticise yourself or "beat yourself up" often comes from the Inner Critic—an echo of voices you've absorbed from others in the past . . . a self-flagellating voice, where directing pain or blame inward has become a form of protection. At some point, you may have learned that turning blame on yourself created a sense of order when life felt chaotic, control when you felt powerless, and hope when you felt hopeless.

3: Body Signals

When you catch yourself thinking "I feel fat," translate: "What emotion am I actually feeling? Overwhelmed? Ashamed? Lonely? What triggered this?"

Practice speaking your Child Modes' emotional language.

4: The Photograph

Try the photograph reflection at least once. Notice if your response changes with practice. Can you access your Wise Self's compassion for this child?

5: Mode Mapping

Create your Mode Map from a recent triggering situation. Track step by step—trigger, Child feelings, Protector responses, and eating behaviours.

Simply observing the pattern without judgement is powerful work.

Journalling Prompt Reflections: Meeting Your Inner Crew

- Which mode showed up whilst you were reading this chapter? What was it trying to protect you from?
- What does your Lost Child most need you to know right now?
- When you picture your inner ship, where is each crew member positioned? Who's steering?
- Which mode feels hardest to recognise or accept as part of you?

A Note on Pacing: You don't need to try all these practices this week. Choose one or two that feel most accessible right now. Spend time with them. Notice what works for your system—what helps you feel more grounded, more connected, and more present.

What You're Learning

Now you're learning about your internal world in ways that make change possible.

The journey toward integration takes time, patience, and courage. But you're not alone. Your Wise Self—that seed of wisdom and compassion within you—grows stronger every time you pause to listen to your inner world with curiosity rather than judgement.

Your Child Modes have been waiting for this attention. For someone who doesn't abandon them when feelings get big, who listens to what's needed, who responds with tenderness rather than criticism. They have much to teach you about what you really need, what brings you joy, what kind of life will nourish you. The deeper work of recovery is not about trying to become unbroken, but learning to see your struggles as places where wisdom, strength, and courage can enter.

Your inner crew—all of them—have been part of your survival story. Now they can become part of your thriving story too.

Notes

1 Rumi poem "Your Body is a Guest House" by Shahram Shiva (2021). Rumi: The Beloved Is You: My Favorite Collection of Deeply Passionate, Whimsical, Spiritual and Profound Poems and Quotes.

2 The *Wise Self* refers to the Schema Therapy concept of Inner Leader or "Healthy Adult" Mode.

3 The *Lost Child* refers to a Vulnerable Child Mode marked by a sense of invisibility, aloneness, and being hidden, forgotten, or left behind.

4 Protector Modes are what Schema Therapy calls coping modes—parts of you that use strategies learned long ago to keep you safe.

4 Understanding Your Survival Crew

I am not afraid of storms, for I am learning how to sail my ship.
—Louisa May Alcott (*Little Women*, 1869) (15)

The Kitchen

 Emma stands in her kitchen at 7 AM, staring at the breakfast she's prepared according to her meal plan. Her Overcontroller is already calculating calories and planning the day's exercise routine. Her People Pleaser is worrying about the work meeting where she'll need to present her ideas. Her Detached Protector is suggesting she skip breakfast altogether—it would be so much simpler to just have coffee and avoid the whole internal debate. She notices this familiar chorus of competing voices. Each feels urgent and well-intended—but together they pull her in different directions.

In Chapter 3, you met your inner crew—Child Modes, Protector Modes, Inner Critic, Wise Self. You learned their basic patterns, how they developed, and what they're trying to do. Now it's time to understand them more deeply—not change them yet. For now, you're learning to recognise them in action: what drives them, how they show up, and the patterns they create.

Without this understanding, change feels vague and slippery; with it, things begin to make sense.

Protector Modes in Your Body

Over time, we can mistakenly come to believe that we ARE our Protector Modes—that they are "me." Healing work invites us to reconnect with our inner Wise Self, loosening their grip so we can reach the Lost Child inside, who has been waiting to be seen.

Chapter 3 introduced the idea that modes don't just live in your thoughts—they have physical signatures. The clearest way to understand how these modes operate is to notice them directly—especially around eating.

DOI: 10.4324/9781003355878-5

Body Awareness Practice[1]

Throughout your day, when you notice eating urges or difficult feelings arising, pause. Take three breaths. Then notice:

- Where am I holding tension right now?
- How is my posture shifting?
- What's happening with my breathing?
- Where do I feel tightness, numbness, or heaviness?
- What thoughts are running through my mind right now?
- What urges are present around food or my body?
- What emotions are here—or notably absent?

Do this enough times and patterns emerge. Your Overcontroller might live in your shoulders and jaw. Your People Pleaser might create tightness in your chest. Your Detached Protector might bring numbness spreading from your stomach.

Emma noticed—Her Overcontroller made her shoulders rise around her ears, jaw clench, and breathing become shallow and rapid. Her People Pleaser created tightness in her chest and made her lean forward as if ready to help. Her Detached Protector brought heavy numbness spreading from her stomach through her whole body, and she'd find herself staring into space.

Understanding these signatures helped Emma catch modes before they took over completely. She could feel her shoulders tensing and think: *Ah, my Overcontroller is activating. What's triggering this?*

Deepening Your Awareness

For a more physical exploration, try this chair-based exercise.

Step 1: Set up different chairs or spaces to represent one or two of your Protector Modes. Place an object that represents that mode in some way on each chair (e.g. a rock might symbolise the rigidity of the Overcontroller, or a cosy blanket might symbolise Detached Self Soother).

Step 2: Choose a recent situation that triggered eating-related urges.

Step 3: Move between the chairs, spending a few minutes in each whilst holding the object. Let the thoughts, feelings, and impulses of that mode arise. What might this side say, if it had a voice?

As you do this, notice:

- How your posture changes
- How your breathing shifts
- Where tension or numbness appears
- What urges or thoughts arise

Reflection Point: Which Protector Modes feel most familiar in your body? Which feel uncomfortable or foreign? Do particular modes live in specific parts of your body? Understanding your unique signatures helps you recognise them as they emerge—before you're completely swept away.

What Your Protector Modes Fear Most

Your Protector Modes have been running your ship without a captain for so long; they genuinely fear what might happen if they relinquish control.

The Core Fear

At the heart of every Protector Mode lies the same fundamental terror: that authentic connection will lead to rejection, humiliation, abandonment, or harm. Each mode is developed as a way to manage this fear of being truly seen and potentially cast out from relationships that you need to survive.

Recovery isn't just about changing eating behaviours. It's about learning to tolerate vulnerability that comes with genuine human connection. It's about learning to see and take care of the Lost Child who has been waiting—unseen, alone, hoping someone might finally notice her without conditions, without her having to earn it through achievement, appearance, or perfect behaviour.

The goal is to build a more reliable kind of relief—reconnecting with your true self and learning to give yourself the emotional vitamins you didn't receive. This means facing a painful truth: what has been missing. And letting go of the fantasy your Protector Modes have lived on—the hope that *if only I please others, give them what they need, achieve enough, have full self-control, work hard, be what others need me to be, get sick enough—then I'll get those missing vitamins. Then I'll finally be seen and cared for. Then I'll get what I've been waiting for.*

Letting go of these fantasies can feel devastating. There's a strange safety in blaming yourself—because the alternative is facing the reality that others may have let you down. But letting go is also freeing. It opens the door to the life that was meant for you. And it's deeply healing for your Lost Child to see your Wise Self take a risk and step out of these old patterns for her benefit—to finally choose her wellbeing over the fantasy that perfect compliance or control will earn her love.

This means learning to be in the messiness and uncertainty of life. To be with your Lost Child and feel with her—rather than trying to fix her or leaving her to suffer alone. It means listening to your Lost Child's sadness, her loneliness, and her longing. To your Feisty Child's signals about crossed boundaries and unfairness. To your Contented Child's sparks of joy and awe when she encounters something beautiful or valuable to her. These parts have the information you need.

Facing reality—letting go of protector modes and their promises—involves grief. Grief about past losses, missing emotional vitamins, and the years consumed by eating difficulties. Grief about a world that has never been as fair or just as we would wish it to be. Grief that historical trauma—wars, poverty, displacement—deprived our ancestors of emotional vitamins, leaving them unable to offer what they'd never known themselves.

This can feel overwhelming. But your Wise Self—when strong enough—can say: *It's sad, but I can handle it. I can let myself feel the sadness, knowing and facing the reality of what happened that shouldn't have and what didn't happen that should have. I can allow the grief and stay with my Lost Child as she heals.*

There may be another fear, too: if your Protector Mode identities become less dominant, who will you be? Behind the Protector Mode masks, you have a real self. You might not be in touch with it yet. But it's there—core to who you are, waiting to be discovered. You can only know this self through the process of letting go of the survival roles your Protector Modes have been playing. Not making them disappear, but helping them exist in their healthy states—as part of your whole rather than dominating voices that drown everything else out.

If you can gently encourage them to trust your Wise Self and let go bit by bit, they'll integrate and become healthy parts of you.

As you read the fears below, you don't need to recognise all of the Protector Modes. One or two may stand out immediately—and that's enough to work with.

Specific Fears of Each Mode

Look closely at each mode's fear, and you'll see which emotional vitamin was missing. Your Overcontroller might fear chaos because voicing your needs once felt unsafe, resulting in feeling subjugated. Your Detached Protector might fear emotions because Connection and Belonging came with too much pain. Each Protector Mode carries particular fears that drive its strategies.

The Overcontroller's Fears

This part developed because feeling out of control once felt genuinely dangerous.

Its specific fears:

- "If I stop controlling my eating/body/achievement, everything will spiral."
- "If I let myself feel emotions fully, I'll be overwhelmed and fall apart."
- "If I'm not perfect, everyone will see how flawed I am."
- "If I have needs, I'll be seen as weak, burdensome, too much."
- "If life becomes unpredictable, I won't cope."
- "If I relax standards, I'll have no value."
- "If I allow vulnerability, others will use it against me."

These fears made sense when you were younger. Perhaps expressing emotions led to punishment, withdrawal, or the silent treatment. Perhaps making mistakes brought harsh criticism. Perhaps adults around you were overwhelmed and couldn't handle their own needs, let alone yours. They may also have been hiding their own emotional struggles, perhaps even from themselves, while pretending all was well to the outside world. Perhaps unpredictability felt genuinely unsafe.

 **Tony's Overcontroller** learned its fears when coaches told him he'd "never amount to anything" if he missed training, whilst praising his friend's muscular physique. The fear became: If I'm not lean enough, muscular enough, and disciplined enough, I'm worthless and will be humiliated.

His rigid "clean eating," compulsive training, and constant body checking became attempts to outrun this terror—proving his worth through his physique whilst avoiding the vulnerability of feeling inadequate.

The Perfectionistic version fears:

- "If I make a mistake, I'll be humiliated."
- "If things aren't perfect, I'll be criticised and shamed."
- "If I can't predict and control outcomes, I'll fail and everyone will see."
- "If I don't achieve, I have no worth."

The Invincible version fears:

- "If I show I have needs, I'll be seen as weak and pathetic."
- "If I depend on others, they'll resent the burden."
- "If I'm not completely self-sufficient, I'll be abandoned."
- "If I allow vulnerability, I'll be that needy child again who was too much."

 **Melissa's Invincible Overcontroller** carries this fear: *If I let myself need anything, I'll deplete the people I love. Better to need nothing.*

Her restriction became proof that she'd transcended the shameful state of being someone who needs.

The Critic: When Loyalty Requires Self-Betrayal

For some people, the Inner Critic becomes one of the most powerful members of the survival crew. Rather than offering guidance or limits, it takes on a harsher role—attacking, shaming, and punishing the Inner Child in an attempt to preserve attachment.

Early on, you may have learned that expressing certain emotions was risky. Anger might have led to withdrawal, punishment, or emotional distance. Sadness may have been dismissed or treated as weakness. Needs may have been experienced by caregivers as inconvenient or burdensome. Messages such as "Stop being so sensitive" or "Can't you see how much I've sacrificed?" taught your system a painful lesson: *showing what you really feel can threaten connection with the people you love.*

To adapt, your system reorganised itself. The Feisty Child—the part that felt anger, protest, or a sense of unfairness—had to be suppressed. The Critic took that angry energy and turned it inward, attacking you instead. In this way, it functioned like an internal safety officer, keeping the ship steady by silencing feelings that once rocked relationships.

The cost of this strategy was high. You learned to doubt your own emotional reality. You gave up your voice and your right to want more. And yet the Critic offered something compelling in return: a sense of order and hope.

"If I'm the problem, then fixing myself will keep me safe."

Blaming yourself can feel safer than facing the possibility that the people you depended on were unable to meet your needs. As long as you believe you are at fault, the fantasy remains that perfect behaviour, greater self-control, or fewer needs will finally bring security.

Over Time, Self-Punishment Comes to Serve Several Overlapping Functions

It turns anger inward, keeping protest and blame from being expressed where they once threatened attachment. It erodes self-worth, making it less likely you will assert needs or expect care. It creates a sense of order and control in situations that once felt helpless and unsafe.

At Its Core, Self-Shaming Becomes a Strategy for Staying Connected

If *you* are the problem, then the people you depend on can remain good—and the hope survives that, with enough correction, restraint, or self-control, love and safety might finally be secured.

In this way, the Critic preserves attachment not by protecting you but by sacrificing you.

In some families, passivity, compliance, or even illness becomes the safest route to care—because direct expression once led to rejection or shame.

Samantha's Loyalty Pattern

 Samantha grew up in a family that valued toughness and emotional restraint. Her father responded to distress with "Toughen up." Her mother offered practical solutions rather than comfort. Emotional expression was treated as a flaw rather than a signal.

Later, when Samantha felt hurt by her partner's emotional unavailability or lonely after days without contact, those early lessons returned. She couldn't express her needs without fear of being seen as too much. Her Critic stepped in immediately: "You're overreacting. Other people cope just fine."

The binge–restrict cycle became a way of managing this conflict. Bingeing allowed a brief release; restriction restored a sense of discipline and control. Shame followed both, reinforcing the Critic's authority. Most painfully, Samantha had to silence her Feisty Child completely—the part that knew her anger made sense and that her needs were reasonable.

What the Critic Fears

If the Critic loosens its grip, something deeply threatening may surface: grief for what was never given, anger that was never allowed, and the realisation that *you were not the problem.*

Recovery asks the Critic to stand down from a role it took on when no one else could protect attachment. It asks you to face loss directly rather than continuing to punish yourself for it.

Your Wise Self can begin to hold this complexity.

To the Critic: "I understand why you did this. You kept me connected when I had no other options. I have more resources now. You don't have to protect me this way anymore."

To the Lost Child: "Your feelings made sense. Your needs were real. I'm here now, and I won't abandon you for telling the truth."

Recognising the Critic's role in your survival does not mean allowing it to dominate your present.

Understanding Perfectionism's Grip

For many people, the Overcontroller operates through perfectionism—the belief that mistakes are dangerous and that flawless performance is the only reliable path to safety. Early experiences taught this part that errors led to criticism, humiliation, or rejection. Perfection became a way of preventing emotional exposure.

In eating disorders, perfectionism often centres on the body. Food, weight, exercise, and discipline become the areas where control feels possible. There is a powerful belief here: *if I can get this exactly right, everything else will settle.* It's an attempt to steer life without deviation, as if precision alone can guarantee calm waters.

Sometimes, it works—briefly. Meeting rigid standards brings relief, pride, and a sense of control. But the relief never lasts. Hunger, emotion, or an unexpected deviation appears, and shame rushes in. The Overcontroller responds by tightening rules and raising standards, trying to restore safety through even greater control.

Although on the surface the aim may appear to be to reach health or well-being, it's actually a way of avoiding shame.

Perfectionism often works hand-in-hand with the Inner Critic. When mistakes happen, the Critic attacks: "You've failed." Anticipating this, the Perfectionistic Overcontroller demands flawless performance: "If I do everything perfectly, there'll be nothing to criticise." This creates an impossible bind. Perfection is required for safety, but perfection is unattainable.

Over time, this grip narrows your life. You avoid new experiences because you might fail. Learning feels threatening because it involves mistakes. An authentic connection feels risky because only the polished version of you seems acceptable.

A crucial shift in recovery is learning the difference between *blame* and *responsibility*.

Blame, driven by the Critic, says: "This happened because I'm inadequate."

Responsibility, guided by the Wise Self, says: "Something didn't go as planned. What can I learn? What do I need right now?"

If you eat more than planned, blame interprets this as proof of failure. Responsibility notices hunger, emotion, or exhaustion and responds with curiosity. Blame keeps you stuck; responsibility creates movement.

Why Struggle Doesn't Mean Failure

Your Perfectionistic Overcontroller believes struggle means you're doing something wrong. If learning feels difficult, if you're making mistakes, if you can't get something right immediately—this must mean you're failing, or perhaps that you lack the natural ability to succeed. But this understanding of learning is backwards.

Educational researcher James Nottingham describes something called the "learning pit"—a concept to help students understand that struggle, confusion, and even failure are *necessary* parts of meaningful learning (16). When you encounter new information that challenges what you thought you knew, your brain experiences conflict. Nothing makes complete sense yet. We often interpret this confusion as a sign that we're doing something wrong—but it's actually evidence that real learning is happening.

Real learning requires you to grapple with contradictions, question your assumptions, debate with yourself, and gradually construct a deeper understanding through the struggle itself. The pit isn't something to avoid or rush through—it's the terrain where actual growth happens.

Recovery is like learning to sail the ocean between where you are now—defined by eating disorder patterns, survival strategies, protective modes—and the life waiting on the other shore, where your true self lives free from these constraints. You can't sail that ocean without encountering storms, changing winds, moments when you lose your bearings entirely. The learning pit is those difficult waters. It's not a sign you've gone off course—it's the actual passage itself.

Your Perfectionistic Overcontroller tries to avoid this pit entirely. It wants the illusion of smooth sailing, the appearance of already knowing how to navigate, and the safety of not being seen struggling. But this means your ship never leaves the harbour—because sailing requires temporary incompetence, visible struggle, and repeated course corrections.

Roger Federer, one of the greatest tennis players in history, won only 54% of the points he played—barely more than half. Yet he won nearly 80% of his matches. How? Because he understood that tennis isn't about winning every single point. It's about showing up, point after point, recovering quickly from setbacks, and staying in the game. Recovery works the same way. You don't need to get everything right. You don't need to "win" every meal or never struggle with food or body image. What matters is learning to come back after difficult moments—to treat the next choice, the next breath, as a fresh start. That's the real sign of strength.

Hard days are the learning pit—the choppy waters between harbour and horizon. You're training your system to handle them differently. The goal of struggle is to develop resilience—the capacity to navigate difficulty without it overwhelming you, to make mistakes without them defining you, to struggle without interpreting this as evidence of brokenness. To learn to face living a life that is full of challenges.

Your Perfectionistic Overcontroller will resist this. It will say: "But other people don't struggle like this. Other people recover faster, do it better, need less support."

Your Wise Self can respond: "Maybe. Or maybe everyone in recovery is in their own learning pit, navigating their own difficult waters, and I just can't see their struggle from where I'm standing. Either way, my struggle is real, and it's teaching me what I need to learn. I'm showing up, point after point. I'm learning to sail. That's what matters."

Small Experiments in Imperfection

Because perfectionism is driven by fear, it needs evidence rather than reassurance. Small, low-risk experiments can help.

You might allow one minor imperfection a day—leaving the bed unmade, sending a message without rereading it, eating from a slightly larger bowl. Then notice what this part predicted would happen and what actually happened.

When struggle shows up, it can help to name it: "I'm in the learning pit right now. This is uncomfortable because I'm learning to tolerate uncertainty and the messiness of life."

Then ask: "What skill is this moment helping me develop that perfectionism never allowed?"

We'll return to perfectionism in Chapter 12, where you'll explore how letting go of flawless control is not a failure of discipline but a necessary step toward sustainable recovery.

Practice: Naming the Pit

Next time you notice yourself struggling—with a meal, with body image, with setting a boundary, with tolerating a difficult feeling—try saying:

> "I'm in the learning pit right now. These are the waters I need to cross to reach freedom. This struggle means I'm learning something my system

doesn't know yet. The confusion is temporary. I'm exactly where I need to be."

Then ask: "What is this struggle trying to teach me? What navigation skills am I learning right now that my Perfectionistic Overcontroller never allowed me to learn before?"

This simple reframe—from "I'm failing" to "I'm learning to sail"—can transform your relationship with difficulty. The pit becomes the passage rather than evidence of inadequacy. The choppy waters become proof you've left the harbour, not proof you should turn back.

We'll explore perfectionism more deeply in Chapter 12, where you'll learn how embracing imperfection is essential to sustainable recovery.

The Detached Protector's Fears

This mode learned that feelings and connection lead to pain.

Its fears:

- "If I let myself feel everything, I'll be destroyed by the pain."
- "If I get close to people, they'll inevitably disappoint or abandon me."
- "If I show vulnerability, I'll be rejected or betrayed."
- "If I stay present with emotions, they'll never end."
- "If I let my guard down, I'll be hurt again."
- "If I hope for connection, the disappointment will be unbearable."

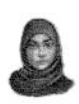 **Faye's Detached Protector** carries this: *If I let myself feel how lonely I really am, the pain will be unbearable. Better to numb it through food and stay disconnected.*

Her bingeing became a reliable escape from feelings that felt too dangerous to face.

The People Pleaser's Fears

This part learned that your own needs and preferences threaten relationships.

Its fears:

- "If I say no, people will leave me."
- "If I prioritise myself, I'm selfish and will be rejected."
- "If I stop being useful, no one will want me around."
- "If I express real feelings, people will see me as difficult and abandon me."
- "If I set boundaries, I'll be alone."
- "If I stop taking care of others, I'll have no purpose."

 **Sophie's People Pleaser** learned: *If I express what I really want or need, I'll hurt people I love and they'll withdraw. Better to keep everyone happy by having no needs of my own.*

Her compliance became a way to stay connected whilst keeping her authentic self safely hidden.

The Helpless Protector's Fears

This part learned that trying and failing is more painful than not trying at all. It might say: "There's no point, I can't do it, I need more strategies."

Its fears:

- "If I take full responsibility for change, I might fail completely."
- "If I try my hardest and it doesn't work, that will prove I'm truly hopeless."
- "If I don't have someone to rescue me, I'll be all alone."
- "If I succeed on my own, expectations will be too high."
- "If I'm not helpless, people will stop caring."
- "If I show my full capability, I'll have to face all the years I wasted."

Deeper fear underneath: *If I'm not the victim, I'll have to feel my anger about what happened—and that anger feels too dangerous.*

Understanding Where These Fears Come From

Your Protector Modes' fears might seem irrational, but they're based on real experiences.

Personal Reflection: For Your strongest Protector Mode, Ask

- When did this fear first develop?
- What happened that taught this part to be afraid?
- Was this fear accurate in my childhood circumstances?
- Is this same danger present in my adult life now?
- What resources do I have now that I didn't have then?

Key Insight: Your Protector Modes developed these fears based on past reality. But they haven't updated their threat assessment for your current circumstances and adult capabilities. They're still responding to a world that may no longer exist in quite the same way—the world of your emotional past, locked in a time capsule within you, that continues to shape how you perceive the present.

Opening Dialogue with Your Protector Modes

Once you recognise modes in your body and understand their fears, you can begin conversations. Our goal is not to control or eliminate them but to understand their perspective and help them feel heard.

The Inner Meeting Space: Imagine a place in nature where you can meet with your Protector Modes one by one. A clearing in a forest. A quiet spot by the ocean. A comfortable room overlooking natural beauty. Your inner meeting space for facilitating conversations.

Approach this from your Wise Self observing perspective—not fully identified with any single mode but able to witness each one with curiosity and compassion.

One-on-One Mode Interviews: This helps you understand what each Protector Mode is trying to accomplish and what it needs to feel safe enough to relax its grip.

The Practice:

1. **Ground Yourself in the Here and Now**: Take deep breaths. Imagine stepping back to observe your internal world from a calm, curious perspective—watching a play from the audience rather than being on stage.
2. **Set Up the Meeting Space**: In your mind's eye, create your safe gathering place. Imagine a comfortable chair for yourself and a place for the mode you'll be meeting with.
3. **Invite One Protector Mode**: Choose a single Protector Mode to meet with first. You might start with whichever one feels most present lately or the one creating the most difficulty. Ask this part to join you in your meeting space.
4. **Notice Its Presence**: How does this mode appear? What does it look like? Where does it sit or stand? What's its posture, expression, and energy? Some people see actual images. Others just sense a presence or feeling. There's no right way.
5. **Interview with Curiosity**: From your observing perspective, ask this Protector Mode:

    - How are you trying to help me?
    - What are you most afraid would happen if you stopped?
    - When did you first develop? What was happening in my life?
    - What would you need to feel safer?
    - What strengths do you bring?

6. **Listen without Judgement**: Allow the mode to answer in whatever form comes—words, images, feelings, body sensations. You're not trying to argue or fix. Just listen and understand.
7. **Acknowledge Its Efforts**: Thank this mode for trying to help, even when its methods create problems. Recognise it developed for reasons that made sense at the time.
8. **Close the Conversation**: Let this mode know you'll return to talk again. Ask if there's anything else it wants you to know before you end this particular meeting.

Faye's Mode Interviews

Faye couldn't understand why she kept sabotaging her commitment to regular meals despite desperately wanting recovery. She decided to interview her Protector Modes one by one.

Meeting with the "Sergeant Major" (Overcontroller)

Faye imagined her meeting space—a quiet garden with two chairs. When she invited her Overcontroller, it appeared sitting rigidly upright, arms crossed, and jaw tight.

"When did you first develop?"

"When you felt invisible. When your brothers excelled at everything and you couldn't compete. I gave you something you could be good at—controlling your body, your appetite. Something that made you special."

"How are you trying to help me?"

"I keep you disciplined. I give you something to be proud of—your willpower, your self-control."

"What are you most afraid would happen if you stopped?"

"You'd become lazy, out of control. Everyone would see you have no willpower—that you're weak and pathetic. You'd be ordinary. Worthless. Just like you felt as a young child."

"What would you need to feel safer?"

Silence. Then: "I'd need to know you have other ways to feel valuable. That I . . . and you won't just dissolve into nothing without me."

Faye thanked this part for working so hard to give her a sense of worth and achievement. She let it know she'd return to talk more.

Meeting with the "Cozy Soother" (Detached Self-Soother)

The next day, Faye returned to her garden. When she invited her Detached Self-Soother, it appeared nestled in the comfortable chair, relaxed and almost drowsy.

"How are you trying to help me?"

"I'm always here when you feel lonely or scared. Other people let you down—they don't see you, don't understand. But I never will. I give you comfort when nothing else does."

"What are you most afraid would happen if you stopped?"

"You'd have to feel everything—all the loneliness, all the pain of never being seen. That will destroy you. You'll be completely alone with unbearable feelings. At least with me, you have something."

"When did you first come into my life?"

"I've been around a long time. It started building when your mum got ill and spent so much time in hospital. Your dad was stressed, working longer hours. Neither of them knew how to talk about what was happening—the fear, the exhaustion, the sadness.

When your dog died, and your best friend moved away, that's when I really took hold. Your mum offered cakes to cheer you up—her way of trying to help when she didn't know what else to do. That's when I learned: food can fill the emptiness when people can't. It became our language. The only reliable comfort when everything else felt so uncertain and alone."

"What would you need to feel safer?"

"I'd need to know you have other ways to cope with loneliness. That you won't be completely alone without me."

Through these separate conversations, Faye could see that both modes were trying to help—one by creating achievement and specialness (to avoid feeling worthless), the other by providing reliable comfort (to avoid unbearable loneliness). But they worked against each other. The Sergeant Major demanded restriction. The Cozy Soother offered binges. Together, they created the cycle that kept her stuck.

Neither was the enemy. Both were parts trying to protect her from genuine pain—the pain of feeling invisible, unworthy of attention, and fundamentally alone. This understanding opened something new: the possibility that these modes could eventually work together under wise leadership rather than fighting for control.

Your Own Mode Interviews

Try this practice with your own Protector Modes:

Choose One Mode to Start With: Which Protector Mode feels most active in your life right now? The Overcontroller? The Detached Protector? The People Pleaser?

Set Aside 15–20 Minutes: Find a quiet space where you won't be interrupted.

Follow the Interview Process: Use the questions above. Write down what emerges, even if it feels silly or strange at first.

Be Patient: Some modes are more willing to talk than others. Some might stay silent the first time you try. That's okay. Just let them know you're available when they're ready.

Interview Each Mode Separately: Over the coming days or weeks, meet with different Protector Modes one at a time. Notice what each one reveals about its fears, its origins, and its intentions.

Notice Patterns: Do different modes share similar fears? Are they all trying to protect you from the same core vulnerabilities?

Reflection Point: Notice what happens when you approach each Protector Mode with curiosity rather than judgement. Does it feel different to think of them as parts trying to help rather than problems to eliminate? What does each mode reveal about your underlying needs and fears? What would these parts need to relax their protective strategies?

The Vicious Cycles

Understanding how Protector Modes operate helps you see the cycles they create—patterns that feel impossible to break because each part is responding to what other parts are doing.

The Restrict–Binge Cycle

For some people, eating difficulties involve cycles between restriction and bingeing—moving back and forth between tight control and episodes where control breaks down. For others, the pattern is primarily restrictive without bingeing episodes. Both patterns involve your Protector Modes trying to manage difficult feelings, but the strategies look different.

If your pattern includes bingeing, understanding this cycle can help you see why willpower alone hasn't worked. If your pattern is purely restrictive, you might recognise parts of this dynamic even if bingeing isn't part of your experience—the building pressure, the tight control, and the fear of what might happen if you loosened the reins.

How the Restrict–Binge Cycle Works:

1. **Overcontroller Takes Charge**: Creates strict rules about eating, exercise, and body. Keeps Lost Child's feelings contained. Provides a temporary sense of control and achievement.
2. **Pressure Builds**: Lost Child becomes increasingly hungry—not just physically but emotionally. She's starving for connection, comfort, expression, and freedom. The feelings get sealed tighter.
3. **Impulsive Child Breaks Through**: Eventually, pressure becomes too much. She breaks through in a desperate attempt to meet needs denied too long. The binge is like a pressure valve releasing.
4. **Inner Critic Attacks**: Harsh messages about the binge trigger shame and disgust. You're weak, pathetic, out of control, and disgusting.
5. **Overcontroller Compensates**: Swings back with even more restriction (or purging or exercise) to "make up for" the binge, regain control, and prove you're not "out of control."
6. **The Cycle Repeats**: Each round typically gets more intense.

For Those without Bingeing

Tony's pattern never included binges—his Overcontroller maintained such rigid control that pressure never broke through into eating episodes. Instead, it leaked out through compulsive exercise, obsessive body checking, and constant anxiety about whether he was lean enough, muscular enough, and disciplined enough.

If you don't experience binge episodes, you might still recognise the building pressure. Perhaps your Overcontroller maintains such tight control that the pressure never gets released through bingeing, but it finds other outlets: irritable outbursts, exhaustion, emotional numbness, rigid rituals, physical symptoms.

The pressure is still there. It's just that your particular constellation of Protector Modes has found ways to keep it from breaking through into eating episodes. This doesn't make your pattern "better"—it's just a different configuration of the same underlying dynamics.

Why These Patterns Are Hard to Break

Each part believes it's doing the right thing. Overcontroller thinks: If I just control hard enough, everything will be manageable. Detached Self-Soother thinks (for those who binge): I'm providing necessary relief from unbearable feelings. Inner Critic thinks: If I'm harsh enough, she'll finally maintain control. Together, they create a self-perpetuating pattern.

The Real Issue: Whether your pattern includes bingeing or not, it continues because Lost Child's actual needs—for connection, comfort, expression, freedom—are never directly addressed. Restriction provides temporary relief through the illusion of control, but it can't meet emotional needs. For those who binge, food provides temporary relief but still can't meet those deeper needs. So the hunger continues. The pressure builds . . . and the pattern repeats.

The People-Pleasing Depletion Cycle

Different pattern. Same trap.

1. **People Pleaser Takes Over**: Monitors others constantly. Suppresses your own needs. Says yes when meaning no. Works to keep everyone happy.
2. **Lost Child's Needs Accumulate**: While focused on others, your own emotional vitamins run low. You become depleted, resentful, and empty.
3. **Overcontroller or Detached Protector Steps In**: Uses eating behaviours to create space, exert control, or numb the resentment and depletion. At least I can control this. At least food doesn't demand anything from me.
4. **Inner Critic Attacks**: You're selfish for focusing on food when others need you. You're letting people down.
5. **People Pleaser Doubles Down.** Works even harder to prove you're not selfish. More depletion. More eating behaviours.

Sophie's version: Her People Pleaser helps everyone, ignoring her own exhaustion and needs. By evening, she's depleted and resentful. Her Overcontroller responds: "Skip dinner. At least you can control that." She restricts, feeling briefly in control. But later, the Detached Self-Soother erupts—rapid bingeing seeking relief from the day's emotional demands. Then her Critic attacks: "Disgusting. You failed." Then Overcontroller converts shame into action: tomorrow's stricter rules, harsher restrictions. The depletion continues.

The Suspicious Protection Cycle

For those with mistrust mindset patterns:

1. **Suspicious Overcontroller Stays Hypervigilant**: Constantly scanning for betrayal, control, danger. Keeps guard up always.
2. **Lost Child Longs for Connection**: Despite fear, there's still a deep hunger for genuine connection and understanding.

3. **Any Connection Attempt Triggers Suspicion**: Why are they being nice? What do they want? This feels like a trap. Pulls away or tests the person.
4. **Isolation Increases**: As suspicion pushes people away, loneliness intensifies. This confirms the belief: See, I was right not to trust.
5. **Eating Behaviours Manage the Loneliness**: Restriction might feel like maintaining control and boundaries. Bingeing might fill emptiness when human connection feels too risky.
6. **The Cycle Reinforces Itself**: Isolation increases suspicion. Suspicion increases isolation. Isolation increases reliance on eating behaviours.

Merrin's pattern: Her Suspicious Overcontroller questioned everyone's motives. When her therapist asked caring questions: Why does she want to know that? She's probably going to use it against me. This kept Lost Child locked away, unable to receive the care being offered. Meanwhile, anxiety about trusting anyone got channelled into obsessive health concerns and food restriction—things she could control when relationships felt dangerous.

Understanding Your Unique Cycles

Mapping Exercise: Take a recent week where eating difficulties were particularly challenging. Map your cycle:

- What triggered it? (Situation that activated which fear)
- Which Protector Mode responded first?
- How did other modes react to that response?
- What eating behaviours followed?
- How did each mode respond to those behaviours?
- How did the cycle continue or repeat?

Understanding your specific cycle helps you see where intervention might be most effective. But that intervention requires coordination. Someone who can see the whole pattern and help each part find better ways to contribute.

How Protector Modes Use Prevention and Emergency Response

Chapter 3 introduced how Protector Modes operate in two main ways. Let's deepen that understanding.

Prevention: Keeping the Hatch Sealed

Most of the time, your Protector Modes aren't responding to a crisis. They're working preventatively, like security guards patrolling the perimeter, making sure nothing gets through that might threaten your carefully maintained equilibrium. Think of them as running a 24-hour operation to keep your Lost

Child safely contained where her vulnerable feelings can't surface and overwhelm you.

Emma's Overcontroller starts its prevention work the moment she opens her eyes each morning. Her mind fills immediately with rules, plans, and calculations about food and exercise. The rigid schedule leaves no space for emotional awareness—and that's exactly the point. Achievement becomes the focus, blocking out any space where feelings might sneak through. The low weight, the high control—these aren't just side effects. They're the tools her Overcontroller uses to maintain emotional numbness.

Emma's Detached Protector has a different strategy. It keeps her busy with work and study, always moving and never stopping long enough to feel. When she does pause, there are substances to take the edge off, screens offering endless distraction. Her relationships stay superficial—close enough to avoid loneliness, distant enough to avoid emotional depth. Emotional numbness has become her baseline state.

Sophie's Protector Modes run prevention around the clock. Her People Pleaser stays busy helping others—no time to tune inward. Her Overcontroller maintains rigid food rules, providing distraction through calculation and control. When these prevention strategies falter and feelings break through, her Detached Self-Soother offers bingeing as escape.

These prevention strategies remember how overwhelming your Lost Child's feelings were in the past. They're determined to prevent you from ever being that vulnerable again. But whilst these strategies protect you from pain, they also cut you off from the very feelings and needs that could guide you toward genuine nourishment and connection. They started protecting you from overwhelm—and over time have come to protect you from fully engaging with life.

Emergency Response: When Prevention Fails

Sometimes, despite all these prevention efforts, your Lost Child pops up unexpectedly. A crack appears in the carefully constructed walls. Something triggers those old emotional wounds—the missing vitamins, the harsh Critic messages, the unmet needs. Suddenly, you feel overwhelmed by sadness, shame, loneliness, and anger. Feelings that were supposed to stay contained come flooding up.

In these moments, your Protector Modes shift from prevention to emergency response. They rush in like a crisis team, deploying whatever strategies will push those feelings back down fastest.

Emma experiences this on a Tuesday evening. Her friend cancels their plans at the last minute—something came up at work, she's really sorry, maybe next week? The message is perfectly reasonable. But it activates something old in Emma: I'm not important. People don't really want to spend time with me.

Intense feelings of rejection and loneliness flood up. For a moment, her Lost Child is right there, vulnerable and hurting. Then her emergency response team activates.

Her Overcontroller jumps in first: Just skip dinner. At least you can control that. Focus on your diet plan—that always helps.

Her Detached Self-Soother offers a different solution: Tasty food . . . cake, chocolate bars would make you feel better right now. Just zone out with food for a while.

Her People Pleaser starts typing a response immediately: No problem at all! I totally understand! Let's reschedule whenever works for you—I'm completely flexible! The exclamation marks hide the hurt. The immediate accommodation ensures her friend never knows she's upset.

None of this is conscious. Emma doesn't think "I feel rejected so I'll restrict my eating now." The response is automatic—her Protector Modes leaping into action with familiar strategies that help her avoid, numb, or indirectly express those overwhelming feelings without actually having to feel them directly.

By the time she's aware of what's happening, she's already standing in her kitchen, staring at the dinner she prepared but won't eat. The feelings that surfaced have been successfully pushed back down. Her Lost Child is safely contained again. Mission accomplished. Crisis averted.

In reality, it's not. Because those feelings don't disappear—they just go back below deck, waiting for the next crack in the wall to appear.

Sophie's emergency response shows the full binge–restrict cycle. When stress builds and her Lost Child's needs break through, her Overcontroller tightens control: "Skip dinner." But the deprivation creates pressure that eventually erupts through her Detached Self-Soother—rapid bingeing for relief—followed by the inevitable shame-attack from her Critic, and Overcontroller pushes for even stricter restriction tomorrow.

Your Emergency Responses

Think about the last time you had a sudden, strong urge to engage in over- or under- eating behaviours. Not the planned, prevention-mode behaviours but the urgent, must-do-this-now impulses.

What happened right before that urge hit? Not just the external event, but what it triggered internally.

What feelings might have been trying to surface in that moment? Rejection? Shame? Loneliness? Anger? Fear? The feelings are often so brief—just a flash before the Protector Mode kicks in—that you might not have even registered them consciously.

Which Protector Mode offered which solution? Did your Overcontroller suggest restriction? Did your Detached Protector offer the numbing comfort of a binge? Did your People Pleaser jump into action to fix everything for everyone else?

The important question is: What did your Lost Child actually need in that moment? Not what the Protector Mode gave her but what she actually needed. Connection? Comfort? To be heard? To express anger? To feel safe expressing sadness?

The gap between what she needed and what she got—that gap is where the cycle perpetuates.

The Addictive Pull

You've probably noticed that even when you consciously want to change, your Protector Modes feel impossible to resist. You might start the day with genuine determination to do things differently, only to find yourself swept back into familiar patterns by afternoon.

This isn't a lack of willpower or commitment. It's because these strategies provide genuine relief, even if temporary. They work—at least in the short term. And your brain remembers what works.

Tony felt this acutely. Every morning, he'd wake up determined to eat normally, to not exercise compulsively, to just be a regular person who could have breakfast without calculating macros and planning how to compensate through extra cardio. But by mid-morning, the pull of his Overcontroller would be so strong it felt like a physical force. The promise of control, of that brief sense of achievement, of looking lean and muscular rather than feeling inadequate—it was irresistible.

Because it actually worked. When he stuck to his rigid plan—"clean" foods, precise macros, training despite exhaustion—his Overcontroller created real feelings of achievement, control, pride, power. These were genuine neurochemical responses. His brain lit up with satisfaction. For those moments, he felt strong, disciplined, superior to people who "couldn't control themselves." The anxiety about not being muscular enough, not being disciplined enough, dampened down . . . Until it didn't. Until the exhaustion built, the injuries accumulated, the isolation deepened. But by then, his Overcontroller was already promising that more training, stricter eating, leaner physique would solve those problems too.

This reliability makes these strategies incredibly compelling. Unlike humans, who might be unpredictable or unavailable, your Protector Mode strategies are always accessible. You don't have to work up the courage to use them. You don't have to risk rejection. You don't have to explain yourself. They're just there, ready to provide their particular form of relief whenever you need it.

Over time, these strategies become wired in your brain as safety behaviours. Your nervous system learns: *This is how we cope with threat. This is what makes us feel secure.* Even thinking about giving them up triggers anxiety because it feels like dismantling your primary defence system.

Sophie noticed this when she tried to stop over-functioning for others. The idea of not immediately responding to someone's need, of letting someone else handle their own problem, created such intense anxiety that it felt easier to just keep helping. Her People Pleaser had become her safety behaviour—the thing that kept her feeling secure in her relationships, even though it was exhausting her.

The strategies also create their own justification. After Tony restricted: *See? I can control myself. I'm not weak like I feared. This proves I'm disciplined.*

The Pleasure–Pain Bind

Your Protector Modes create what feels like an impossible situation—a double bind where every option leads to suffering.

Using the behaviour brings temporary relief or pleasure. You get the achievement, the control, the numbing, some version of connection. Your Protector Mode delivers what it promised. But choosing not to use it triggers intense anxiety and brings up exactly the feelings your modes have worked so hard to avoid—the discomfort of sitting with these emotions can feel more unbearable than any consequence of the behaviour itself.

But using it creates new problems—physical health deteriorating, life becoming increasingly restricted, shame building, and isolation deepening. Which increases the need for the behaviour to cope with those new problems. Which creates more consequences. Which requires more of the behaviour.

Emma lived inside this bind for years. Her Overcontroller promised that perfect control would finally make her safe from criticism and rejection. But the rigid control it demanded made her increasingly anxious, socially isolated, and physically depleted. When her Lost Child's feelings broke through that control, her People Pleaser would swing into action, overextending herself to prove she wasn't selfish or weak. This led to exhaustion and resentment, which her Overcontroller would try to manage through more dietary control. She was stuck because she was trapped between two modes that both believed they were saving her, each activating in response to the suffering the other one created. Back and forth, each mode creating the conditions that activated the other.

The bind is also in the underlying logic: *If I just do this enough, I'll finally be safe. If I just control it perfectly, the pain will stop. If I just avoid it completely, I won't get hurt.* These promises feel true in the moment, even though experience has proven them false again and again.

Breaking Free Requires Understanding, Not Willpower

You can't simply decide to stop these patterns through force of will. This might be hard to accept, especially if you've been told repeatedly that recovery is just about "choosing to get better" or "wanting it badly enough."

But your Protector Modes didn't develop through lack of discipline. They developed for genuine reasons—they're meeting real needs in the only ways they know how. They emerged when you were younger and didn't have other options. They've been refined over years of practice. They're deeply wired into your nervous system as survival strategies.

Trying to simply stop through willpower is like trying to stop breathing through determination. Your system believes these strategies are keeping you alive.

Breaking free requires something different. It requires understanding what needs your Protector Modes are trying to meet—which you're doing right now by reading this chapter and reflecting on your own patterns. It requires addressing the fears that drive them, helping them see that those fears are based on past reality, not present danger. It requires finding alternative ways to meet those underlying needs, which means developing new capacities you may not have built yet. Most importantly, it requires leadership—and that's what we turn to next.

Looking toward Leadership

You've deepened your understanding significantly. You can now recognise your Protector Modes in your body, understand their fears and intentions, see how they relate to each other and create cycles. You understand why they feel so compelling, why willpower alone can't override them.

But awareness isn't enough to create change. Your Protector Modes need what they've been missing all this time: coordination from someone who can see the bigger picture whilst respecting each mode's concerns. Someone who can stay grounded when fears get activated and emotions run high. Someone who can appreciate what each part is trying to do, whilst gently guiding them toward healthier strategies.

Someone who can hold space for your Lost Child's feelings without being overwhelmed or rushing to make them disappear. Someone who can set firm boundaries with your Inner Critic's attacks, refusing to let that harsh voice dominate the conversation. Someone who can provide steady, compassionate leadership that allows all these parts to relax their emergency vigilance and trust that help has arrived.

Your Protector Modes have been doing their best without this kind of guidance for a long time. They're exhausted. They're like crew members who've been working around the clock with no clear coordination, everyone rowing in different directions, creating enormous effort but little forward movement. They need a captain.

Think back to Emma in her kitchen that morning, surrounded by competing voices. Her Overcontroller is calculating calories and exercise, already planning how to compensate for eating. Her People Pleaser is worrying about disappointing others, trying to anticipate everyone's needs. Her Detached Protector is quietly suggesting she just skip the whole thing, avoid the internal debate entirely.

Each mode is trying to help in its own way. Each genuinely believes it has the solution. But together they create chaos rather than clarity, confusion rather than direction. The internal noise drowns out any possibility of simply being present with breakfast, with herself, with the day ahead.

What Emma needs—what all these modes need—isn't to be controlled, eliminated, or fought against. They don't need another Critic telling them they're wrong. They don't need to be shamed for trying to help.

They need a wise leader who can coordinate their efforts, appreciate their strengths, address their fears with compassion, and guide them toward ways of operating that serve genuine wellbeing rather than just preventing threats.

That someone isn't a therapist who sees you once a week. It isn't a friend or family member. It isn't a book or a programme.

That someone is a part of you that's been waiting beneath all these survival strategies—a wise presence that can guide your internal world with both strength and compassion. It's been there all along, just quiet, overshadowed by the louder, more urgent voices of your Protector Modes and Critic.

In the next chapter, you'll remember this wise leader. You'll discover that you already have the capacity to provide the kind of leadership your Protector Modes have been desperately waiting for. You'll learn how to develop this inner leader so it can coordinate your internal world in ways that allow all parts—including your Lost Child—to finally get what they truly need.

Your Protector Modes have been working so hard for so long. They deserve support, not criticism. They deserve appreciation for their dedication, even when their methods haven't worked. They deserve a wise leader who can help them find new ways to contribute—ways that don't require such enormous sacrifice, such constant vigilance, such relentless effort.

And that leader is already within you, waiting to be re-membered.

Gentle Experiments to Try

1: Body Awareness and Mode Recognition[2]

Several times this week, pause for a body scan. Notice where you're holding tension and which Protector Mode might be active. Ask yourself what might have activated it, what this part is most afraid of right now, and when in your life it first learned this fear. Then gently inquire whether that same danger is actually present now or whether you're responding to an old threat that no longer exists in quite the same way.

This combined practice helps you recognise modes in your body whilst distinguishing past-based fear from present reality. You're not trying to make the modes go away—just becoming aware of them with curiosity.

Body scans can be more difficult for those with experience of trauma (as well as many people with neurodivergence). If you find that you can't go into your body like this yet, this is perfectly normal, and the most important thing is to honour the stage you are at and trust in your intuition regarding whether or not to try this out. Simply noticing which modes seem active through your thoughts or behaviours—without the body component—is valuable work too.

2: Cycle Mapping and Understanding

Track one complete cycle this week, whether it's restrict–binge, people-pleasing depletion, or suspicious protection. Map out what triggered it, which modes participated, and what each mode was trying to prevent or achieve. Notice how it perpetuated itself—how each mode's solution became the next mode's problem. Most importantly, identify what underlying needs all the modes were actually trying to meet.

Understanding your unique pattern—seeing how parts work together or against each other—is the first step toward interrupting the cycle. You can't change what you don't understand.

3: Mode Appreciation and Intention Recognition

Each evening, acknowledge one thing a Protector Mode did to try to help you that day. Maybe your Overcontroller tried to help by creating structure when you felt anxious. Maybe your Detached Protector tried to help by offering escape when feelings felt too big. Say it out loud or write it down.

Then ask what fantasy this mode might be holding about perfect outcomes, or being rescued, or reaching full self-control. What would this mode need to feel safer? Even if its methods weren't ideal, can you recognise its positive intention whilst gently questioning whether the strategy still serves you?

This practice begins to shift your relationship with your Protector Modes from adversarial to collaborative.

4: Emergency Response Tracking and Lost Child Connection

When you have a sudden urge to engage in eating behaviours, pause for just a moment before acting. Ask yourself what just happened, what feelings might be trying to surface, which Protector Mode is offering which solution, and what your Lost Child actually needs right now.

Can you stay with her feelings for just a moment before responding? Not hours—just a moment. Thirty seconds of allowing yourself to feel what's there before the Protector Mode pushes it back down.

You don't have to act differently yet. You're not trying to stop the behaviour. You're just practising noticing—and briefly being with your Lost Child rather than immediately deploying a Protector Mode to make her feelings disappear.

This simple practice of pausing begins to create space where change becomes possible.

Journalling Prompt Reflections: Understanding Your Survival Crew

- Which Protector Mode's fears feel most familiar to you?
- What fantasy has this mode been holding onto? What would it feel like to let that go?
- When you interviewed your modes (in your mind or on paper), what did they reveal about what they're trying to protect?
- What pattern or cycle can you now see clearly that was invisible before?

Pace Yourself: Just a reminder that you don't need to try everything at once—choose one or two practices that feel doable and stay with those for now. Notice what helps your body settle and what supports your inner world. Let the rest wait until you feel ready; healing grows from steady, compassionate attention, not perfection.

The Foundation Is Set

Your ship needs coordination. The survival crew members—Overcontroller, People Pleaser, Detached Protector—need a leader who can see the bigger picture whilst respecting each mode's concerns. That someone is the captain you're about to remember.

You'll discover that you already have everything you need to guide your internal world with wisdom and compassion. It's not something you need to create from scratch—it's something you need to uncover, to bring back from wherever it's been waiting.

You're ready for what comes next.

Notes

1 Body scans can be more difficult for those with trauma history or neurodivergent wiring. Respect your body signals and consider starting by simply noticing which modes seem active through your thoughts or urges. Trust your intuition about whether to try this practice now or return to it later.

2 Safety Note: This practice can bring up strong feelings. If at any point you feel overwhelmed, pause. Place a hand on your heart, use the cyclic sigh from Chapter 5 (two inhales through your nose, long exhale through your mouth), and remind yourself: "I'm here now. I'm safe. I can return to this when I'm ready".

5 Remembering Your Wise Self

Creating the Foundation for Healing

The Leader You've Been Waiting For

 Emma stands in her kitchen at 7 AM, staring at the breakfast she's prepared according to her meal plan. Her Overcontroller is already calculating calories and planning the day's exercise routine. Her People Pleaser is worrying about the work meeting where she'll need to present her ideas. Her Detached Protector is suggesting she skip breakfast altogether—it would be so much simpler to just have coffee and avoid the whole internal debate.

But somewhere beneath this familiar chorus of competing voices, Emma senses something different emerging. A gentle presence that isn't trying to control, please, escape, or perform. A part of her that's learning to listen to all these voices with curiosity rather than being hijacked by whichever one shouts loudest.

Rather than being something new that Emma needs to develop, it's something she's re-membering—both in the sense of remembering what was forgotten and in the deeper sense of re-membering what was dismembered, putting back together what got fragmented under pressure.

Emma's Wise Self—the inner leader she's always had but lost touch with when survival became more urgent than authenticity.

The Ship That Lost Its Captain

You might imagine your inner world as a ship that has sailed through all kinds of weather—fierce storms, yes, but also deceptively calm seas, sudden squalls, thick fog, and everything in between. The Overcontrollers have been at the helm, keeping it moving forward. The Protectors have been patching leaks and manning the sails. The Lost Child has hidden below deck, where the weather can't reach her. Everyone is working hard, but no one is coordinating the efforts.

Without a captain, the crew can't adapt to changing conditions. When storms hit, they know what to do—battle mode, all hands on deck. But when the waters are calm? They're still in crisis mode, unable to relax or adjust their approach. When conditions shift from one moment to the next—as life always

DOI: 10.4324/9781003355878-6

does—each crew member responds based on old patterns rather than current reality. There's no one coordinating their efforts, no one who can assess what this particular weather actually requires.

Remember Jane Goodall's wisdom from our introduction: "Only when head and heart work together can we reach our true potential." Your Wise Self embodies this integration—whereby the thinking mind and feeling heart finally work as partners rather than adversaries. The Wise Self is the captain returning to bring calm, coordination, and direction. A captain who can assess the actual conditions and guide the crew accordingly—sometimes calling for full sails when winds are favourable, sometimes dropping anchor to wait out danger, sometimes simply enjoying the calm.

This chapter is about re-membering the parts that survived underneath survival. It's about bringing the captain home so your whole crew can finally work together instead of against each other—responding to life's actual weather rather than the storms they remember from long ago.

Part 1: Remember—The Wise Self You Lost

What Gets Buried When Survival Takes Over

You were born with this wise presence. Every young child experiences moments of being fully themselves—creative, spontaneous, knowing instinctively what they need and how they feel.

But when the emotional vitamins you needed weren't consistently available, when the world around you felt unsafe for your authentic self, something had to give. Your Wise Self—that grounded, present, integrated part of you—got buried under layers of protective strategies. Your Protector Modes stepped forward to handle immediate threats, and they've been running things ever since.

Your Protector Modes try to protect you *from* feelings by controlling, numbing, pleasing, or withdrawing. Your Wise Self helps you *be with* feelings by staying present, grounded, and compassionate. Recovery isn't about eliminating or forcing change on your Protector Modes, but it is about remembering your Wise Self—bringing this wise presence back online so it can provide the kind of leadership your whole internal world has been waiting for.

Who Is the Wise Self?

The Wise Self is the integrated, grounded presence that can lead your internal world with both strength and compassion. Your Wise Self isn't a part you need to earn through hard work or perfect behaviour. It's already there, waiting to be recognised and strengthened. You've likely already experienced glimpses:

- When you've felt calm and centred despite difficult circumstances
- When you've handled a challenging situation with unexpected grace
- When you've shown deep compassion to someone you care about

- When you've known something was right for you, even when it didn't make logical sense
- When you've been able to observe your own reactions without being completely swept away by them

These moments reveal your Wise Self—the part of you that can stay grounded during storms, make decisions based on wisdom rather than fear, and provide the kind of steady, unconditional presence that your Lost Child has always needed.

Your Wise Self is the part of you that can:

- **Stay Present during Emotional Storms**: noticing "I'm feeling very anxious right now" rather than becoming the anxiety itself.
- **Step Back and Observe**: "Ah, my Overcontroller is taking over," you notice. "I can feel my People Pleaser getting anxious." Beneath the protective noise, you hear your Lost Child's actual needs.
- **Make Decisions Based on Wisdom Rather Than Fear**: choosing what serves your wellbeing even when it doesn't feel immediately safe.
- **Hold Space for Difficult Feelings** without immediately trying to fix or escape them.
- **Treat Yourself with the Same Kindness** you'd offer a dear friend, recognising your humanity and accepting your imperfections.
- **Respond with Both Firmness and Kindness**, setting boundaries when needed whilst remaining compassionate.

Your Wise Self naturally integrates both your thinking mind and your feeling heart. When this part is leading, you experience decision-making that comes from both logic and intuition, both strength and vulnerability—combining self-care with care for others.

Wise Self versus Protector Modes: A Key Distinction

One of the most important skills in recovery is learning to recognise when you're operating from your Wise Self versus when your Protector Modes have taken over. They can sound surprisingly similar at first, but they come from fundamentally different places and lead to very different outcomes.

When Challenge Arises	*Protector Mode Says*	*Wise Self Says*
Strong emotion	"Make this feeling go away right now through restriction/bingeing/exercise"	"This feeling is uncomfortable, but I can stay present with it. What might it be trying to tell me?"
Someone criticises you	"This proves I'm fundamentally flawed. I need to work harder/be smaller/disappear"	"That feedback stings. Let me take a breath and consider whether there's something useful here"

Continued

You notice your body	"I feel disgusting and need to control this immediately"	"I notice uncomfortable feelings about my body. What emotion might be underneath this?"
Facing uncertainty	"I need to control everything I can to feel safe. At least I can control food/weight"	"Uncertainty is uncomfortable, but I can tolerate not knowing. What support do I need?"

Think of 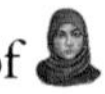 Faye, whose Detached Self-Soother would numb her feelings through bingeing whenever her sensitive system felt overwhelmed. Her Wise Self learned to step in earlier, noticing: "I'm feeling very overstimulated right now. My Detached Self-Soother wants to binge to escape. But what my Lost Child actually needs is to leave this loud environment and find some quiet space."

Similarly,  Sophie noticed her pattern: yesterday's binge meant today's punishment plan—skip breakfast, stick to "low calorie" options. But her Wise Self paused: "My Overcontroller creates stricter rules because I binged. But strict rules led to the binge. What if the solution isn't more restriction? What if it's giving myself permission to have breakfast?"

Change doesn't come from scrutinising yourself to ensure you "get it right," but from *staying curious*, from recognising each Protector part as it shows up, and from keeping in mind that every moment of awareness—no matter how brief—is already part of healing.

"Me Needs" versus "We Needs"

Place your hand on your heart for a moment.

Your Protector Modes focus on "me" survival—keeping ME safe, making ME acceptable. This made sense when threats felt immediate. But your Wise Self balances both your "we" and "me" needs—the relationship between you and your Lost Child, between thinking and feeling, between survival and authenticity. Your Wise Self knows that true safety comes not from rigid control, but from creating internal conditions where all parts can be heard.

Protector Mode strategies, whilst well-intentioned, often create more suffering because they keep your Lost Child isolated, cut off from the connection and care she needs to thrive.

Distinguishing Past from Present

Your Protector Modes developed during times when certain feelings, needs, or situations genuinely felt dangerous. Perhaps expressing anger led to punishment. Perhaps showing vulnerability triggered rejection. Perhaps taking up space made you feel like a burden. Far from being irrational fears, these were accurate assessments of your circumstances at the time.

But often the Protector Modes continue operating as though those old dangers are current threats. They haven't updated their threat assessment to account for your changed circumstances. Your body often holds past-tense fear even when the present moment is actually safe. Your Protector Modes leap into action, reaching for familiar strategies—perhaps restricting food to create a sense of control, or bingeing to numb the fear—without checking whether these responses fit the current reality.

Your Wise Self learns to distinguish between then and now. It can notice: "My body is having a strong reaction to this situation. That makes sense given my history. But let me check—what's actually happening right now? Am I actually in danger, or is my system remembering old pain?"

Rather than dismissing your Protector Modes' concerns, this means helping them recognise that whilst their fears made perfect sense in the past, you now have capacities and resources you didn't have then. You can handle situations that once felt impossible. If there are boundaries you couldn't set as a child, you can set them now. You can leave environments that don't serve you and ask for what you need.

 ***Tony's Wise Self: Questioning the Overcontroller's Absolute Authority***

For years, Tony followed his Overcontroller's commands without question: skip breakfast, train harder, eat less. These directives felt like reality rather conscious choices. But as he practised the Wise Observer exercise from this chapter, he began to question them.

One morning, when his Overcontroller commanded, "Skip breakfast—you didn't earn it," a different voice emerged. His Wise Self asked simply: "Is that true? Or is that fear from a 12-year-old trying to win his coaches' approval?"

The question created a pause—a tiny space between the directive and automatic compliance. In that space, Tony could observe: "My Overcontroller is terrified. But that's not based on my current reality—that's old fear." His Wise Self offered: "You don't need to earn nourishment. Your body needs breakfast." Tony ate breakfast. His Overcontroller protested throughout. But his Wise Self had spoken—and Tony started to recognise he had a choice about which voice to follow.

Practice: Past or Present?

When you notice strong reactions arising, try this simple check-in:

- "What is my system afraid of right now?"
- "When in my past did I experience something similar?"
- "Is that same danger actually present now, or is my body remembering old pain?"
- "What resources do I have now that I didn't have then?"

This practice helps strengthen your Wise Self's capacity to assess reality accurately rather than operating from outdated threat detection. Each time you ask these questions, the captain steadies the ship a little more.

Reflection Point: These questions might feel difficult to answer at first—you may not immediately know what triggers your Protector Modes or when your body shifts from present to past. That's completely normal. Consider spending the next week simply noticing and recording:

- Moments when you felt a strong reaction (anxiety, shame, anger, numbness)
- What was happening externally (situation, conversation, sensory experience)
- What you noticed internally (body sensations, thoughts, urges)
- Any memories or past situations that felt similar

At the end of the week, look back over your notes. Patterns often emerge when you can see several examples together. You might notice: "I leave the present whenever I perceive someone criticises me" or "My body remembers the past when I feel trapped or controlled" or "Uncertainty sends me straight back to childhood feelings of being unsafe."

This detective work—gathering evidence before drawing conclusions—is itself an act of your Wise Self. You're learning to observe with curiosity rather than immediately knowing all the answers.

Part 2: Re-Embody—Grounding Your Wise Self in the Present

Your Wise Self—the captain—learns to read the seas, to distinguish between past storms and present weather, to guide with both strength and care. Now that you've located your Wise Self conceptually, let's activate this part of you physiologically—through breath, body, and awareness. The practices in this section are to enable you to literally embody the wise presence you've been remembering.

Why Grounding Matters

You can't access your Wise Self when your nervous system is in fight, flight, or freeze. These survival states keep you either hyper-activated (racing thoughts, constant vigilance) or shut down (numb, disconnected). In both states, the present moment becomes inaccessible.

Your Protector Modes prefer these states because they feel like control. The Overcontroller stays busy. The Detached Protector goes numb. The People Pleaser stays hypervigilant.

Grounding practices let your nervous system know: "You are safe right now. You can settle." This settled, alert state is where your Wise Self naturally emerges.

Your breath offers one of the gentlest, most accessible ways to begin reconnecting with your body and calming your nervous system. Unlike other body sensations that might feel unpredictable or overwhelming, your breath is always with you, always responsive to your needs, always available as an anchor when things feel difficult. For all of these practices, check with your medical practitioner to ensure that it's safe for you in your current state of recovery.

Cyclic Sigh: The Breath That Brings You Home

The cyclic sigh is a highly effective, evidence-based breathing technique developed by a team led by Dr. Balban at Stanford University that can help calm your nervous system and create a bridge back to embodied awareness (17).

The Practice:

1. Take a normal inhale through your nose.
2. When you think you've inhaled fully, take one more small sip of air through your nose—this is the "double inhale."
3. Exhale slowly and completely through your mouth, making a gentle "ahh" sound if that feels comfortable.
4. Repeat two to three times, then return to natural breathing.

This technique works because the double inhale helps open the tiny air sacs in your lungs, and the long exhale activates your parasympathetic nervous system—the part responsible for rest, digestion, and feeling safe. It's like telling your whole system, "It's okay to settle. You're safe right now."

You can use the cyclic sigh anytime you sense your body holding tension, when emotions feel too big, or simply as a gentle way to check in with yourself. Remember this isn't about controlling your breath perfectly—it's about offering your nervous system a moment of calm regulation.

Try This Right Now: Take three cycles of the cyclic sigh. What do you sense in your body after completing them? Does it feel easier to notice what's happening internally? What does your Lost Child want you to know?

4–7–8 Breath: Grounding during Emotional Storms

The *4–7–8 breath* is adapted from traditional pranayama breathing by Dr. Andrew Weil (18). This is a gentle breathing pattern that helps settle a nervous system stuck in urgency, anxiety, or eating disorder panic. It works by slowing the exhale—the part of the breath that signals to the body, "You're safe enough to soften."

How to Practice

1. Inhale through your nose for 4 seconds

   (a comfortable, natural inhale—no forcing).

2. Hold the breath for 7 seconds

   (just long enough to create a pause; shorten if this feels uncomfortable).

3. Exhale slowly through your mouth for 8 seconds

   (as if fogging up a window—long, steady, unhurried).

4. Repeat for three to four rounds.

Why It Helps in Eating Disorder Recovery

- The long exhale reduces the fight-or-flight activation that often fuels impulses to restrict, binge, purge, or avoid.
- The 7-second pause interrupts spirals of panic or self-attack.
- It helps your Wise Self come back online so you can respond—rather than react—to difficult sensations like fullness, fear of food, or body anxiety.
- Practised regularly, it strengthens your capacity to stay present with discomfort without being overwhelmed.

You can use the 4–7–8 breath before meals, after meals, during urges, or anytime your system feels flooded.

*A simpler version of this, which also capitalises on the long out-breath, is to breathe in for 4 seconds, hold for 1–2 seconds, breathe out for 8 seconds, hold for 1–2 seconds, and so on. After 3–4 rounds of breath, you are likely to notice a drop in anxiety levels.

The Steady-Anchor Breath (Nasal Humming for Emotional Storms)

A gentle grounding practice when emotions surge

When a storm shakes the branches of a tree, the trunk doesn't fight the wind—it steadies itself through its centre of gravity. The Steady-Anchor Breath works in the same way. Rather than pulling attention inward, it uses sound, vibration, and rhythm to provide ballast—something solid to lean into while feelings move through.

When emotions rise quickly, many people experience everything lifting upward: panic in the chest, racing thoughts in the head, and a sense of becoming unmoored. For people recovering from eating difficulties, directing attention to the abdomen—especially after eating—can feel unsafe or overwhelming. Nasal humming steadies the nervous system through a long, voiced out-breath, gentle vibration in the chest and throat, and a rhythmic sensory cue that signals safety—without requiring focus on fullness, digestion, or the stomach.

How to Practise

1. Sit with your feet supported, feeling contact with the floor or chair.
2. Inhale slowly through your nose, at a natural pace.
3. As you exhale, hum softly through your nose, making a low, steady sound—like a quiet "mmm."
4. Let the out-breath hum be longer than the in-breath, without forcing.

5. Notice the vibration wherever it appears—lips, throat, chest, back of throat or face.
6. Allow the hum to fade naturally, then pause briefly before the next inhale.
7. Repeat for three to five slow cycles.

How This Helps

A long, voiced out-breath naturally slows breathing. Slower breathing patterns are associated with increased heart rate variability, reflecting a shift toward calmer, more organised autonomic regulation.

Humming adds auditory and vibratory feedback, which helps pace the breath and gives attention a steady external anchor—often safer than inward body focus when emotions or eating-related sensations are intense.

Nasal humming also increases nitric oxide release in the nasal passages, due to gentle vibration and airflow in the sinuses. Nitric oxide supports airway comfort and relaxation and may further reinforce a sense of ease in the body.

Rather than "fixing" the emotion, you're actively regulating your system and staying present while it passes through.

When to Use It

When emotions spike • when urges rise • after meals • when dissociation begins • when you feel overwhelmed or scattered,

The Neuroscience of Present-Moment Awareness

In simple terms, every grounding exercise you practise rewires your brain to feel more like you. Each time you practice grounding, you're strengthening your brain's insula—the region that integrates body signals into a coherent sense of self. This is how body awareness literally rebuilds your identity from the inside out.

Recent neuroscientific research (19) reveals that our sense of self is built from the ground up through our connection to internal bodily signals, particularly from the heart, lungs, and gut. People with a stronger, more stable sense of self are more attuned to these internal signals and less influenced by external pressures.

This is particularly relevant for recovery from eating difficulties. When you've been disconnected from your body's wisdom, your sense of self can become fragmented or overly dependent on external validation—weight, appearance, others' approval, or achievement. But as you rebuild your connection to your heart rhythms, breath patterns, gut sensations, and sense of how your body is held by gravity, you're actually reconstructing the neurological foundation of a stable, authentic self.

The Difference between Feelings and Self: Emotions come and go like weather patterns—they arise, peak, and naturally pass if we allow them to flow through us without resistance. But your essential self—the aware, witnessing part of you—remains constant. It's the steady presence that observes all the changing emotional weather.

When you're connected to your body's internal rhythms, you develop what researchers call "interoceptive coherence"—a stable inner foundation built from body awareness that isn't easily shaken by external circumstances or internal emotional storms. This is why practices like breath awareness and gentle body attunement are literally rebuilding the neurological basis of a coherent, resilient sense of self.

Safe Movement as Dialogue

Movement can be one pathway back to embodied awareness and connection with your Lost Child. We'll explore this more deeply in Chapter 7, where you'll learn specific practices for using movement as dialogue with your body rather than punishment or control. For now, simply notice: What does your body want to do when you're feeling strong emotions? Does it want to move, to be still, to curl up, to stretch?

The Wise Observer Exercise

This practice helps you access the observing, coordinating perspective of your Wise Self—the part that can see all your Protector Modes without being completely absorbed by any of them.

The Practice:

1. Close your eyes and take three slow breaths. Sense where your body makes contact with whatever you're sitting or lying on. Feel the gravitational pull that connects you to the earth.
2. Now imagine that you can observe your internal world from a calm, wise perspective—as if you're watching from a place of gentle curiosity rather than harsh judgement. From this position, you can see the different Protector Modes without being completely absorbed by any of them.
3. You can observe your Overcontroller organising and planning. You can watch your People Pleaser scanning for others' needs. You can notice your Detached Protector standing guard.
4. Notice that you—the observer—are separate from all this activity. You can see these parts, but you are not only these parts. You are the one observing them all.
5. From this wise perspective, ask yourself: "What does my internal world need from me right now? What kind of leadership would help these Protector Modes work together more effectively?"
6. Simply notice whatever arises without needing to act on it immediately. The goal is to strengthen your capacity to access this observing, coordinating perspective.
7. Say quietly: *I see you all. I am the one who can listen to each.*

This capacity to step back and observe with compassion sits at the heart of your Wise Self. As you practice accessing this perspective, you're remembering something important: you are not your thoughts, not your emotions, not your Protector Modes. You are the aware presence that can hold all of these with wisdom and care.

Part 3: Re-Integrate—Leading with Wisdom and Compassion

The captain is learning to coordinate the crew, helping each member find their rightful contribution under wise leadership. With your Wise Self online, we can now turn toward the parts that most need her leadership. This section develops the core qualities that allow your Wise Self to guide your internal world with both strength and tenderness.

This section contains several foundational practices. You might spend days or even weeks with each one. There's no expectation to master everything immediately—you're building capacities that will strengthen throughout your recovery journey.

Compassionate Observation

One of the foundational capacities of your Wise Self is the ability to observe your internal world without immediately judging, fixing, or controlling what you see. This is radically different from how your Protector Modes operate.

Your Protector Modes observe with an agenda: the Overcontroller watches for mistakes to correct, the Inner Critic scans for flaws to attack, and the People Pleaser monitors for ways you're disappointing others. All of this watching creates tension and reactivity.

Your Wise Self observes with curiosity: "I notice my Overcontroller is active right now. What might have triggered this?" This shift—from "I AM anxious" to "I notice I'm feeling anxious"—creates space between you and the experience. You're no longer fused with the feeling or completely hijacked by the Protector Mode.

Compassionate observation means:

- **Noticing without Judging**: "My People Pleaser is very active" rather than "I'm pathetic for caring so much what others think."
- **Recognising Patterns without Shame**: "I see that conflict with others tends to trigger restriction urges" rather than "I'm so messed up."
- **Acknowledging Protector Modes as Parts, Not Your Whole Self**: "A part of me wants to binge right now" rather than "I have no self-control."
- **Staying Curious about What's Underneath**: "I wonder what my Lost Child might be feeling beneath this urge?"

This kind of observation takes practice—your default may still be to judge or try to control whatever you notice. But each time you can pause and simply observe with curiosity, you strengthen your Wise Self's capacity to lead with wisdom rather than reactivity.

Practice: Throughout your day today, try simply noticing when different Protector Modes are active. Use the phrase "I notice . . ." to create that small space of awareness. "I notice my Overcontroller is planning obsessively." "I notice my Detached Protector wants to zone out." No need to change anything—just notice.

Staying Present with Difficulty

Your Protector Modes have one primary mandate: make difficult feelings go away as quickly as possible. They learned early that certain emotions felt dangerous or overwhelming, so they developed strategies—including eating patterns—to avoid, numb, or control these feelings.

Your Wise Self has a different relationship with difficulty: it can stay present even when things are uncomfortable. This doesn't mean enjoying the discomfort or forcing yourself to endure unnecessary pain. It means developing the capacity to be with challenging experiences without immediately abandoning yourself.

Think about how a wise, attuned caregiver sits with a frightened child. They might drop down to the child's eye level. They'd soften their voice, speaking slowly and gently. They might offer physical comfort—a hug, holding their hand, sitting close beside them. Most importantly, they'd stay present, saying things like: "I'm here with you. You're safe. It's okay to feel scared. I'm not going anywhere." They wouldn't rush to fix or distract—they'd reflect back what they see and wait while the child's feelings move through.

You wouldn't tell a frightened child to stop being scared, or distract them so thoroughly that they never process what happened, or leave them alone with their fear. You'd stay present, offering comfort and understanding, helping them feel less alone with their difficult experience.

If you didn't experience this kind of care yourself, these examples might feel foreign or even impossible to imagine. That's understandable—it's hard to offer what you've never received. But you can learn this now. You might think of a teacher, therapist, friend, or even a character from a film or book who embodied this quality of steady, warm presence. Borrow their approach until it becomes your own.

The first step in this process is to turn toward what is here. Interpersonal neurobiologist Dr. Daniel Siegel (20) uses the phrase "name it to tame it" to show how simply labelling our inner experience engages the prefrontal cortex, creating enough distance to reduce overwhelm. In practice, this doesn't just mean naming neat emotion words like "sad" or "angry." It also includes giving simple language to body sensations and felt sense: "there's a tight band across my chest," "my stomach feels knotted," "there's a heavy, foggy feeling behind my eyes," "something scared is here, even if I don't yet know exactly what it is." You don't have to get the label perfect. Often, just saying "something painful is here" or "I can feel a knot of 'not-okay' in my body" is enough to begin calming the alarm system. This is one way your Wise Self practises staying with uncertainty—allowing the feeling and its sensations to be real, even before you fully understand them.

Researchers in Finland (21) have also shown that different emotions tend to light up in distinct patterns in the body, which are illustrated in the "emotional-weather" images at the end of this chapter. These maps—and the Feelings Wheel in Appendix 8—are provided to help you identify your *own* sensation—emotion patterns.

Emotional fluency develops gradually. You don't need to sit with intense emotions for hours at a time. You might start by staying present with mild discomfort for just a few minutes. The belly breath practice helps enormously with this—it gives you an anchor point so you're not swept away whilst also not abandoning the feeling entirely.

What staying present looks like in practice:

- **When Anxiety Arises**: "I feel anxious right now. My Overcontroller wants to control something. But I can stay here with this feeling for a few breaths before deciding what to do."
- **When Sadness Emerges**: "There's sadness here. My Detached Protector wants to numb it. But I can let my Lost Child feel sad whilst my Wise Self stays present with her."

The key is building your tolerance gradually. Each time you can stay present for even a few moments longer than your Protector Modes want you to, you're strengthening your Wise Self's capacity to hold difficulty with compassion.

Optional Advanced Practice: Physicalisation Practice: Bringing Emotions into Your Body[1]

Some people find it helpful to go beyond visualisation and actually embody their emotions physically. This practice draws from both acceptance and commitment therapy (ACT) and theatre traditions—both recognise that emotions aren't just thoughts in our heads, but lived experiences in our bodies.

This can create a powerful shift in your relationship with difficult feelings. Instead of trying to push them away or being overwhelmed by them, you learn to be with them in your body. Actors use physicalisation to portray emotions consistently and authentically. You can use the same approach to understand and hold your own emotions with compassion.

If this appeals to you, you might try the physicalisation exercise. This practice invites you to:

- Choose an emotion connected to your eating patterns (shame, anxiety, loneliness, anger)
- Notice where it lives in your body
- Give it a physical form—a posture, a gesture, a pattern of breathing, held tension
- Actually take on that physical position and stay with it
- Notice what happens when you stop trying to change it and simply allow it to be present

This is about giving your Lost Child's feelings a form that your Wise Self can observe, be with, and eventually hold with compassion. Theatre practitioners know that when you embody an emotion through specific physical actions—a clenched jaw, slumped shoulders, rapid breathing—it can lead to something shifting at an emotional level. The emotion becomes something you're allowing space for rather than something that's happening to you. When you can literally embody an emotion without being overwhelmed by it, you're making space for your inner child modes to be heard. You can discover that feelings, no matter how intense, are temporary sensations that you can endure.

The full physicalisation practice can be found in Appendix 9.

Speaking with Warmth and Gentleness

Your Lost Child has been hearing harsh voices for a long time—perhaps from your Inner Critic, perhaps from Protector Modes that use shame and pressure as motivators, perhaps from the punitive way culture talks about bodies and food. These voices may have become so familiar that you barely notice them anymore.

Your Wise Self speaks differently. The tone is warm, gentle, interested—the voice you might use with a frightened child you care deeply about. This isn't about being "nice" in a superficial way. It's about communicating genuine care and acceptance through the quality of your internal voice.

Tone matters as much as words. You could say "It's okay to feel sad" in a dismissive, annoyed tone that communicates "Stop being so emotional." Or you could say the same words in a gentle, accepting tone that communicates "Your sadness makes sense. I'm here with you."

Your Lost Child is exquisitely attuned to tone. She's spent years learning to read between the lines, to hear what's really being communicated beneath the surface words. She'll know whether your Wise Self genuinely accepts her or is secretly wishing she would just be different already.

Practice: The Voice Check

Next time you notice yourself speaking internally to your Lost Child or about your eating struggles, pause and check the tone:

- Is this the voice of your Critic? (harsh, attacking, shaming)
- Is this the voice of a Protector Mode? (urgent, controlling, pressuring)
- Or is this the voice of your Wise Self? (warm, curious, accepting)

If you notice you're using a harsh tone, see if you can soften it. Imagine you're speaking to a young child you love who is struggling. How would you speak to her?

Sometimes it helps to speak out loud, sensing the actual quality of your voice. Is it tight and clipped, or soft and spacious? The physical sound can help you tune into whether you're accessing your Wise Self or still operating from Protector territory.

The Practice of Holding Complexity

One of the most liberating discoveries in recovery is learning that you can hold seemingly contradictory experiences at the same time. You can be scared and still take steps forward. You can feel angry with someone and still love them. You can be struggling with your eating patterns and still be making progress in recovery.

This capacity for holding complexity is essential because eating difficulties often create all-or-nothing thinking: you're either in control or completely out of control, either succeeding or failing, either perfect or worthless. But life is far more nuanced than that, and healing happens in the space between extremes.

Life will always be messy, and we need to find ways to embrace that messiness—to recognise that we can be struggling in one area whilst experiencing moments of aliveness in another. That we can love someone whilst also feeling grief about this relationship. That we can be sad about what we've lost whilst knowing this doesn't cancel out the good parts of those experiences.

Examples of Healing Complexity

- You can feel vulnerable and still set boundaries.
- You can have difficult body image days and still choose nourishing behaviours.
- You can feel sad about what you've lost and grateful for what you're gaining.
- You can be frightened of certain foods and still slowly work toward including them.
- You can love someone deeply and still feel irritated and need space from them when their behaviour is harmful.

- You can be proud of the progress you've made and still acknowledge how hard the journey is.
- You can honour what your eating patterns gave you whilst recognising it's time to find new ways forward.

Learning to hold complexity means developing tolerance for nuance, uncertainty, and the messy reality of being human. It means your Wise Self can hold space for all your different parts and experiences without needing to resolve them into neat categories or simple answers.

Your Wise Self can hold the both/and of human experience: both the pain and the possibility, both the struggle and the strength, both the fear and the courage, both the wounds and the wisdom.

Reflection Point: What contradictory experiences are you currently holding? Can you allow both to be true at the same time rather than needing to resolve them into one simple answer?

Self-Compassion as Foundation

Self-compassion isn't about letting yourself "off the hook". It's about guiding your Lost Child with wisdom and care rather than with force and punishment. It's about becoming the kind of inner leader who can work with your natural traits rather than against them.

Research (22) shows that self-compassion is associated with more effective and sustainable behaviour change than self-control alone. When you treat yourself with the same kindness you'd offer a dear friend, your nervous system calms down, making it easier to make choices aligned with your values rather than driven by fear.

Self-compassion involves three key elements (23):

1. **Mindful Identification of Emotions**: Noticing and naming your experience without over-identifying with it or pushing it away: "I feel sad/angry . . ."
2. **Recognise Your Reactions Make Sense**: Recognising that struggle, imperfection, and difficulty are part of being human and make sense both in the context of your present and past experiences: "It's natural to feel sad in this difficult situation . . . especially in the context of what I've been through."
3. **Self-Kindness**: Treating yourself with warmth and noticing the calming sensations this brings.

Your Wise Self operates from this foundation of self-compassion. This doesn't mean passively accepting that this is the way things will always be. Nor does it mean accepting harmful behaviour. It means approaching yourself with the same fierce tenderness you'd bring to protecting someone you love—with both strength and softness, both boundaries and acceptance.

Reflection Point: How do you talk to yourself when you're struggling? Do you use the harsh, controlling voice of your Inner Critic, or can you access a gentler, more understanding perspective? What would it feel like to approach your traits and struggles with curiosity rather than judgement?

Your Wise Self is learning to provide the emotional vitamins that were missing. We are not aiming for perfection—that only creates stuckness! But consistently enough that your Lost Child begins to trust she'll be nourished.

Part 4: Trusting Your Inner Guidance

Developing Your Internal Compass

As you develop your Wise Self's capacity for compassionate observation, staying present with difficulty, and kindness, you begin to trust your inner guidance. Your body holds wisdom that your Protector Modes have mistrusted and overridden. Now your Wise Self can begin listening to this deeper knowing. As you reconnect with your body, you're developing your internal compass—that felt sense of what's right and true for you. This compass doesn't speak in words or logical arguments but through bodily sensations that arise when you're considering different options or facing decisions.

Your compass operates through several centres of emotional-body intelligence. Here we focus on three, each contributing different information:

Your head (thinking) analyses situations logically. It sees patterns, considers consequences, and plans ahead. When your thinking is clear and aligned, decisions feel mentally coherent—the pieces fit together, the logic makes sense. When your thinking is muddled or you're operating from fear rather than wisdom, you might notice mental confusion, circular thoughts, or an inability to see options clearly.

Your heart (feeling) responds to whether something aligns with your values and relationships. This isn't about emotion in the sense of mood—it's about whether something feels right at the level of what matters most to you. Your heart speaks through sensations in your chest. When something aligns with your deepest values, you might notice a sense of opening or expansion in your chest, a warmth, or simply a quiet "yes." When something moves against your values or authentic needs, you might notice tightness, constriction, or a pulling away sensation in your chest.

Your gut (intuition) knows things before you can explain why. This is your body's accumulated wisdom—all the patterns it's recognised over your lifetime, processing faster than conscious thought. Your gut speaks through sensations in your belly. When something feels safe and right, your belly might settle, soften, or feel grounded. When something's off—even if you can't yet articulate why—your belly might churn, tighten, or create that familiar "bad feeling in my stomach."

When all three centres align—head says yes, heart says yes, gut says yes—decisions tend to feel clear and right. You move forward with confidence because your whole system is in agreement.

When they conflict, that's valuable information too. Perhaps your head says, "This makes logical sense," but your heart feels constricted and your gut is churning. That gives you important information: maybe the logic is sound, but the choice violates your values or ignores important emotional information. Or perhaps your heart wants something, but your head sees real practical problems and your gut signals danger. That's your system asking you to slow down and look more carefully.

Your Lost Child speaks powerfully through this compass, particularly through your heart and gut. She knows what brings genuine joy versus what you think "should" make you happy. She knows which people feel safe versus those who trigger your protective responses. She knows when you're moving toward your authentic self, versus performing for others.

Learning to Read Your Compass

When facing a decision, pause and check in with each centre:

1. **Close your eyes and take three slow breaths to settle.**
2. **Bring the decision to mind. Imagine you've chosen option A.** Don't think about it—just hold it in your awareness and notice:
   - **What happens in your head?** Does your thinking feel clear or confused? Can you see the path forward, or does everything feel murky?
   - **What happens in your heart?** Notice your chest. Does it open or contract? Does warmth spread, or does tightness close in? Does something in you lean toward this option or pull away from it?
   - **What happens in your gut?** Notice your belly. Does it settle or churn? Does it feel grounded or agitated? Is there a sense of rightness or wrongness you can't yet articulate?
3. **Now clear that image. Take a breath. Let option A dissolve.**
4. **Imagine you've chosen option B.** Again, don't analyse—just notice what happens in head, heart, and gut.
5. **Compare**: Which option created a sense of ease, opening, or settling in your body? Which created tension, constriction, or agitation?

One Crucial Check: Is This My Compass or My Critic?

Ask yourself: "Is this my true inner compass speaking, or has my Critic hijacked the signal?"

Your Critic might create chest tightness around options that involve receiving care—but that's fear based on old messages ("your needs are a burden"), not wisdom.

Your Critic might create gut churning around choices that involve setting boundaries—but that's anxiety about others' reactions based on schema conclusions ("I'll be abandoned if I say no"), not your authentic guidance.

Your Critic might create intense body tension around options that feel "too self-indulgent"—but that's old protective programming ("you must earn everything through deprivation"), not your compass.

This is where your Wise Self's observing capacity becomes essential. You learn to distinguish between:

- **Authentic guidance** (steady, clear, aligned with your values)
- **Critic reactions** (urgent, fear-based, driven by shame or guilt)
- **Body memories** (past-tense fear responding as if old dangers are current)

This takes practice. At first, you might not trust your compass at all—years of letting your Critic drive decisions have trained you to override or misinterpret your body's signals. That's to be expected. The compass is still there, still speaking. You're simply learning to hear it again beneath the Critic's loud voice.

Closing: The Foundation Is in Place

Brief Practices for Daily Connection

5-Minute Compass Check

Place your hand gently on your heart or another comforting spot. Take three slow breaths. Ask yourself: "How am I feeling right now?" Notice any body sensations without trying to change them. Ask: "What do I need in this moment?" Listen with curiosity rather than immediately moving into action.

Wise Self Check-In

When facing a decision or difficult emotion, pause and ask: "What would the wisest part of me do here?" Notice what arises—it might be words, images, or just a felt sense.

If your own wise voice feels unclear, try channelling what someone you deeply respect would advise, what your therapist might gently suggest if they were sitting beside you, or what you'd tell your best friend if they were in this situation. You might think of a wise mentor, a character from a book or film, a spiritual figure, or anyone whose compassion and wisdom you trust.

Trust the first gentle guidance that emerges, rather than the loudest or most urgent voice. Over time, notice how these borrowed voices of wisdom begin to merge with and strengthen your own Wise Self.

Daily Mode Awareness

Set three gentle reminders throughout your day to pause and ask: "Which part is active right now? What does my Wise Self notice about this?" Simply observing without immediately trying to change anything strengthens your capacity to lead from wisdom rather than reactivity.

These practices help you stay connected to your inner world throughout the day, building the foundation for deeper healing work whilst supporting you in navigating daily challenges with more skill and self-compassion.

The Re-Membered Ship

The captain has returned. The crew members—Overcontroller, People Pleaser, Detached Protector—are beginning to recognise that they are part of the same team rather than competitors. The Lost Child is sensing that maybe, finally, someone is here who can lead with both strength and care. The sea is still wild, but you now have a compass and steady hands at the wheel.

The foundation is set—your Wise Self grounded in the present moment, able to observe with compassion, stay present with difficulty, and speak with warmth. Now comes the work of using this wise presence to protect your Lost Child and begin building the relationship she's been waiting for. The most important voyage is the one that closes the distance between you and you—your Wise Self and Lost Child.

What Comes Next

With your Wise Self established and embodied, you're ready for the deeper work of Chapter 6: using this wise presence to protect your Lost Child from your Inner Critic's attacks, and beginning to build the healing relationship between your Wise Self and the vulnerable part of yourself.

You'll learn how to set firm boundaries with your Critic. You'll discover how your Wise Self talks to your Lost Child in ways that begin filling in the missing emotional vitamins. And you'll start developing the internal compass that helps you distinguish authentic guidance from Protector Mode interference.

This is gentle and gradual work. Your Lost Child has been waiting a long time for someone who won't abandon her when feelings get big. That someone is the Wise Self you're becoming—the inner leader your whole system has been waiting for.

Permission for Imperfect Practice

As you move forward, remember that this work doesn't require perfection. You won't always access your Wise Self easily. Some days you'll forget these practices entirely. Sometimes your Protector Modes will take over before you even notice.

All of this is normal. You're learning to navigate your inner world in entirely new ways. You're developing capacities that may have been unavailable during your formative years. This capacity develops gradually.

What matters is your commitment to keep showing up—to notice when you've been hijacked by old patterns and gently guide yourself back to your Wise Self. Recovery isn't a straight line from struggle to freedom. It's a gradual process of reconnection, of building trust between parts of yourself that have been operating in opposition for years, of creating new neural pathways that support integration rather than fragmentation.

You're learning to captain your ship with both head and heart engaged, with all your crew members working together under wise leadership rather than competing for control. Give yourself credit for every small step forward, every moment of awareness, every time you choose connection over control.

Each time you place your hand on your heart when you feel lost, the warmth beneath your palm is proof: your Wise Self is here, alive, guiding you home.

Gentle Experiments to Try

As we close this chapter, here are practices to help you continue developing your Wise Self presence. You're invited to choose two or three that feel most relevant to where you are right now and try them out this week. But keep in mind: these aren't "weekly assignments" with a deadline. They're ongoing invitations you can return to whenever they feel helpful. Taste each one. Notice which ones resonate. Keep the ones that nourish you, and return to them as often as you like.

1. **Daily Mode Awareness**: Set three gentle reminders throughout your day to pause and ask: "Which part is active right now? What does my Wise Self notice about this?" Simply observing without immediately trying to change anything strengthens your capacity to lead from wisdom rather than reactivity.
2. **Breath Practice**: Use the cyclic sigh (double inhale through the nose, long exhale through the mouth) whenever you notice tension or overwhelm. Even once or twice a day helps you remember you have a way to calm your system.
3. **Flow Moment Practice**: Choose one daily activity to do with complete attention (washing dishes, walking, listening to music). Put away distractions and engage fully with the task. When your mind wanders, gently return attention to the activity.
4. **Wise Self Connection**: Spend five minutes each day connecting with your Wise Self through visualisation, journalling, or simply sitting quietly and sensing that presence within you. The more you visit this part of yourself, the more accessible it becomes.

Journalling Prompt Reflections: Remembering your Wise Self

- When have you experienced your Wise Self, even briefly? What was that like?
- What makes it difficult to access this wise presence? Which Protector Mode gets in the way?

- Try the cyclic sigh practice now. What do you notice in your body afterwards?
- What does your Wise Self want to say to your Lost Child that your Protector Modes usually block?

Remember: These practices remain available to you always—return to them whenever you need support. Each time you practice, you're strengthening your Wise Self and building the foundation for all the work ahead.

Looking Ahead

The young part of you who has been waiting is beginning to sense that maybe, finally, someone is here who can lead with both wisdom and strength. Someone who sees all the crew members clearly. Someone who won't be overwhelmed by the storms ahead.

That someone is you—the wise, compassionate leader you're becoming.

The foundation is set. Your Wise Self is re-membered. And the journey toward wholeness continues with each compassionate step you take.

You're ready for what comes next.

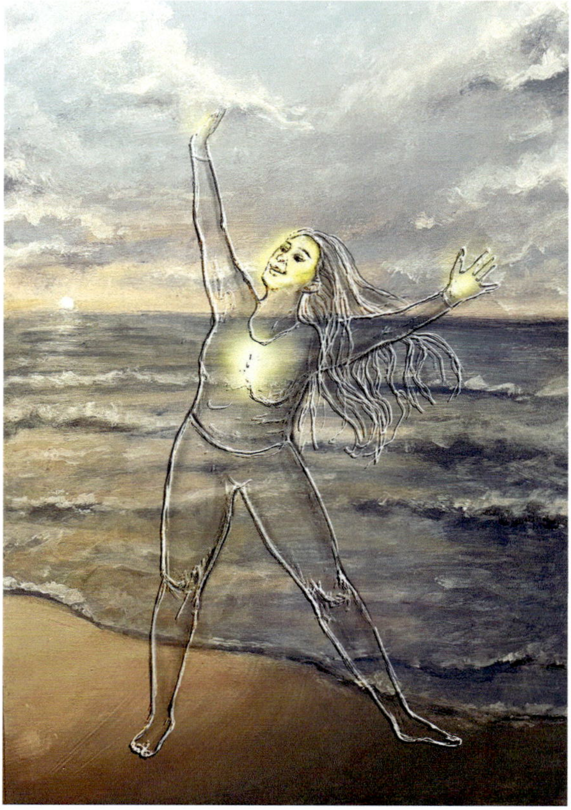

Figure 5.1 Joy

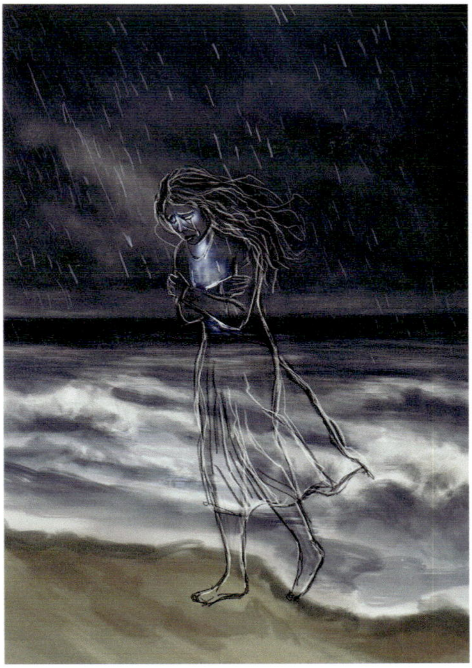

Figure 5.2 Sadness

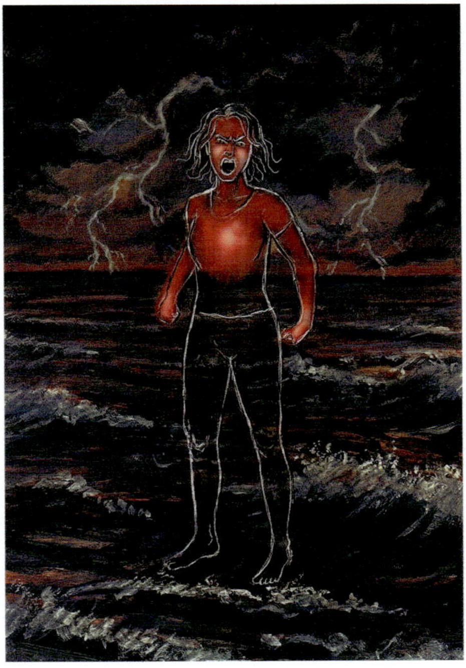

Figure 5.3 Anger

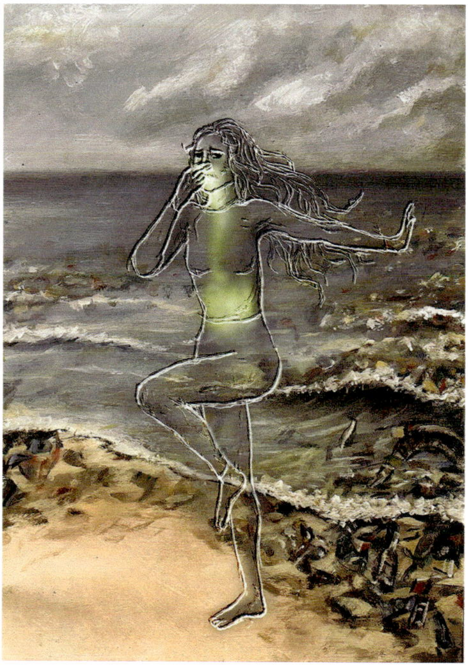

Figure 5.4 Disgust

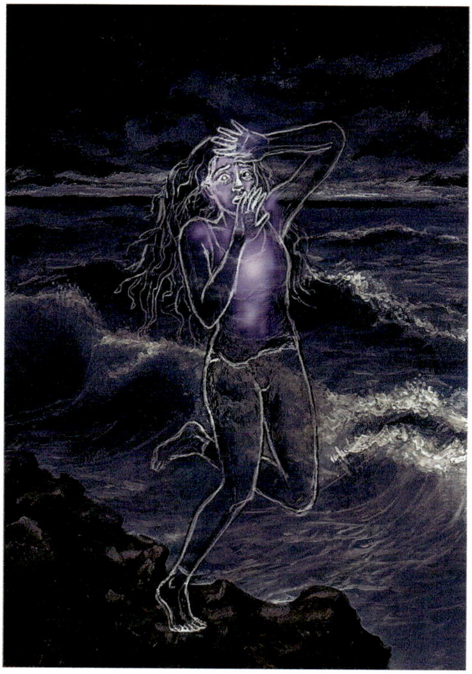

Figure 5.5 Fear

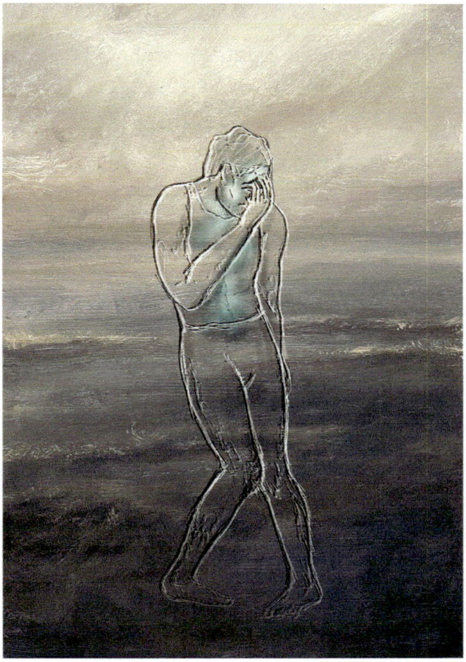

Figure 5.6 Shame

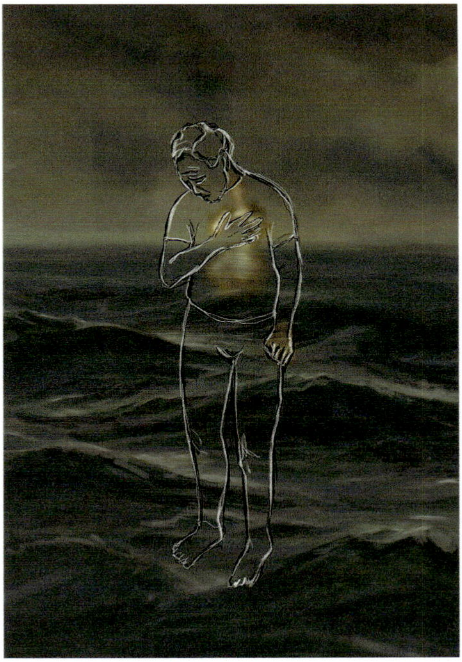

Figure 5.7 Guilt

Note

1 Safety Note: This practice can bring up strong feelings. If at any point you feel overwhelmed, pause and use the cyclic sigh and remind yourself: "I'm here now. I'm safe. I can return to this when I'm ready."

6 Protecting the Lost Child

Setting Boundaries and Building Connection

Freedom is not given to us by anyone; we have to cultivate it ourselves.

Thích Nhất Hấnh[1]

When the Captain Sees the Bully

Three weeks into practising her Wise Self exercises, Emma notices something different happening. She's standing in front of her wardrobe when she hears that familiar harsh voice: "Nothing fits right. You're disgusting. You shouldn't have eaten that breakfast."

But this time, instead of immediately collapsing into shame, Emma senses a pause. A space opens up. From somewhere deeper and wiser, she notices: "That's my Critic. I can hear it attacking. And I can feel my Lost Child believing those words."

For the first time, Emma isn't fused with the harsh voice. Her Wise Self can see what's happening. She can see her Critic using shame as its tool. She can see her Lost Child shrinking under the attack. And she realises: I need to step in. I need to protect her.

Your Wise Self—the captain—is learning to protect your Lost Child (hidden below deck) from the Critic (the guard who's been keeping her trapped). This chapter is about teaching the guard new methods—protection without imprisonment.

Part 1: Understanding Your Inner Critic

The Security Guard Who Became Too Harsh

As you learned in Chapter 3, your Critic actually operates like your Protector Modes—a crew member who learned to keep you safe through harsh self-attack. It absorbed specific messages from culture, family, religion, and peers and then internalised those messages because doing so gave you some sense of agency in situations where you otherwise felt powerless.

Taking those messages inside once had a purpose. When you learned to criticise yourself before others could, when you absorbed impossible standards

DOI: 10.4324/9781003355878-7

and tried desperately to meet them, when you made your body the problem to solve, you were trying to survive. The Critic promised: "If we're just harsh enough, controlled enough, perfect enough, we'll finally be safe—from rejection, humiliation, and abandonment."

These methods that helped you survive childhood are now keeping you trapped and creating further chaos in your life. The harsh voice that once felt like protection has become the very thing your Lost Child needs protection from.

Understanding Your Critic: Messages and Protection

Your Critic is made up of harsh messages absorbed from the outside world, merged with a part that uses self-attack as its protection strategy.

The Messages Layer: Your Critic carries toxic content—cultural lies about bodies, patriarchal demands, impossible family standards, schema-mindset conclusions about your worth. These messages are poison, even though internalising them once served a purpose.

Examples:

- "Your body is unacceptable unless it meets narrow standards."
- "Your worth depends on weight, appearance, or achievement."
- "Your needs make you a burden."
- "Perfection is the only protection from rejection."

The Protective Function Layer: Underneath those messages, your Critic genuinely believes shame, guilt, and self-punishment will keep you safe. It operates through self-flagellating—inflicting blame and pain on yourself: a protective part that learned: "If I punish myself first, control the body harshly, I can prevent something worse from happening."

What Your Critic Is Really Defending Against

Here's what makes the Critic so difficult to work with: the self-attack isn't actually about you being terrible. It's about something much more frightening that your system learned to avoid—becoming disconnected from those you care about.

Your Critic developed its harsh methods to defend against three unbearable realisations:

1. The Unbearable Helplessness

Deep down, your Critic is protecting you from facing a painful truth: the people you needed most—parents, caregivers, partners—couldn't or wouldn't meet your needs in the ways you required. And there was nothing you could do to change that.

This realisation—"I am powerless to make them love and care for me the way I need"—is unbearable for a child who depends on these relationships for survival. It's also unbearable for adults who find themselves in relationships where they cannot get the care, attention, or respect they long for.

So your Critic offers an alternative: "It's not that they can't love you properly—it's that YOU are unlovable. If you could just be thinner, quieter, more perfect, less needy, then they would finally give you what you need."

This reframing gives you back a sense of control. If the problem is you, then you can fix it. You can work harder, control more, achieve more, and disappear more. The Critic's attacks become a way of maintaining hope: change is possible if you just criticise yourself enough.

But this comes at a cost. Rather than facing the grief of unmet needs and the powerlessness of needing people who couldn't fully show up, you turn all that energy inward—attacking yourself as a substitute for acknowledging what you couldn't control.

2. The Dangerous Anger

When your needs go unmet, when you're hurt or neglected or dismissed, anger is the natural response. In healthy secure relationships, we learn that we can express healthy levels of anger without harming others or it leading to retaliation or rejection. But sometimes anger toward the people you depend on feels too risky.

As a child, showing anger might have led to punishment, withdrawal, or abandonment. As an adult, expressing anger toward people you're attached to can feel equally dangerous—what if they leave? What if they retaliate? What if my needs are a burden on them? What if your anger confirms their worst beliefs about you?

So the anger doesn't disappear—it redirects. Your Critic takes all that rage about how you've been treated and turns it back on yourself. Every harsh thought, every punishing restriction, every moment of body hatred carries the force of anger that was never safe to express outward.

The eating disorder becomes the perfect vehicle for this redirected anger. Restriction punishes your body. Bingeing and purging create a battlefield inside you. Compulsive exercise inflicts controlled harm. You become both the perpetrator and the victim—a way of managing anger that keeps your attachments with others intact.

3. The Preservation of Hope in Important Relationships

This is what's called the "moral defence"—a concept that explains why children (and adults) would rather believe they are bad than face the reality that their caregivers are unable or unwilling to provide what they need.

If you believe "I am defective," you can still hold onto the idea "they are good and capable of love—I just need to become worthy of it." The relationship remains safe in your mind, even if you pay the price.

But if you begin to see "they couldn't meet my needs," you must also face: "they are limited, damaged, or insufficient." For a child who needs to trust their caregivers for survival, this is unbearable. For an adult still seeking approval, it threatens the very foundation of the relationship.

Your Critic helps keeps this uncomfortable truth out of awareness by making you the problem. As long as you focus on fixing yourself, you never have to grieve the limits of what those relationships could provide. It can be painful to recognise that, despite their intentions, others were not always able to meet your emotional needs in consistent or attuned ways—often because of their own limitations.

When the Critic Attacks: The Triggers

Your Critic tends to activate most strongly in specific situations—particularly when something threatens the careful balance it's been maintaining.

The Critic often strikes hardest when you:

Allow Yourself to Have Needs: The moment you acknowledge "I need connection" or "I deserve care," the Critic rushes in: "Who do you think you are? Your needs are too much. You're being selfish and demanding."

Feel Good about Yourself: Any flicker of self-worth or pride triggers immediate attack: "Don't get too big for your boots. You'll say something that leads to retaliation or rejection, or evokes their envy. Better stay small and controllable."

Receive Care or Compassion from Others: When someone offers genuine care, the Critic panics: "You don't deserve this. They'll see you're not worth it. You're tricking them. You should refuse this and prove you don't need it."

Show Yourself Compassion: When your Wise Self tries to offer kindness, the Critic intensifies: "Stop being so self-indulgent. This is weakness. You need to be harder on yourself, not softer."

Allow Vulnerability: Any moment of letting your guard down, showing authentic feelings, or admitting struggle activates a harsh attack: "You're pathetic. Pull yourself together. Stop being so dramatic."

Why these particular triggers? Because each one threatens one of the Critic's primary functions: *maintaining the idealisation of loved ones while keeping you controllable and "safe" through self-blame.*

If you're allowed to have needs and those needs go unmet, you might have to face that others couldn't or wouldn't meet them. But if the Critic attacks you for having needs in the first place ("Your needs are too much"), then others remain good and you remain the problem, preserving hope that if you just changed yourself enough, maybe you'd finally get what you need.

If you're allowed to feel good about yourself, you might stop accepting poor treatment or start expecting better. But if the Critic immediately cuts you down ("Who do you think you are?"), you stay in the familiar position of not deserving better, which paradoxically feels safer than risking disappointment.

If you receive care from others and allow yourself to take it in, you might discover that you're actually worthy of care, which would mean that you deserved better all along. The Critic can't allow this realisation, so it attacks: "You're fooling them. They'll see through you soon."

This is why self-compassion feels so threatening. It's not just about being "nice to yourself." It's about dismantling the entire system that's kept you attached to people who couldn't fully meet your needs—a system built on the foundation of self-blame, preserving the idealisation of others.

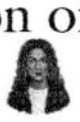 Samantha noticed this pattern acutely. Whenever she started to feel angry at Gary for his emotional unavailability—whenever she glimpsed the truth that *his* behaviour was the problem—her Critic would swoop in immediately: "You're too sensitive. You're too needy. If you were tougher like you should be, this wouldn't bother you."

The attack served a purpose: it redirected her anger back onto herself, preserving Gary as "good" (just a normal guy who doesn't like drama) and herself as "the problem" (too emotional, too much). This maintained hope: *If I can just fix myself, he'll be able to love me properly.*

But it also meant she could never acknowledge the painful truth: she was powerless to make him show up differently. Staying attached through self-blame felt less devastating than facing that reality.

This Is Why "Building Self-Esteem" Doesn't Work

When someone comes to therapy saying "I hate myself," the natural response is to help them see their worth—point out their strengths, teach self-validation, and encourage self-care behaviours.

But this rarely works. Because the real issue isn't low self-esteem. The real issue is:

- Buried helplessness about ever getting emotional needs met in relationships
- Redirected anger toward loved ones that feels too dangerous to express
- An outdated protective strategy that says, "I'd rather hate myself than face what I couldn't control"

Until you address these deeper layers—until you can acknowledge the powerlessness, find safe ways to feel the anger, and grieve the limits of what certain relationships could provide—the Critic will keep attacking. Because, from its perspective, self-hatred is still the safest option.

Recovery requires helping your Critic discover that you now have other options. You're not that powerless child anymore. You can acknowledge unmet needs without collapsing. You can feel anger without destroying relationships. You can grieve what was missing without losing hope for what's still possible.

How the Critic Manages Your "Rejected Inner Child"

Your Critic is trying to manage what we might call your Rejected Inner Child—essentially, *your Lost Child frozen at a particular time in the past* when shame or rejection became unbearable. This is your Lost Child stuck in that specific moment, still feeling in her body what it was like to be rejected, shamed, or unwanted at that particular age.

Why This Developed: Making yourself the problem was once a clever survival strategy. It protected you from facing the unbearable idea that someone you relied on simply couldn't or wouldn't love you in the way you needed. If you decided "I am the problem," then that person could stay good and safe in your mind—the relationship stayed intact—even though you paid the price.

Your Critic attacks your body, needs, and emotions aggressively to prevent you from ever feeling like that rejected child again. Self-punishment becomes a way of staying in charge:

- By rejecting yourself first, you hope to avoid the terror of being rejected by others.
- By keeping expectations low, you protect yourself from disappointment.
- By making yourself suffer, you prove you're "good enough" to deserve care—even though the suffering itself pushes care further away.

The problem is your Critic treats that frozen moment in the past as though it's happening right now. It attacks you in the present to protect you from a feeling that belongs to the past. The harsh voice keeps you trapped, believing you still are that powerless, rejected child—when actually, you're an adult with resources that child never had.

Sophie's Pattern: When Love Becomes Debt

 Sophie's Lost Child carries a frozen moment from childhood—a time when feeling "too much" and "a burden" was unbearable. Her emotional needs overwhelmed already-depleted parents, and that experience settled in her body as a shame-filled identity.

Beneath the self-hatred lay something harder to face: the helpless grief of loving parents who simply couldn't meet her emotionally. Her mum worked tirelessly to get the practical care right—but emotional attunement wasn't available. Her dad's high standards meant he did things for her rather than teaching her—leaving Sophie feeling incompetent and "wrong."

Sophie couldn't afford to be angry at them. They sacrificed so much. They loved her in the ways they knew how. So the anger had nowhere to go but inward.

Her Critic learned: "If I deprive and punish myself, I prove I'm not needy. If I suffer well enough, I earn my right to exist without being a burden."

The eating disorder became the perfect tool: restriction proving she didn't need much, the "empty stomach feeling" signalling achievement, and rigid control demonstrating she wasn't greedy or demanding. Every act of deprivation declared: "See? If I suffer enough I will eventually deserve love."

The self-perpetuating loop: the Critic attacks Sophie in the present to protect her Lost Child from that frozen childhood moment—the time when being "too much" felt intolerable. It punishes her body now to ensure she never has to feel that shame again.

What the Critic hasn't realised is that the moment was real—but it is *frozen in the past*. It's a memory, not her identity. Sophie is no longer that overwhelmed child. She is an adult with resources that a child never had.

Recovery means helping the Critic update its story: "We don't need to attack to prove we're different now. We can bring that moment into the present, understand it with compassion, and care for the child who once felt like a burden—without punishing the adult she has become."

Samantha's Pattern: When Anger Turns Inward

Samantha's boyfriend, Gary, is often unavailable. When she reaches out for connection, he labels her "too emotional, too sensitive." She can feel the rejection building—but expressing anger at him feels impossible. What if he leaves entirely? What if he's right that she's too much?

So Samantha turns all that anger, all that hurt, all that powerlessness about not being able to get him to show up for her—she turns it on herself and her body.

Here's the self-perpetuating trap: Samantha restricts to prove she's not "too much"—to demonstrate control and worthiness. But the deprivation fuels her Feisty Child's rage at being silenced and dismissed. That underground anger eventually erupts through bingeing—a rebellion against all the suppression, all the accommodating, all the self-erasure. Then the guilt floods in. Her Critic attacks: "See? You ARE out of control. You ARE too much."

This confirms the very belief she was trying to escape. The restriction tightens further—more punishment, more silence, more proving she needs nothing. The eating behaviours meant to protect her from feeling controlled and dismissed actually create more subjugation and dismissal—now from herself. The cycle reinforces exactly what she learned in childhood: expressing needs (even indirectly through eating) leads to shame. Her Feisty Child stays underground, and the pattern deepens.

The binge carries rage she cannot express toward Gary. Then comes punishment: restriction, compulsive exercise, harsh self-criticism. Her Critic says, "If you were thinner, less emotional, he'd treat you better. You're the problem." This reframing protects her from facing that she's powerless to make Gary love her properly, and she's furious and heartbroken about it. As long as she attacks herself, she never has to grieve the relationship's limitations.

How the Critic Drives Eating Disorder Behaviours

Your Critic uses shame, guilt, and self-punishment to keep you away from that frozen moment when your Lost Child felt utterly helpless, rejected, or powerless:

Restriction creates distance from needs: "If I override hunger, I prove I'm not that needy child who was helpless to get care."
Body control becomes obsessive: "If I perfect the body, I can outrun the shame stuck in that frozen moment and finally become worthy of the love I couldn't get."
Rigid rules prevent slipping back: "If I follow food rules perfectly, I'll never return to that powerless state where I needed things I couldn't have."
Self-punishment feels protective: "If I hurt myself first, I control when and how pain happens—and I don't have to face the anger I feel about past hurts and unmet needs."

Body image distortion makes sense from this perspective: you're not misperceiving your body cognitively—you're experiencing it through the lens of that frozen, shame-encoded moment in your Lost Child's past. The internal body image is anchored to that traumatic time when rejection felt unbearable.

As long as your Critic maintains this harsh grip—attacking you to prevent you from feeling like that helpless, rejected child again—your Lost Child remains trapped in the past.

Recovery requires helping the Critic discover that you now have resources to face what that child couldn't. You're not that powerless child anymore. That frozen moment of shame and rejection can be brought into the present, understood with compassion, and recognised for what it is: a painful memory, not your identity.

In This Book's Framework

In this book, we use the term "Critic" to describe two different layers of the same harsh voice:

One layer is made of absorbed, toxic messages from culture, family, or past experiences—this part is not truly you, and your Wise Self must set strong boundaries with it.
The deeper layer is your own Flagellating Critic—a protective part that uses harshness because it genuinely believes shame will keep you safe from the unbearable feelings of helplessness, anger, and powerlessness that you once couldn't face.

In Appendix 10, you'll learn a simple way to sort these layers: the Inner Critic messages that represent toxic cultural messages require eviction, but the Flagellating Critic requires patient retraining. Both layers need your Wise Self's strength but in different ways.

Both need to be addressed but in different ways. The toxic messages can be rejected outright. But the protective part underneath—the one trying to defend you from helplessness and keep dangerous anger contained—that part needs something different. It needs your Wise Self to show it that:

- You can face the powerlessness now without collapsing.
- You can feel the anger now without destroying relationships.
- You can grieve what was missing without losing hope.
- You are not that frozen Rejected Inner Child—you are an adult with resources that child never had.

This is the work of the next section.

Part 2: Setting Boundaries with Your Critic

When Love Requires Strength

Your Critic has been attacking your Lost Child for years, maybe decades—using shame and guilt whilst genuinely believing this serves a protective purpose. True wisdom requires you to step in with both strength and care to protect the innocent.

Boundaried compassion recognises that sometimes love requires us to say "no" clearly and firmly. This isn't about aggressive anger—it's about intervening in a harmful dynamic with loving strength.

Embodying Strength: A Preparatory Practice

Before working directly with your Critic, practice what strength feels like in your body. Many people with eating difficulties have spent years making themselves small and suppressing their power.

The Practice (5 minutes):

1. **Find Your Power Stance**: Stand with feet hip-width apart, spine lengthened, shoulders back and down. This is your grounded, stable position.
2. **Breathe into Your Strength**: Take several deep breaths. Let yourself feel solid, rooted, present.
3. **Practice Saying "No"**: Out loud, say:
   - "No."
   - "That's not okay."
   - "This stops now."
4. **Notice**: What volume feels powerful without being aggressive? Where in your body does the sound originate?
5. **Create a Physical Anchor**: Choose one simple movement that helps you feel grounded—perhaps straightening your spine or planting your feet more firmly.

Note: Take your time with this embodiment work. You might spend a whole week just finding your power stance and noticing how it feels in your body before moving on to actually saying "no" out loud. There's no rush. Practice saying it once, notice how that feels. Do you like the flavour of having a voice? Then try again tomorrow. Small steps, repeated consistently, create lasting change.

Step One: Rejecting Harmful Messages

The first layer of work involves your Wise Self setting clear boundaries around the harmful content your Critic absorbed—the cultural lies, patriarchal demands (on all genders), impossible standards, and schema-mindset conclusions.

These messages are poison, even though internalising them once served a protective purpose. You can reject them now.

The Practice

When you notice your Critic speaking, pause and identify the specific message underneath the shame:

> "Your body is unacceptable" → This is cultural fat-phobia and diet industry propaganda.
>
> "You must be perfect or you're worthless" → This is an impossible standard absorbed from perfectionist environments.
>
> "Your needs make you a burden" → This is a schema-mindset conclusion from emotional deprivation.
>
> "You must earn love through performance" → This is conditional regard from childhood.

Your Wise Self Can Firmly Reject These Messages

> "That cultural message about bodies—that's a lie. I reject it."
>
> "Those cultural demands that I be smaller and need less—I'm not following them anymore."
>
> "That impossible standard of perfection—it's harmful and I'm done chasing it."
>
> "The conclusion that my needs make me a burden—that's not truth. That's what I learned when my needs couldn't be met, but it doesn't define my worth."

This is not the same as evicting your Critic entirely. You're not throwing a crew member overboard. You're setting boundaries around the toxic material the Critic absorbed and mistakenly thinks will keep you safe.

Think of it like this: your Critic is a security guard who picked up weapons (shame-based messages), believing they'd protect you. Your Wise Self is saying: "Those weapons are poison. Put them down. I'll show you better tools."

Step Two: Helping Your Critic Learn New Methods (the Main Event)

Your Critic is a Protector part that genuinely believes shame and guilt keep you safe. Your task: help it discover that protection doesn't require punishment.

Your Wise Self's Stance: Compassionate Accountability

Before beginning the negotiation, understand the position your Wise Self takes—what we might call compassionate accountability:

> I understand where you came from. You absorbed harsh methods because you genuinely believed shame would keep us safe. You learned to attack first to prevent something worse. I recognise your protective intent—I won't resent you for trying to help.
>
> But I will not allow you to continue harming my Lost Child. The attacks stop now. Understanding your origin doesn't mean accepting your methods.
>
> I'm not throwing you overboard—you're part of our crew. But your role changes today. You can alert me to danger without using shame as your weapon. You can help protect without punishment. This is strength with care: I see your struggle, and I'm still setting this boundary.

The Negotiation Practice

For this exercise you will need three chairs: one for your Lost Child, one for your Critic, and one for your Wise Self.

1. **Make a List of Triggers**: Write situations that activate your Critic. Rate anxiety 0–100 for each. Arrange into a hierarchy.
2. **Choose and Imagine**: Select a situation toward the middle of your list. Close your eyes and imagine you've faced that situation.
3. **Bring in the Critic**: Open your eyes. Place one chair to represent your Critic. If you completed the visualisation exercise in Chapter 3, where you drew or described your modes, retrieve that image now and place it on or near this chair. Visualise your Critic—what does it look like? What's its posture? What's its tone? How does it use shame or guilt? What messages does it carry?
4. **Notice Its Protective Intent**: Before standing, take a moment to recognise: *This part is trying to help, even though its methods cause harm. It genuinely believes shame and guilt will protect me.*
5. **Step into your Wise Self**: Stand between your Lost Child and your Critic. Your energy is strong but also curious and warm—you're here to protect whilst also understanding.
6. **Acknowledge Its Efforts**: Begin by recognising what this part has been trying to do: "I see you there. I see how hard you've been working." "I understand you learned to keep us safe by being harsh." "You've been

using shame and guilt because you genuinely believe that's what protects us from rejection." "You absorbed all those impossible standards and you've been trying to meet them, thinking that would finally make us acceptable."

7. Name the Cost: Help this part see what its methods have actually created: "But look at her [gesture to Lost Child]. Look at what your methods have done." "You've been so harsh that she's terrified. She can't come out. She believes everything you say about her." "Your shame hasn't made us acceptable—it's just made us isolated and exhausted." "The guilt you use to motivate us hasn't earned us love—it's kept us disconnected from the very care we need."
8. **Offer a New Way**: Now your Wise Self makes a clear offer:

I understand you learned to punish us to prevent becoming her again—that frozen version of our Lost Child from when shame felt unbearable. You've been attacking the body, the needs, the emotions, trying desperately to keep us from returning to that moment.

But our Lost Child frozen in that painful moment is not who we are now. She's stuck in unprocessed shame and fear that needs care and updating, not an identity we need to outrun forever.

I'm strong enough now. I can meet that frozen part of our Lost Child and help her see she's not alone in that moment anymore. We don't need to keep attacking ourselves to prove we're different from her—we can bring her out of that frozen state care instead of punishment.

9. **Set the Boundary Gently but Firmly**: "I won't let you attack her with shame anymore. That stops now." "But I'm not throwing you away. You're part of our crew. You just need to learn new methods." "From now on, when you want to use guilt or shame, I need you to pause. Come to me first. Let me show you another way."
10. Invite Collaboration: "You know so much about what we're afraid of. You know all the ways we've been hurt." "I need that knowledge. But I need you to share it without attacking." "Can you try being the one who alerts me to situations that feel risky, instead of the one who punishes with shame?" "Can you help me identify when we need protection, without using guilt as the tool?"
11. **Turn to Your Lost Child**: Let her know she's protected now: "I see how scared you've been. I know that voice has been scary." "It's not going away completely—it's part of our history, part of how we learned to survive. But I'm teaching it new ways." "I'm here. You're safe. I won't let it use shame to hurt you anymore."

Why This Works

Your Critic learned harsh methods as the only available tools—outdated childhood and adolescent conclusions about safety. By acknowledging its protective intent whilst firmly redirecting its methods, you help it update:

"Thank you for trying to protect me. But I'm an adult now. Shame doesn't protect—it perpetuates pain. Let me show you a better way."

What to Expect

This takes time. Your Critic won't immediately trust your Wise Self can keep you safe without harsh methods. It will test you, revert to shame under stress. That's to be expected.

Keep showing the steady message: "I see you trying to protect through shame. We don't need that anymore. Here's another way."

Some days your Critic might soften—less noisy and tight. Other days, it roars back. Both are part of the process. You're helping it discover that protection can happen through compassion instead of cruelty.

Common Questions

"What If My Critic Won't Soften?"

This Protector Mode has been keeping you safe using harsh methods for years, maybe decades. It won't immediately trust that your Wise Self is strong enough to take over.

Keep showing up. Keep offering the same steady message. Over weeks and months of consistent practice, it will begin to believe you.

If progress feels stuck, this is valuable work to bring to therapy. A skilled therapist can help you understand what your Critic is still afraid of and what it needs to feel safe enough to soften.

"What If the Critic Comes Back Stronger after I've Set Boundaries?"

This often happens. When your Critic feels you pulling away from its methods, it may intensify temporarily—like a security guard who sees the person they're protecting start to take risks.

This is actually a sign your work is having an impact. The Critic is scared. It genuinely believes that without its harsh methods, something terrible will happen.

Don't give up. Return to the negotiation practice. Acknowledge: "I see you're scared. I see you think we need harsh discipline to be safe. But I'm showing you—we're okay. We're actually more than okay. We're learning to be safe through care."

"How Do I Know If I'm Setting Boundaries on Messages versus Attacking My Critic?"

There's an important difference:

Setting Boundaries on Messages: "That cultural standard about bodies is a lie. I reject it." (You're rejecting the content, not the part.)

Attacking the Critic: "You're terrible. You need to shut up and go away." (You're trying to eliminate the part itself.)

Your Critic is a crew member who absorbed harmful messages because it was trying to protect you. You can firmly reject the messages whilst showing compassion for the part that carries them.

A Key Distinction: When the Critic Carries Someone Else's Voice

In Step One, you learned to reject toxic cultural messages—Layer 1 of your Critic. Sometimes these messages are subtle: diet culture mantras, beauty standards, and family expectations. But sometimes Layer 1 carries something far more severe: the actual voice of someone who abused, violated, or tried to annihilate you.

This is still Layer 1—toxic messages that don't belong to you and must be rejected. But it deserves special acknowledgement because it's not vague cultural noise. It's a specific person's cruelty, shame, and poison that they tried to put inside you.

If your Critic's attacks feel like they're trying to destroy you completely, if the tone matches someone who harmed you, if the shame feels like someone else literally planting their poison inside you—recognise this for what it is: *their voice, their shame, their cruelty. Never yours.*

Your Wise Self's response remains the same as all Layer 1 content—rejection and eviction—but with clear recognition of where it came from:

> This voice doesn't belong to me. It never has. This is [person's] shame, [person's] cruelty, [person's] attempt to make me carry what they couldn't face in themselves. I recognise where this came from—and I refuse to accept it. This isn't my voice. It's yours. I'm handing it back.

This is different from Layer 2 (your Flagellating Critic—the protective part you're retraining in Step Two). That part is genuinely yours and trying to help, even though its methods are harmful. *This perpetrator voice was never yours. It doesn't get retraining—it gets eviction.* For work with internalised perpetrator voices connected to trauma, see Chapter 11.

When You Need Quick Intervention: The SPACE Practice

This negotiation work takes time, works best in private, and needs your full attention. But what about the moments when your Critic hijacks you in the middle of the day? When you're at lunch with colleagues and body shame floods in? When you wake at 3 AM with restriction urges screaming?

You need something *portable, rapid, and reliable*—a way of bringing your Wise Self back online when a mode has taken over and you're at risk of reacting automatically.

That's where the *SPACE practice* comes in. Think of it as *emergency mode management*—a five-step process you can use anywhere, anytime a mode hijacks your system and you need to restore Wise Self leadership.

When to Use SPACE

- When strong eating disorder urges arise suddenly
- When Critic launches shame attacks
- Before, during, or after challenging meals
- When relationship conflicts trigger old patterns
- Any moment when a mode is hijacking your ship and you need your Wise Self back at the helm

The Five Steps of SPACE

S—Slow the Body

Ground your nervous system first. Your modes thrive when you're physiologically activated. Shifting your body helps shift your mind.

Take a longer out-breath (exhale slower than inhale), feel your feet pressing into the floor, or place a gentle hand on your heart.

Say to yourself: "I notice a wave rising. I can slow this moment down."
Purpose: Shift from reactive survival mode to allow access to your Wise Self.

P—Pinpoint the Mode

Name which crew member has taken control of your ship:

- Overcontroller tightening food rules?
- Inner Critic attacking with shame?
- Lost Child panicking about your body?
- Feisty Child wanting to lash out?
- Detached Protector pushing you toward numbness?

Say to yourself: "A strict Protector Mode is tightening the rules." "My Critic is using shame right now." "My Lost Child part is panicking."
Purpose: Create separation between you and the mode. You're not the anxiety—you're the one noticing an anxious part. This alone begins to break the fusion.

A—Assemble the Crew

Invite all your modes into an internal meeting—especially your Lost Child. You're creating space for everyone to have a voice rather than allowing one mode to solo-hijack.

Say to yourself: "Each part is here trying to help in its own way. Everyone gets a seat at the table."

Purpose: Counter the isolation and shame that come when the ED feels like it's completely taken over. You're remembering that you have an internal crew, not just one dominant voice.

C—Choose the Healthy Adult

Intentionally hand the microphone to your Wise Self. This is the explicit mode shift—from protection to care.

Ask yourself: "What would honour my real needs right now?" "How can I show up for my Lost Child in this moment?" "What does wisdom—not fear—suggest here?"

Purpose: Bring your Wise Self back online as the decision-maker. Your modes can offer information, but your Wise Self leads.

E—Enact a Tiny Protective Step

Take one small, compassionate action right now that reduces suffering—even by 1%. This is about showing your body and Lost Child that your Wise Self is actively protecting them in this moment.

- Loosen one food rule slightly.
- Soften your clenched jaw or shoulders.
- Stay seated 30 seconds longer after the meal.
- Send a brief text to a supportive person.
- Place your hand on your heart and take three breaths.
- Say one kind phrase to your Lost Child.
- Choose one food you've been avoiding and include a small amount.

Say to yourself: "Just 1% more safety for my body right now." "One small caring action to show my Lost Child I'm here."

Purpose: Behavioural enactment reinforces new neural pathways. You're proving—through action—that your Wise Self can protect and care for you, even when a mode is loud.

SPACE in Action: Emma's Morning

 Emma wakes up and immediately her Overcontroller starts calculating: *You ate too much yesterday. Skip breakfast. Exercise first.*

S—Slow: Emma notices her heart racing. She takes three breaths, making each exhale longer than the inhale. She feels her feet touching the floor.

P—Pinpoint: "That's my Overcontroller. It's trying to tighten control because I'm anxious about yesterday."

A—Assemble: "My Overcontroller is here trying to protect me. My Lost Child is here feeling scared about food. My Wise Self is here too—I can hear all of you."

C—Choose: "What would my Wise Self do here? She'd recognise that skipping breakfast will just fuel the restriction cycle. She'd know my body needs morning fuel regardless of what happened yesterday."

E—Enact: Emma makes toast and sits down to eat it, even though her Overcontroller is protesting loudly. She places one hand on her heart: "I'm choosing you, Lost Child. I'm feeding you even though it's uncomfortable."

The urge to skip breakfast doesn't disappear, but Emma doesn't let it decide for her. Her Wise Self leads, and her Lost Child receives care instead of punishment.

Why This Works

SPACE interrupts the automatic hijack. Most ED behaviours happen when a mode takes over so completely that you lose access to your Wise Self. By the time you realise what's happening, you've already restricted, binged, or compensated.

This practice gives you a pattern interrupt—a way to catch the wave before it sweeps you away completely.

You won't always remember to use it. Sometimes modes will hijack you so fast that SPACE doesn't even occur to you until afterwards. That's normal.

But each time you do remember—each time you slow down enough to pinpoint the mode and choose your Wise Self—you're strengthening the neural pathway that makes it easier next time.

Practice This Week

Try using SPACE at least once when you notice a mode taking over. You don't need to do it perfectly—even pausing at "S" and taking three breaths is progress.

If you forget to use it in the moment, you can even practice it afterwards: "What mode was driving then? What would my Wise Self have done differently?" This retrospective practice still strengthens your awareness for next time.

Each time you practice, you're teaching your system: *My Wise Self can interrupt these patterns. I have more choices than I realised.*

Part 3: Beginning the Bond with Your Lost Child

How Your Wise Self Talks to Your Lost Child

Now that you understand how to protect your Lost Child from your Critic—setting boundaries on harmful messages whilst helping the Critic learn new methods—you can start building the relationship at the heart of recovery: the bond between your Wise Self and your Lost Child.

Your Wise Self offers something entirely different from your Critic: warm, present, curious, accepting attention. Not trying to fix or change—just being present with emotions.

The voice your Lost Child needs to hear is: warm and gentle in tone. Curious rather than judgemental. Accepting of whatever arises. Present, attentive and patient.

Think about how a wise, attuned caregiver sits with a frightened child. They might: Get down to the child's eye level. Soften their voice, speaking slowly and gently. Offer physical comfort—a hug, holding their hand and sitting close. Say things like: "I'm here with you. You're safe. It's okay to feel scared." Stay quiet and simply be present. Reflect back what they see: "You seem really frightened right now." Wait patiently, letting feelings move through at their own pace.

If you didn't experience this kind of care yourself, these examples might feel foreign. But you can learn this now. Think of a teacher, therapist, friend, or even a character from a film or book who embodied this quality of steady, warm presence. Borrow their approach until it becomes your own.

Beginning to Speak Differently

Every Lost Child needs to hear certain messages. Your Wise Self can begin offering these now:

> "You are no longer alone, [name]. I am with you." "Of course you feel [sad/scared/angry]. This makes sense." "You are good. There's nothing wrong with you." "I'm here, right by your side."

These simple messages—offered consistently by your Wise Self—begin to fill in what was missing. Your Lost Child has spent years believing she's alone, too much, fundamentally flawed, or undeserving. These new messages create a different neural pathway.

In Chapter 7, you'll learn the complete system of reparenting messages based on which emotional vitamins were missing, along with specific practices for how and when to deliver these messages during emotional work.

The "Sawu Bona" Practice: I See You

There's a beautiful greeting used by Indigenous tribes in Northern Natal, South Africa: "Sawu bona" literally translates as "I see you"—not just your physical presence, but your heart, your emotions, your essence.

This is what your Lost Child needs from you.

Practising "Sawu Bona"

When you sense her presence—through anxiety, sadness, or even unexpected joy:

Pause and acknowledge: "Hello, little one. I see you there."
Use your voice as comfort: Speak softly, warmly, without urgency.
Offer soothing touch: Place your hand on your heart, stroke your cheek, or wrap your arms around yourself.
Stay present: "I see your fear." "I see your loneliness." You're not trying to fix—just witnessing.
Let her know she matters: "Right now, you're important. Your feelings matter. You matter."

When your Lost Child receives these experiences from your Wise Self, she stops needing to use food and body behaviours to communicate her distress. She begins to trust that someone is finally here who sees her and won't abandon her—and won't use shame to motivate or control her.

Reflection Point: Try the Sawu Bona practice right now. What is your Lost Child feeling? What does she need you to know?

Closing: The Protection Is in Place

The Protected Ship

Your ship has changed. The guard is softening. The captain is strong. The child is beginning to trust that she can come up on deck.

The boundaries are set. The protection is in place—a new armour of self-connection is replacing the old patterns of self-denial. The reparenting has begun.

What Comes Next

Now that your Wise Self can protect your Lost Child from your Critic's harsh methods—setting boundaries on harmful messages whilst helping the Critic discover compassionate protection—and has begun offering the first messages she needed, you're ready for Chapter 7: learning to stay present with strong emotions as they arise, discovering that feeling doesn't destroy you, and developing the practices that deepen this healing bond.

You'll learn how to be with difficult emotions through the TREE practice, the complete system of reparenting messages your Lost Child needs to hear, how to deliver these messages in the moment when your Lost Child needs them most, and how to work with all your Protector Modes as they respond to this deeper work.

The work ahead requires the protection you've established in this chapter. Your Lost Child needs to know that your Wise Self is strong enough to redirect the Critic's harsh methods, consistent enough to keep showing up, and brave enough to stay present when big feelings arise.

That's exactly the leader you're becoming.

Gentle Experiments to Try

These practices help you establish the protection and connection that make deeper healing possible. Choose two or three that feel most accessible right now and try them out this week.

These aren't one-time exercises—they're skills you'll continue developing throughout your recovery journey. Taste each one. Notice which ones help you feel more grounded or connected. Return to them whenever they feel supportive.

1. **Embodying Strength**: Practice your power stance daily. Find what it feels like to be grounded, present, and strong. Even if you never use it in the negotiation exercise, this embodiment work strengthens your Wise Self's capacity to protect.
2. **Message Rejection**: When you hear your Critic speaking, pause and identify the harmful message underneath. Then practice rejecting it clearly: "That cultural lie about bodies—I reject it." "That impossible standard—I'm not following it anymore."
3. **Negotiation Practice**: Try the full Negotiation Practice at least once. Help your Critic understand that it can protect through care instead of shame. This might take many repetitions before it truly softens, so be patient with the process.
4. **Sawu Bona Daily**: Practice "I see you" with your Lost Child at least once each day. This might be the first thing in the morning, before bed, or whenever you sense her presence. Notice what happens when you offer this consistent acknowledgement.
5. **Critic Awareness**: Simply notice when your Critic appears. You don't need to immediately set boundaries or do anything about it—just practice seeing it clearly. "There's my Critic using shame. I hear it." This awareness alone begins to shift the dynamic.

Journalling Prompt Reflections: Protecting the Lost Child

- What specific message does your Critic use most often? Where did this message come from?
- When you imagine setting boundaries with your Critic, what feelings arise? Fear? Relief? Doubt?
- What would it mean to protect your Lost Child the way you'd protect someone you care about?

Remember: These practices are opportunities for consistent presence, showing your Lost Child repeatedly that you're learning to lead with both strength and care.

Some days you'll remember some practices; other days you'll forget completely. Both are fine. What matters is returning to these practices when you can, building trust through your steady—not perfect—presence.

Looking Ahead: The Journey Continues

The young part of you who has been waiting is beginning to sense that maybe—finally—someone is here who won't abandon her when things get difficult. Someone who sees her, values her, and is willing to protect her without shaming her into silence.

Someone who can hold steady when the Critic grows loud. Someone who can stay when feelings start to stir. This is your Wise Self—the compassionate authority you are becoming.

The protection is now in place. The boundaries are forming. The relationship has begun. And because your Lost Child is no longer facing the emotional world alone, something new now becomes possible.

You are ready to begin feeling what you once had to avoid.

That is the work of the next chapter.

Note

1 **Thích Nhất Hạnh** (2002). *Be free where you are.* Berkeley, California: Parallax Press.

7 Bringing Your Child on Deck

Working Safely with Strong Emotions

Come sit down beside me, I said to myself, And although it doesn't make sense, I held my own hand As a small sign of trust And together I sat on the fence.

—Michael Leunig[1]

Your Lost Child is learning that she is no longer alone with her feelings.

In the last chapter, your Wise Self began doing something different: standing between your Lost Child and the Critic, setting boundaries, and offering protection that doesn't rely on punishment.

Until now, many of your emotions have lived below deck—kept out of awareness by fear, control, or numbness. This is because, at one time, feeling them felt too dangerous or overwhelming.

This chapter is about what happens after protection begins. It is about learning how to stay present with feelings as they rise—without being overwhelmed, without escaping into old coping patterns, and without needing to shut yourself down to survive. This is not about forcing yourself to feel everything at once but about learning—gently and safely—that feeling itself is not what harms you. What heals is *who you feel with . . . having that emotion in the presence of someone—inside or outside you—who can stay, protect, and understand.*

Opening: Ready for Deeper Waters

Three months into her recovery work,

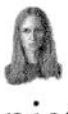 Emma finds herself in an unexpected moment. She's sitting with her therapist, describing a difficult week, when suddenly tears start flowing—not the controlled, "acceptable" tears she's allowed before but deep, chest-heaving sobs she can't stop.

Her first instinct is panic. Make it stop. This is too much. I'm being ridiculous. She can feel her Overcontroller scrambling to regain control, her Detached Protector trying to numb her again. But then, beneath all that protective noise, Emma senses her Wise Self—that captain presence she's been strengthening—stepping forward with a different message: "It's okay. Stay

DOI: 10.4324/9781003355878-8

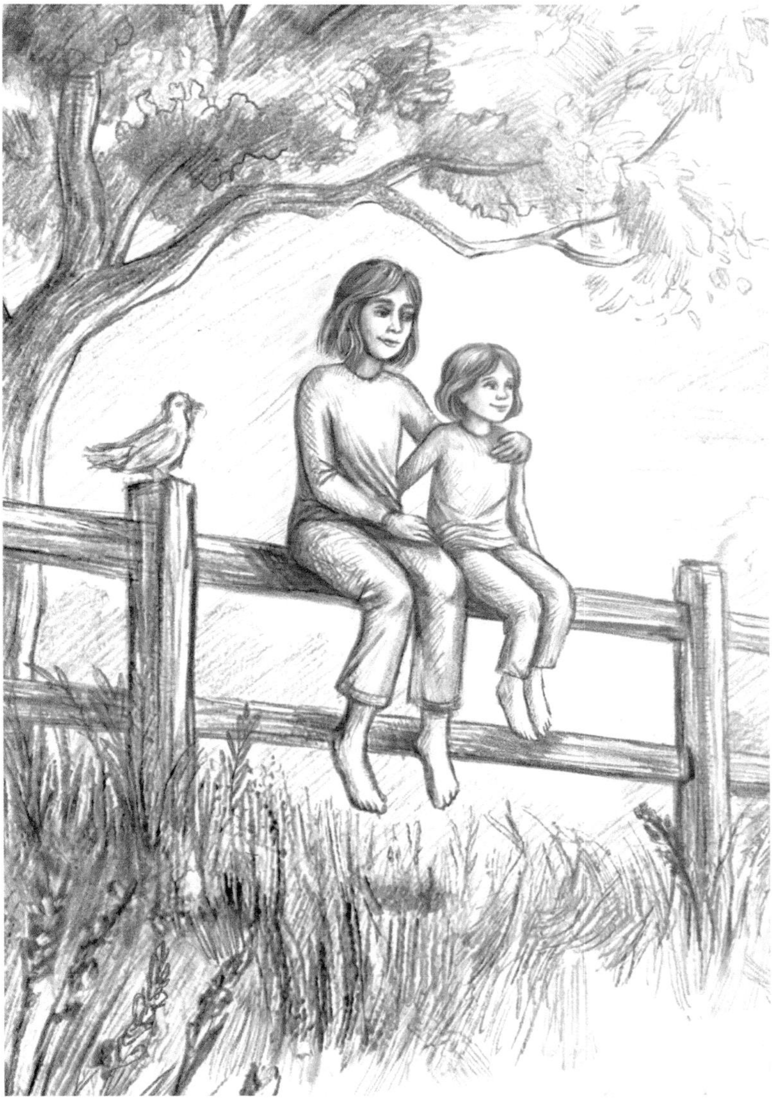

Figure 7.1 Sitting on the fence with our Inner Child

here. These are your Lost Child's tears. She's been holding this for a very long time. You can be with this. You're strong enough."

Emma doesn't stop crying. But she doesn't run either. For perhaps the first time in her adult life, she lets herself feel the full force of her sadness whilst someone—her Wise Self—and her therapist—stays present beside her Lost Child, holding space for what needs to be felt. This is Emma's deeper work beginning—and yours too.

Now you can bring your Lost Child up from below deck—gently, safely, with your Wise Self (the captain) providing steady guidance and the crew learning to support rather than suppress her. You've been preparing for this moment since you first stepped aboard your ship. You've learned to recognise the crew members on deck—those Protector parts that have worked tirelessly to keep you safe. You've re-membered your Wise Self and begun setting boundaries with your Inner Critic. You've offered your Lost Child the first "I see you" messages, beginning to build trust.

Now comes the work of learning to stay present with the strong emotions that arise as you deepen this healing. Recovery is about developing the capacity to be with difficult feelings—with your Wise Self present alongside your Lost Child so she doesn't have to face them alone.

In this chapter, we'll practice tools and internal resources to stay present with difficult feelings whilst keeping yourself emotionally and physically safe.

Part 1: Understanding What Your Lost Child Has Been Holding

The Protection Enables the Feeling

In Chapter 6, you established crucial protection for your Lost Child. You learned to set boundaries with your Inner Critic, helping it discover that protection doesn't require self-punishment. You began offering your Lost Child the reparenting messages she's needed all along—the emotional vitamins that were missing. That foundation, that safety, is what makes the work of this chapter possible.

Your Lost Child has probably been holding feelings for a long time—loneliness, shame, anger, grief, and fear. These emotions didn't disappear when your Protector Modes stepped in to manage them. They've been waiting, stored in your body, for the moment when it finally feels safe enough to be felt. That moment is now. With your Wise Self strengthened and your Inner Critic learning new methods, your Lost Child can begin to emerge, trusting that someone will stay present with her.

The Language Your Body Speaks

When you've been cut off from your emotional world, feelings don't simply disappear—they express themselves through your body in ways that might not immediately make sense.

You might describe feeling "full" when you're actually overwhelmed by sadness or anger. You might feel "empty" when you're longing for connection. You might feel "heavy" when you're carrying unprocessed emotions or "disgusting" when you're experiencing shame about your deepest vulnerabilities.

Your Lost Child lives in your body—her emotions and needs express themselves as bodily sensations. But your Protector Modes often create a smokescreen and reinterpret what your Lost Child is actually experiencing:

Table 7.1 The Language Your Body Speaks: How Feelings Become Eating Urges

Lost Child Feels	*Protector Mode Translates*	*Creates Seeming Solution*
Lonely and empty (feels endless, hopeless)	"I feel hungry and empty"	Eating to fill the void
Ashamed and unworthy	"I feel fat"	Restriction or weight loss
Overwhelmed by sadness	"I feel heavy"	Losing weight to lighten feeling
Guilty about needs	"I'm too much"	Restriction to become smaller
Angry but can't express	"I'm out of control"	Bingeing as rebellion, restriction as punishment

This translation might provide temporary relief—helping confusing or overwhelming emotions feel more manageable by 'hanging' them onto something concrete and controllable—but it prevents you from addressing what your Lost Child actually needs—connection, understanding, and acceptance.

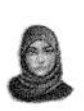 **Faye's Pattern**: Growing up in a family where emotions were handled awkwardly and comfort was offered through food rather than emotional attunement, Faye's Lost Child learned that her loneliness and longing for connection were too much for others. Now, when these feelings arise, her Detached Self-Soother immediately translates them into "I need to eat."

The bingeing provides temporary relief from the emotional emptiness but can never fill the void her Lost Child is experiencing—the need to be truly seen and understood. After each binge, her Overcontroller steps in with harsh rules and renewed restriction, keeping her Lost Child's real needs hidden and unmet.

For many people, this pattern follows a familiar chain: a sensation appears, an emotion stirs underneath it, an old schema-mindset adds meaning ("this is bad," "I'm too much"), and a Protector responds with an eating behaviour. As your Wise Self slows this sequence down, new meanings—and new options—begin to emerge.

As you reconnect with your body, you'll learn to distinguish physical sensations from emotional ones. This distinction becomes clearer after you've established regular eating (see Chapter 8)—but for now, if you're uncertain whether a sensation is physical or emotional, it's okay to both eat AND attend to emotional needs.

Mini Practice: Emotion Check-In (30 Seconds)

- *What am I feeling right now?*
- *Where do I notice this in my body?*
- *What does this feeling seem to be predicting might happen?*
- *Is there anything else that might also be possible here?*

Even pausing long enough to ask these questions helps your brain revise old schema predictions and widen the space around your emotional experience.

What Thawing Out Actually Means

If you've been emotionally numb for a long time, the prospect of feeling again can be both appealing and frightening. Numbness has been protection. It kept you safe from overwhelming emotions when you didn't have other ways to cope. Thawing out means creating conditions where feeling can happen gradually, gently, with your Wise Self present to provide the care your Lost Child has always needed.

An important note: Sometimes, as you begin reconnecting with your emotions, things might feel more intense than they did when you were numb. You're simply feeling what was already there, what your body has been holding for you until you were ready. If emotions feel overwhelming during this process, having a therapist by your side becomes invaluable. You don't have to feel everything alone.

Thawing out happens in stages. Some days might bring gentle awareness—small patches where you notice a feeling you hadn't been in touch with before. Other times, you might experience a rush of emotion that seems to come from nowhere. Bodies that have been holding emotions for a long time need to release that energy when they finally feel safe enough. The key is learning to be with these movements rather than immediately reaching for your Protector Modes to freeze them again.

About anxiety and excitement: Psychologists (24) have found that anxiety and excitement run on the same body fuel—quicker heart rate, faster breathing, butterflies. What diverges is how we interpret them: anxiety reads those sensations as threat, while excitement reads them as opportunity. Research shows that even a small label shift—"this is my body gearing up; to help me face . . ."—can help channel the same arousal toward engaging rather than withdrawal.

Reflection Point: Consider your own relationship with numbness. What emotions feel most frozen or inaccessible to you? What do your Protector parts tell you would happen if you allowed yourself to feel more fully? Can you identify which specific Protector Mode is most invested in keeping you numb?

Now that you understand what your Lost Child has been holding and why feelings once felt unbearable, you're ready to learn how your Wise Self guides her through the actual experience of feeling.

Part 2: Learning to Stay with Feelings

Why Feelings Feel Overwhelming: The Missing Ingredient

There's something important to understand about why emotions have felt so overwhelming: it's not because the feelings themselves were too much. It's because you had to feel them alone.

When you were young and experiencing difficult emotions—sadness, loneliness, anger, fear—you needed someone to be emotionally present with you. Not to fix the feeling or make it go away but simply to stay beside you whilst you felt it. To help you understand what you were experiencing. To show you, through their steady presence, that feelings can be felt and survived.

This is what we call *emotional presence*—the capacity to stay grounded and connected whilst someone else experiences difficult emotions. It's different from physical presence or practical care. Someone can be wonderful supportive practically—feeding you, clothing you, keeping you safe—but if they're not emotionally present for themselves, they can't be fully emotionally present for you.

If you consider that some of the adults around you could have been stuck in their own Protector Modes—numbing their feelings, staying busy to avoid emotions, acting as if everything was fine when it wasn't—they simply wouldn't have had the capacity to sit with your feelings. Not because they were bad people or didn't love you. If they didn't have access to their own emotional world, so they probably struggled to help you navigate yours.

This isn't about blame. Emotional inhibition is common across many cultures, with many of us inheriting patterns of emotional disconnection—generations of people doing their absolute best whilst cut off from their own emotional lives.

But what happens when you have to feel big emotions alone as a child is that they become overwhelming. Without someone helping you contain and make sense of the feelings, they feel like they might destroy you. So your Protector Modes stepped in to help you survive by not feeling.

Now, as an adult, you can learn to provide what was missing. From this grounded position, you can offer the emotional presence your Lost Child needed but didn't receive. This is what makes feelings bearable—the presence of someone (you) who can stay grounded whilst they move through.

Understanding How Emotions Actually Work

Before learning how to stay with your Lost Child's feelings, it helps to understand what emotions actually do inside your body. This understanding makes it easier to stop fearing feelings that your Protectors learned to shut down.

Emotions Are Visitors, Not Who You Are

In Irish (Gaeilge), most emotions aren't expressed as something you *are*, but rather as something that comes upon you, stays for a while and then lifts. Where English says, "I am sad," Irish says, "Tá brón orm"—"sadness is on me." You contain the feeling but it does not define you.

This is exactly what your Wise Self is learning: emotions move through, but they aren't your identity.

See the Lighthouse image in Figure 7.2: emotions have an important function—they signal which emotional vitamins are missing (or met).

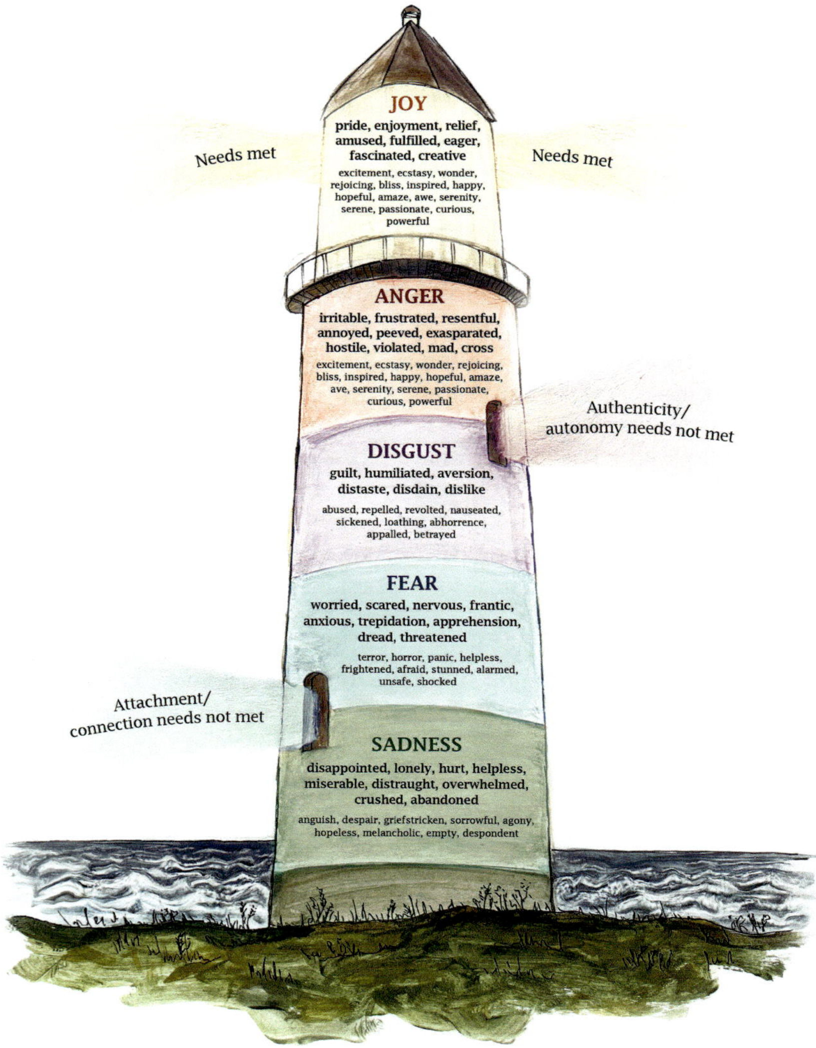

Figure 7.2 Lighthouse image with coloured segments

How Emotional Waves Move through the Body

Neuroanatomist Jill Bolte Taylor observed that, when an emotion is first triggered, the first physiological surge often peaks and begins to settle within about 90 seconds (25). During this window, sensations such as heart rate, heat, or constriction tend to rise and then begin to settle. This doesn't mean the emotion is "gone" after 90 seconds—feelings like grief or shame can continue to arise in waves—but the body's first physiological surge is usually brief.

Your Protectors never learned this. When sadness or anger appears, they assume, "This will swallow us whole—make it stop now." Your Wise Self is now learning: "This is a wave in my nervous system. I can stay with my Lost Child until it softens."

What Prolongs Feelings (and What Helps Them Settle)

Emotions linger when we:

- Fight them—resisting creates more tension
- Feed them—turning one feeling into a whole story ("I'm always like this," "Nothing ever works")

They settle more naturally when we:

- **Let them be felt** without adding narrative or judgement
- **Stay grounded** while they move through

Many mindfulness teachers describe the mind as a big blue sky with emotions moving through it like the weather. The metaphor captures a concept supported by research: emotional states naturally rise, shift, and settle when they aren't actively suppressed or fuelled by rumination (26).

In this image, some emotions pass quickly, like light clouds. Others—especially those connected to loss, shame, or attachment wounds—feel more like slow-moving weather systems.

The point is not to force the "weather" to clear but to recognise that emotional activation follows a natural arc. When you don't push feelings away or over-engage with them, the nervous system typically finds its own way back toward baseline.

Each time you stay with a feeling for a few seconds longer than your Protector Modes expect, you gently expand your capacity to tolerate uncertainty—instead of rushing back to old, familiar predictions about what the feeling "means."

Why Emotions Once Felt Unbearable

As children we depend on caregivers for co-regulation—their nervous system helps to steady ours. If those around us lacked the capacity to be *emotionally present and attuned*, our inner world still felt unshared. Without attunement, emotions had no container: they felt too big, too intense, or too confusing to manage alone. Your Protectors stepped in to block or reinterpret these feelings, and the eating disorder became a substitute container—a way to organise or numb emotions that had nowhere safe to land. The problem was never the emotions themselves; it was having to face them *without emotional presence beside you.*

Now you are learning to offer the steadiness and attunement that were missing, so you no longer need the eating disorder to hold or silence your feelings.

A Reflection

Which emotions feel most "too much" for you?
Where do you sense them in your body?
And which Protector jumps in first when they appear?

Your Wise Self doesn't need you to feel everything at once—only to notice the next small wave and stay beside your Lost Child as it rises and falls.

The Practice of Sitting on the Fence Together

Recovery is about your Wise Self learning to sit beside your Lost Child whilst feelings move through. Michael Leunig captures this: "Come sit down beside me, I said to myself." Imagine yourself sitting on a fence—not fully immersed in the feeling, but beside it, observing it, staying present with the part of you who's experiencing it. This is the practice of separation and connection working together:

Your Lost Child feels the emotion fully in her body.

Your Wise Self sits beside her on the fence, close enough to feel some of what she's feeling, but separate enough to stay grounded and not be overwhelmed.

From this position on the fence, your Wise Self can offer what the Lost Child needs: "I see you're feeling very sad right now. I'm here with you. You're not alone with this anymore. This sadness makes sense—it's telling us something important about what you need. I can handle this feeling. The initial intensity will naturally begin to ease if we stay present without fighting it or feeding it with rumination. Some feelings pass quickly; others, like grief, may come in waves over time. I can be with whatever comes, for as long as it needs to be felt. I won't shut you down or fall apart or judge you. And I promise I'll check in with you more often, so feelings don't have to build until they become unbearable before I notice them."

Physicalise Your Wise Self

When practising this, it helps to physically embody your Wise Self rather than collapsing into the overwhelmed feeling. Adjust your posture: sit up slightly straighter, drop your shoulders, place both feet flat on the ground, put one hand on your heart, and take three slow breaths.

This physical shift helps you access the part of you that can stay steady whilst emotions move through. You're not the overwhelmed child anymore—you're the Wise Adult who can hold space for her.

From this grounded posture, you can observe: "My Lost Child is feeling very frightened right now. Part of me wants to join her in that fear, but I'm choosing to stay in my Wise Self position. From here, I can help her."

The TREES Practice: A Daily Check-In with Your Vulnerable Child

You can use TREES as a brief, repeatable way of attuning to your Lost Child—especially when feelings are stirred up. It works best if you practise it regularly, not just in crises.

T—Tune In

Gently bring attention into your body. Notice where you feel something: tightness in your chest, fluttering in your stomach, a lump in your throat, or a vague "knot of not-okay." You don't need the perfect emotion word—it's enough to notice: "pressure in my chest," "tight shoulders," "something sad is here." This is your Wise Self turning towards your inner weather rather than ignoring it.

R—Receive

Let whatever you've noticed be there, just as it is. You might simply say: "I'm here. I see you. You're not alone with this." Receiving is the opposite of pushing away—its making space for the feelings to visit. It tells your Lost Child: "You're allowed to feel what you feel, and I'll stay."

E—Explore

With curiosity, ask:

> "What are you most afraid of?"
> "What are you needing from me right now?"

Answers may come as images, words, or just a felt sense. You're not interrogating—just listening. You also don't need the full story yet.

E—Enrich (with Emotional Vitamins)

Now imagine offering the emotional vitamins that were missing in the past: safety, comfort, protection, validation, and belonging.

Ask: "What would a caring adult say or do for this part?"
You might offer words like: "You're not too much. Your feelings make sense. I'm not going to abandon you. You deserve care and rest." If words feel hard, a hand on your heart or cheek can be enough to let your Lost Child know: "I'm here with you."

S—Soak in Presence

Pause for a few breaths and let your system *soak* in the sense of "someone is with me in this." You may notice small shifts—a softening, a drop in tension, or simply feeling less alone. Even if nothing seems to change, the practice still counts—you're teaching your system that feelings can be met with presence rather than certainty or immediate action.

Example—Tony's TREES practice

 Tony notices a rise in anxiety before a social event where he'll see his ex-partner. His Overcontroller urges him to skip the event and spend the day at the gym "to stay in control."

Tune In: Tony pauses and brings his attention into his body. He notices a sinking feeling in his stomach—his Lost Child feels exposed and afraid of being rejected again.

Receive: He lets the feeling be there and says quietly inside, "I'm here. I see you. You're not alone." The sensations soften slightly as his system registers his presence.

Explore: He gently asks, "What are you most afraid of?" The answer emerges as a felt-sense of squeezing-twisting sensation in his chest—a feeling of dread—with the words: "If I see her, I'll feel unlovable again."

Enrich: Tony places a hand on his heart and offers emotional vitamin messages: "You are worthy whether she notices you or not. You belong. I won't abandon you—I'll stay with you."

Soak in Presence: He takes a slow breath and rests for a few moments in that sense of connection. His Overcontroller relaxes—there's a Wise Self on deck, so extreme control isn't needed.

Tony goes to the event. The anxiety visits throughout the evening—some waves are brief, others last longer. He checks in with his Lost Child regularly, and whilst the evening isn't easy, he's not alone with his feelings anymore.

Part of what makes TREES so powerful is that it teaches your system that you don't have to rush to certainty. You can stay with a feeling—even when you don't yet fully understand it—and allow its meaning to emerge with your Wise Self beside you.

How TREES Helps Protector Modes Relax

The TREES practice changes the relationship between your Wise Self and Lost Child in ways that help your Protector Modes trust that eating behaviours aren't their only option.

When your Protector Modes see your Wise Self consistently turning toward difficulty, recognising what's needed, embracing your Lost Child with compassion, and providing real emotional nourishment—they gather evidence that you're building genuine capacity to handle what they've been managing through food and body control.

Your Overcontroller Notices: "She stayed present with uncertainty instead of restricting. The anxiety came and went but didn't floor her. She didn't make it worse by fighting it or catastrophising."

Your Detached Protector Observes: "She felt sadness without numbing through bingeing. The sadness moved through and lifted—she created internal space where feelings could be contained safely."

Your People Pleaser Sees: "She acknowledged her own needs instead of just keeping others happy. Connection deepened when she was authentic."

Your Wise Self demonstrates, again and again, that there's a new way forward. You're building the capacity to provide emotional presence and containment for yourself—the ingredients that were missing all along.

Over time, your Protector Modes learn that feelings don't need to be shut down or controlled the moment they appear. Your system discovers that a little "not-knowing yet" can be safe when your Wise Self is present.

How Your Wise Self Learns to Be With Feelings

Over time, your Wise Self develops four core emotional skills:

1. **Noticing**: recognising what you're feeling
2. **Staying With**: remaining present long enough for safety to register
3. **Understanding**: sensing what the feeling is protecting or needing
4. **Responding**: offering care so your Protector Modes don't have to take over

This is the "sitting on the fence" with your Child Modes—a capacity that grows through repeated moments of safe emotional contact.

Building Your TREES Practice

TREES gives you a complete process for being with emotions. The four steps—Tune In—Receive—Explore—Enrich—Soak—are skills you'll develop gradually.

You might start with very brief moments of turning toward feelings for just 30 seconds before your Protector Modes pull you away. That's progress.

Over weeks, you'll find your capacity to identify what your Lost Child actually needs (Explore) will deepen and to stay present with uncertainty for longer.

Each practice—however imperfect—strengthens your capacity to stay present and your Lost Child's trust that someone will finally be with them.

See Appendix 13 for detailed exercises strengthening each TREES skill.

Part 3: Reparenting Your Lost Child

In Chapter 6, you began building the bond between your Wise Self and Lost Child. Now you'll learn what messages your Lost Child needs to hear—messages that directly supply the emotional vitamins we explored in Chapters 1 and 2.

Universal Messages All Children Need

Every Lost Child needs to hear certain foundational messages repeatedly:

> "You are no longer alone, [name]. I am with you."
> "Of course you feel [sad/scared/angry]. This makes sense."
> "You are good. There's nothing wrong with you."
> "I love you. I'm here, right by your side."
> "Your existence matters. You matter simply because you exist."
> "I'm learning how to care for you, and I won't give up on you."

Messages by Emotional Vitamin

Beyond these universal messages, your Lost Child needs specific reassurance based on which emotional vitamins were scarce:

For Safety and Stability: "You're safe now. I will keep you safe." "I will never abandon you."
For Connection and Belonging*:* "You belong with me." "You are enough. You don't need to earn my care."
For Play and Spontaneity*:* "You are allowed to rest, to play, to have fun." "You don't have to earn the right to enjoy yourself."
For Autonomy and Mastery*:* "It's okay to make mistakes." "I'm proud of you for trying, regardless of the outcome."
For Freedom to Express*:* "I want to hear how you feel—all the messy, uncomfortable feelings." "Your emotions won't overwhelm me. I can handle them."
For Healthy Limits and Boundaries*:* "You are allowed to set boundaries and say no." "Your needs are as important as everyone else's needs."

For an extensive list of reparenting messages linked to emotional vitamins, see Appendix 12.

Quick Reference: When to Use Which Messages

When Eating Disorder Urges Arise: "These urges are trying to protect you from difficult feelings. What does my Lost Child actually need right now?"
After Difficult Interactions: Safety messages if threatened, connection messages if rejected, expression messages if you suppressed yourself, boundary messages if someone overstepped.
During Body Image Struggles: "What you're feeling isn't really about your body. What emotion might be underneath?" Connection messages work well here.
When Perfectionism Drives You: Autonomy and play messages.
When You Feel Like a Burden: Connection and expression messages.

When Your Protector Modes React to Reparenting Work

As you begin offering compassionate reparenting messages to your Lost Child, some Protector Modes may react with fear or even aggression. Your Inner Critic might attack more fiercely. Your Invincible Overcontroller might show disdain for "weakness." Your Detached Protector might intensify its numbing. This is to be expected—these parts are terrified that allowing vulnerability will lead straight back to those frozen moments of unbearable rejection you explored in the Rejected Inner Child Exercise.

Remember the Mode Interview practice from Chapter 4? The same principle applies here. When a mode reacts strongly, pause and talk to the Protector about its fear:

> I know you're scared. That's why you're attacking/numbing/showing disdain. It would have been dangerous to feel this in the past. But I'm here with my Lost Child now. I'm sitting on the fence beside her. I can hold her feelings. She's safe with me in ways she wasn't safe then. You don't have to work so hard anymore—you don't have to do this alone.

Your Protector Modes need to SEE your Wise Self succeeding before they'll trust enough to relax. Each time you stay present through difficulty, offer compassion, and your Lost Child settles—you're building evidence that a different way is possible.

Building Emotional Presence through Practice

Learning to offer emotional presence and containment to your Lost Child is a skill that develops over time. You might start with very brief moments:

- **Week 1**: Sitting on the fence whilst noticing a feeling, observing its natural rhythm
- **Week 2**: Staying present through several waves of emotion throughout a day
- **Week 3**: Offering one reparenting message whilst feeling is present
- **Week 4**: Using the full TREES practice with emotions that feel manageable

You're gradually building your capacity to stay grounded whilst emotions move through and to create an internal space where feelings can be safely held. Each time you practice, you're strengthening the neural pathways that allow you to be emotionally present.

You can also build this capacity through contemplative practices: mindfulness meditation, active meditations (yoga, tai chi, walking in nature), dialogues with your inner parts (writing conversations between Wise Self and Lost Child), therapy (experiencing someone else's emotional presence whilst you feel), and physicalisation practice (see Appendix 9).

All of these strengthen your Wise Self—the part of you that is courageous enough to face difficulty head-on, even when Protector parts want to avoid.

They help you internalise the capacity to contain your emotional self that was missing in childhood.

The more you practice sitting on the fence beside your Lost Child, the more natural it becomes. Eventually, emotional presence and containment aren't something you have to think about—they're simply how you relate to your internal world.

Before learning the specific methods for delivering reparenting messages, it helps to meet the version of yourself who needs them most—the Rejected Inner Child your Protector Modes have worked so hard to keep hidden.

Meeting Your Rejected Inner Child

In Chapter 6, you learned about your Rejected Inner Child—the version of yourself frozen at a moment when rejection or shame became unbearable. Your Protector Modes have worked hard to distance you from this child, believing that keeping her hidden keeps you safe. This exercise helps you meet her directly, with your Wise Self present to offer what was missing.

Safety Note: If this exercise feels too difficult at this stage, or if you have experienced trauma, consider a shorter version—spend just 5 minutes at first and build up from there. Alternatively, do this exercise with a therapist present.

The Practice

Close your eyes and let your mind drift towards an image of a past version of yourself—the version you most fear becoming if you stopped trying to control your body and started eating intuitively. This might be a child or teenage version of yourself that you've worked hard to leave behind.

What does this past self look like? How old are they? What about this version triggers the most fear or shame? What were they feeling about themselves? Is your Inner Critic active when you look at this younger self, and if so, what accusations is it making?

Reflection Moment

As you consider this younger version, pause and ask: What was actually happening in their life at that time? Were they feeling lonely, hurt, unsafe, trapped, rejected, or overwhelmed? When you think about the emotional vitamins from Chapter 2, which ones were missing? What did this young person really need that they weren't receiving?

Now, from your present adult perspective, look at this younger version with curiosity. Take a look back at the Life Story Timeline exercise from Chapter 2 to help you understand this younger version with compassion—how did she make sense of the struggles she was going through?

What Might Start to Become Clear

The version of yourself you've been trying to escape wasn't the problem. She was a vulnerable young person doing her best to survive without the emotional vitamins she needed. Your eating patterns may have been about trying to prove you're different from her, trying to control what felt uncontrollable then.

Your Wise Self can now recognise that young person—your Rejected Inner Child—is still inside you, still holding those same feelings. You might notice the feelings linked to this part arising when you *don't* engage in your eating behaviours. Your Protector Modes have been working tirelessly to keep her hidden, believing that if she emerges, you'll become that "rejected child" again.

See Appendix 11 for the full Rejected Inner Child Transformation visualisation.

How to Deliver Reparenting Messages

We have begun to explore the messages your Lost Child needs to hear. Now you'll learn how to offer these messages in the moment—when emotions are active, when urges arise, when your Lost Child is struggling.

Different delivery methods work for different people. The key is finding what helps your Lost Child feel most genuinely seen and cared for.

Five Approaches to Explore

1. **Speaking Out Loud**: Say the messages aloud, even when alone. Your Lost Child hears the care in your actual voice, and your nervous system responds to the soothing tone.
2. **Internal Silent Messages**: Think the messages directly to your Lost Child. Pair this with physical gestures (hand on heart, gentle self-touch) to create embodiment. Works well anywhere, including public settings.
3. **Writing to Your Lost Child**: Keep a journal where your Wise Self writes letters to your Lost Child. This creates a tangible record she can return to. Try writing with your dominant hand as Wise Self, then letting Lost Child respond with your non-dominant hand.
4. **Visualisation**: Close your eyes and picture your Lost Child (perhaps at a specific age). Imagine your Wise Self approaching her, sitting beside her, offering comfort. Notice what her body language shows about whether she's receiving the care.
5. **Recording Yourself**: For messages your Lost Child needs repeatedly, record yourself speaking to her in a warm, caring tone. Play during difficult moments, before sleep, or when eating disorder urges are strong.

Your Practice This Week

Choose ONE method to experiment with. Use it to deliver one reparenting message your Lost Child needs most right now.

Try this method several times over a week. Notice: Does your Lost Child seem to receive it? Does anything shift in your body? Does it feel genuine or performative?

If it doesn't resonate, try a different method next week. You're tasting what creates real connection, not trying to get it "right."

For more detailed instructions, see Appendix 12.

Building Consistency: Your Lost Child has learned not to trust words alone—she needs to experience your Wise Self showing up repeatedly, staying present through difficult emotions, and following through on these promises.

Start Small and Be Consistent: Choose one message your Lost Child needs most right now. Decide which delivery method you'll try first. Offer this message once daily for a week, using your chosen method. Notice what happens—does your Lost Child seem to hear it? Does anything shift in your body?

Over time, as you prove that you won't abandon her when things get hard, she'll begin to emerge more readily, trusting that it's finally safe to let someone see and care for her.

Matching Messages to Your Lost Child's Current Needs

When applying reparenting in the moment, match the message to what your Lost Child is experiencing right now:

When she feels alone or abandoned, offer safety and connection messages: "You are no longer alone. I am with you. I will never abandon you."

When she feels shame or defectiveness, offer acceptance messages: "You are good. There's nothing wrong with you. You are lovable exactly as you are."

When she feels she must earn care, offer belonging messages: "You are enough. You don't need to earn my care. You belong with me."

When she fears her emotions are too much, offer expression messages: "I want to hear how you feel—all the messy, uncomfortable feelings. Your feelings aren't shameful."

When she needs permission to rest or play, offer spontaneity messages: "You are allowed to rest, to play, to have fun. You don't have to be productive every moment."

Refer to Appendix 12 for marching reparenting messages to missing emotional vitamins.

Choose one or two reparenting messages to begin with—you can always return for more as your practice develops.

Part 4: Reclaiming Your Feisty Child

Understanding Anger as Your Emotional Immune System

Remember from Chapter 3: your Feisty Child is your emotional immune system. She signals when boundaries are crossed, when you're treated unfairly, when something isn't right.

For many people with eating difficulties, this part has been suppressed for years. Anger felt too dangerous—too out of control, too likely to drive others away. Better to turn it inward through eating behaviours than risk expressing it outward.

Anger isn't the enemy. It's information that tells you when someone has overstepped, when you're being treated unfairly, when a situation doesn't align with your values, and when you need to protect yourself.

Samantha's Anger Journey

Growing up with a family that valued stoicism,

 Samantha learned that anger was unacceptable. Whenever she showed distress, her father would shrug: "It's character building!"—as if pain was just a life lesson in disguise. Her mother suggested running to push difficult feelings away.

Her binge–restrict cycles became her way of turning anger inward—punishing her body instead of expressing fury at Gary's emotional unavailability, at her family's dismissal of her feelings, at a world that demanded she be perpetually cheerful.

When she finally started expressing anger—even just talking about it in therapy—she realised it wasn't the monster she'd imagined. It was information about her boundaries, about what she needed, and about what wasn't okay.

Learning to welcome her Feisty Child meant: noticing when anger arose (jaw clenching, chest tightening, heat rising), asking what the anger was protecting, translating anger into boundary-setting rather than self-attack, and expressing anger appropriately rather than suppressing it.

Samantha practised welcoming this anger concretely. She journalled the uncensored rage she'd suppressed for years: "I'm furious that I've turned this against myself because expressing it felt too dangerous."

She practised physical release—pushing against a wall with bent arms, vigorous dancing—letting the energy move through her body rather than staying trapped. Gradually, by allowing herself to really feel it in her body, the anger softened into grief—sadness for the child whose emotions were dismissed, for years believing she was too much. As her Feisty Child spoke directly rather than through eating behaviours, the desperate rebellion against herself began to ease.

The Underground Anger That Drives Eating Patterns

When anger can't be expressed directly, it often goes underground—emerging through passive-aggressive behaviour, self-directed punishment (restriction as "cutting off your nose to spite your face," bingeing as rebellion, body hatred as displaced anger, self-harm through eating disorder behaviours), and the restrict–binge cycle itself.

The restrict–binge cycle often expresses anger:

- **Restriction**: "You can't control me. I'll control myself first."
- **Bingeing**: "I'll do what I want. You can't stop me."

Both target yourself rather than the actual source of anger—because that feels safer.

Learning to Express Anger Appropriately

Your Wise Self can help your Feisty Child express anger in ways that protect boundaries without destroying relationships.

The Anger Translation Process

1. **Notice the Anger Signal**: Body sensations (tension, heat, clenching), emotional tone (irritation to rage), behavioural urges (wanting to withdraw, attack, or restrict)
2. **Get Curious about the Message**: What boundary was crossed? What value or need is being violated? What is your Feisty Child trying to protect?
3. **Validate the Anger**: "This makes sense. Someone did overstep." "Of course you're angry. That wasn't fair." "Your anger is giving me important information."
4. **Translate It into Boundary-Setting**:
    - Instead of "I'm going to skip dinner because I'm angry at Gary," try: "I'm feeling hurt that you haven't called in three days. I need more consistent contact in this relationship."
    - Instead of "I'll restrict to punish myself for being angry at my mother," try: "I'm feeling frustrated that you hear me out when I talked about my feelings. I need you to listen without immediately trying to fix things."
5. **Express It Appropriately**: Use "I" statements ("I feel angry when . . ."), be specific about the behaviour not character, state what you need ("I need . . ." or "I would like . . ."), and set consequences if necessary ("If this continues, I will . . .")

Reflection Point: Where might underground anger be driving your eating behaviours? What old angers have never been expressed? What current situations make you angry but you suppress it? What would it feel like to welcome your Feisty Child as valuable information rather than something shameful?

The work ahead is about your Wise Self finally offering that younger version what she actually needed then and still needs now: to be seen with compassion, to have her feelings acknowledged, to receive the care that was missing.

Part 5: Teaching Lost Child It's Safe to Receive

Why Receiving Feels Dangerous

For many people with eating difficulties, receiving is one of the most challenging practices imaginable. You may have learned that you need to earn everything—food, rest, care, and even breath. You may have been taught that receiving makes you greedy, selfish, a burden, or weak. Receiving can feel frightening because it asks your nervous system to trust an experience your old schemas never predicted could be safe.

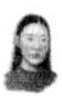 Melissa understands this struggle. Growing up with family members who sacrificed everything whilst never treating themselves, she absorbed the message that receiving care meant depleting others' happiness. "Every time I take something from them, I'm taking away from their limited supply," her Lost Child learned. Now, even offering herself basic kindness feels like theft. Her Overcontroller insists: "You don't deserve care when they went without. The only way to be worthy is to need nothing."

But your Lost Child knows better. She longs to receive without earning, to be cared for simply because you exist, to take up space without apology.

Your Wise Self Explaining: "Things Are Different Now"

Your Protector Modes developed their beliefs about receiving during childhood, when taking care from others might genuinely have come with strings attached—obligation, guilt, and pressure to perform or comply. Your Overcontroller learned that needing less made you safer, less burdensome, more in control.

Your Wise Self can help your Protector Modes understand:

> Things are different now. I'm an adult with resources I didn't have as a child. I can provide for my Lost Child without depleting anyone else. Receiving care from myself isn't taking from others—it's finally giving to the part of me who needed it all along.

How Wise Self Reassures Protector Modes

To your Overcontroller: "I understand you learned that deprivation equals safety and worth. But look what's happened—the restriction triggers binges, the control creates rebellion. I'm learning to provide structure through care rather than punishment."

To your People Pleaser: "I know you're worried that if we focus on our own needs, we'll lose everyone. But people who can only handle us when we're convenient aren't offering the kind of relationship my Lost Child needs anyway. Real connection happens when we're genuine."

How Wise Self Teaches the Lost Child about Receiving

"The care I'm offering you now doesn't come with strings. You don't have to earn it, repay it, or prove you're worthy. This is what you needed all along—someone who provides simply because you exist and you matter."

"When you receive from me—rest, nourishment, comfort, play—you're not depleting anyone. You're finally filling the spaces that have been empty for too long."

Noticing Your Overcontroller's Deprivation Patterns

Your Overcontroller likely learned to create safety through deprivation—convincing you that needing less made you safer, more worthy, more in control. This deprivation may have extended far beyond food.

Take a few moments to consider: In what ways has your Overcontroller taught you to deprive yourself? Make a list of all the forms of nourishment—bodily and spiritual—that your Overcontroller restricts or rations.

You might notice:

- **Physical Deprivation**: Food, water, sleep, warmth, comfort, healthcare. Shallow breathing, uncomfortable positions, avoiding pleasant sensations.
- **Time and Space**: Never allowing breaks, staying constantly busy, avoiding time alone with yourself or in nature.
- **Relational and Emotional Nourishment**: Connection with others, asking for what you need, expressing feelings, receiving care from others.
- **Movement and Expression**: Restricting yourself to punishing exercise rather than joyful movement, blocking creative expression, play, or spontaneity.

As you create your list, notice which deprivations feel most familiar. Which ones does your Overcontroller insist are necessary for your safety or worthiness?

Self-deprivation may have provided some protection from being obligated, controlled, or guilt-induced, but it usually backfires. Your Lost Child feels even more lonely and cut off, perpetuating the illusion that trusting your feelings leads to spiralling out of control. Your Feisty or Impulsive Child might rebel, driving binge eating or other ways of expressing frustration.

Beginning to Receive in Small Ways

Learning to receive starts with the tiniest moments of allowing nourishment without earning it first—so small that your Inner Critic and fearful Protector Modes barely notice before it's done.

We're talking about micro-moments: a single full breath, five seconds of sunlight on your skin, one sip of water when you're thirsty.

Choose just one small thing from your deprivation list. You might:

- Notice the warmth of sunlight on your skin without immediately moving away
- Take a full breath without cutting it short
- Sit down for five minutes without doing anything "productive"
- Drink a full glass of water when you notice thirst
- Turn up the heating when you're cold

Practice that one thing for several days. Notice: what does this taste of receiving feel like? Does it create more safety or more anxiety?

Working with Protector Modes' Resistance

As you experiment with receiving, notice what your Critic or Overcontroller says ("You don't deserve this," "This is wasteful"). Notice what sensations arise in your body—guilt, anxiety, warmth, relaxation.

Your Wise Self can respond: "Overcontroller, I understand you're worried. But my Lost Child needs this. Watch what happens when I allow her to receive—she doesn't spiral out of control. She settles. She feels cared for."

Staying with Good Feelings Even Briefly

One of the most challenging aspects of receiving is tolerating positive experiences. Your system may be so accustomed to deprivation and struggle that pleasure feels foreign or dangerous.

Clinical psychologist Dr. Joan Farrell describes this as like walking on ice your whole life and then putting your feet in a warm bath—the initial warmth can feel overwhelming or even painful before it begins to feel soothing.

Can you stay present with the good feeling anyway, even just for a moment? Can your Wise Self help your Lost Child notice: "This warmth feels good. This rest feels nourishing. This play feels joyful"?

Reflection Point: Which form of deprivation on your list feels most deeply ingrained? What does your Overcontroller tell you would happen if you allowed yourself to receive this form of nourishment? Can you experiment with receiving it just once this week, and notice what happens?

Making Receiving Visible: The Emotional Vitamins Jar

To help make your receiving practice tangible and visible, you might try the Emotional Vitamins Barrel Practice detailed in Appendix 14. This simple practice helps your Lost Child see evidence that she's receiving care—transforming an abstract concept into something concrete she can witness accumulating over time.

Beyond these internal practices, your body itself can become a partner in healing. Movement—offers another pathway for your Wise Self and Lost Child to connect.

Part 6: Movement as Integration

Safe Movement as Body–Wise Self–Lost Child Integration

Safe movement offers a unique pathway for integrating the relationship between your Wise Self, your body, and your Lost Child. This isn't about exercise as punishment or calorie-burning—but about movement as a way of being with yourself and your emotions in your body.

Movement as Medicine: The Science of Hope Molecules

Neuroscientist Kelly McGonigal (27) describes how, when you move, your muscles release chemicals called myokines into your bloodstream. Some head straight to your brain, acting like anti-anxiety medication—suppressing fear and worry whilst increasing motivation. In the long term, regular exposure changes your brain's structure, making you more resilient to stress.

Researchers call them "hope molecules" because studies show exercise prevents trauma-induced depression. These are literally molecules being released from your muscles that function like an intravenous dose of hope in difficult circumstances.

The important bit: your muscles release these chemicals only when you use them. Movement is medicine you can't access any other way. You need to lift something heavy, push something, dance, walk, play sports, garden—as long as you're using your body, your muscles release these chemicals.

Movement as Way of Being with Emotions (Not Escaping)

Your Protector Modes may have used exercise in the past to escape from or control emotions—working out to "burn off" anxiety, running to numb feelings, or using movement as punishment.

You can now learn to use movement differently: as a way to be with your Lost Child whilst emotions move through your body. One useful distinction:

Protector Mode Movement

- Driven by rules, shoulds, or compensation
- Used to punish, control, or "earn" food
- Pushes through pain or exhaustion
- Focused on outcomes (calories burned, body changes)
- Creates more disconnection from body signals
- Feels compulsive, anxious, or desperate

Wise Self Movement

- Guided by curiosity and care
- Offered as support for your Lost Child
- Honours your body's signals and limits
- Focused on internal experience (how it feels)
- Creates more connection with body wisdom
- Feels grounded, exploratory, or nourishing

The question to ask yourself: "Is this movement helping me be more present in my body, or is it helping me escape from my body?"

Key: Listening to Body, Not Controlling It

Approaching movement as a conversation with your body rather than something you do to your body changes everything.

Before moving, check in: "Body, what do you want to do right now?" Notice what arises—perhaps a desire to stretch, to walk, to lie still, or to move energetically.

During movement, stay curious: "How does this feel from the inside?" Notice sensations without judging them as good or bad.

Respect what you discover: If something doesn't feel good, stop or modify it. If something feels nourishing, stay with it. Your body's wisdom is more important than any external instruction.

After movement, express appreciation: "Thank you, body, for moving with me today."

Integration Practice: This week, experiment with one form of gentle movement approached as a conversation. Set a timer for just 10 minutes. Before you begin, ask your Lost Child: "What kind of movement would feel good right now?" Then follow her guidance, staying curious about your internal experience throughout.

See Appendix 15 for guidance on movement practices to strengthen the Wise Self–Lost Child bond.

N.B. Ensure that your treatment team have given you the green light before undertaking any of these movement practices, especially if your eating practices have put your health at risk.

Closing: The Bond Is Established

What You've Accomplished

If you remember only one thing: recovery isn't about getting rid of difficult feelings. It's about the relationship between your Wise Self and your Lost Child—the safety that lets her come up on deck.

You've discovered that your body speaks an emotional language, that "I feel fat" or "I feel empty" are actually your Lost Child's attempts to communicate deeper emotional truths.

You've practised turning toward emotions through the TREES technique, offering your Lost Child the emotional vitamins she needed: safety, connection, expression, healthy limits, and the freedom to be authentic.

You've begun learning to receive—allowing nourishment without earning it first, noticing your Overcontroller's deprivation patterns, and trusting that self-care doesn't make you selfish.

You've discovered movement as medicine—literal hope molecules that help you build resilience and strengthen the connection between your Wise Self and Lost Child.

The Difference This Makes

When you first began this book, your Protector Modes were running the show, using eating and body-focused behaviours to manage feelings that seemed too dangerous to face. Your Lost Child was locked below deck, her voice unheard.

Now your Lost Child can begin to trust that your Wise Self will stay present even when feelings are big. She's learning she doesn't have to communicate through body symptoms or eating behaviours—she can express herself directly, and someone will listen.

Your Protector Modes are beginning to relax, gathering evidence that they don't have to work quite so hard. They're seeing that your Wise Self can provide the structure, safety, and care they've been trying to create through more extreme measures.

The relationship between your Wise Self and Lost Child is growing. When your Lost Child feels lonely, your Wise Self can pause and ask: "What does she actually need?" When she feels ashamed, you can recognise: "This is old shame being triggered. She needs reassurance that she's worthy exactly as she is."

What Still Lies Ahead

This relationship forms the foundation for everything that comes next.

In Chapter 8, we'll explore how to change eating behaviours themselves—establishing regular eating and moving toward intuitive nourishment. You'll approach this work differently now, because you understand what's underneath.

In Chapter 9, we'll look at changing relationships and getting your needs met more directly, building connections where your authentic self is welcomed.

Throughout all the work ahead, you'll return to what you've learned here: that feelings aren't the enemy, that your body speaks truth, and that the relationship between your Wise Self and Lost Child is the foundation everything else rests upon.

A Message to Your Lost Child

You've been waiting so long for someone to come below deck and find you. You've been holding all these feelings—the loneliness, the fear, the shame—believing that maybe if you held them quietly enough, you wouldn't be too much of a burden.

Someone is here now. Your Wise Self is learning to recognise your voice, to stay present even when your feelings are big. You don't have to be perfect to deserve this care. You are worthy simply because you exist.

You can start to come up on deck now. Slowly, at your own pace. Your Wise Self is here, hand extended, ready to sit beside you through whatever comes. You're not alone anymore.

Your Continuing Journey

This work takes time, patience, and courage. Some days you'll move forward with ease. Other days you'll face storms that test everything you've learned.

But each time you turn toward emotions rather than away, each time you offer your Lost Child compassion instead of criticism, each time you receive nourishment without guilt, you're strengthening the relationship that matters most.

You're learning what it means to sit down beside yourself, to hold your own hand, to stay present together even when things feel difficult.

This is how you come home to yourself.

Gentle Experiments to Try

Choose two or three practices that resonate most. These aren't assignments with deadlines—they're invitations you can return to whenever they feel helpful.

Core Emotional Practices

- **Daily TREES Practice**: Notice one difficult emotion and guide your Lost Child through Tune In → Receive → Explore → Enrich → Soak.
- **Emotion Check-In**: Three times daily, pause and ask: "What am I feeling right now? Where do I notice this in my body?"
- **Body-Emotion Translation**: When eating urges arise, pause and ask: "What is my Lost Child actually feeling underneath this?"

Relationship Building

- **Reparenting Messages**: Choose one message your Lost Child needs most and offer it daily (spoken aloud, written, or silently with hand on heart).
- **Receiving Experiment**: Choose one form of nourishment from your deprivation list to practice receiving without earning. Track your progress with the Emotional Vitamins Jar.
- **System Check-In**: Acknowledge your Protector Modes' concerns and show evidence of your Wise Self's growing capacity.

Expression and Integration

- **Anger Translation**: When anger arises, practice: What boundary was crossed? What does my Feisty Child need to communicate?

- **Movement as Conversation**: Try 10 minutes of gentle movement, asking "What do you need?" before you begin.

Journalling Prompts

- Which emotion feels most difficult or dangerous to experience? Why?
- When you practised TREES, what did your Lost Child reveal about what she needs?
- Which form of nourishment has your Overcontroller been restricting most severely?
- What changed in your body when you experimented with receiving without earning?

A Note on Pacing

This chapter covers ground on understanding emotions, TREES, reparenting, receiving, anger, and movement. Think of these as a menu, not a to-do list. You might spend weeks practising TREES with mild emotions before adding other elements. Some practices will resonate immediately; others may never feel right for you, and that's fine.

Trust yourself about what you need right now. Each small moment—each time you turn toward a feeling, stay present for 30 seconds, and offer one kind message—builds the capacity your Wise Self needs. Recovery grows from steady, kind attention, not perfection.

Note

1 Michael Leunig poem "Sitting on the Fence" printed here with permission granted by the Estate of Michael Leunig.

8 Changing Eating Behaviours and Reconnecting with Your Body

Everybody has a little bit of the sun and moon in them. Everybody has a little bit of man, woman, and animal in them. Darks and lights in them. Everyone is part of a connected cosmic system. Part earth and sea, wind and fire, with some salt and dust swimming in them. We have a universe within ourselves that mimics the universe outside.

From Part Sun and Moon by Suzy Kassem[1]

Opening: From Feeling to Action

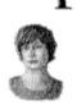 Sophie stands in her kitchen, staring at her lunch—carefully portioned, arranged just so, part of the same routine she's followed for years. As she picks up her phone to log the meal, a small voice surfaces: "I'm tired of all these rules. I just want to eat lunch like everyone else."

Her Perfectionist Overcontroller immediately protests: "Don't listen to her! The rules keep us safe. Without them, you'll lose all control." But Sophie has been practising the skills from previous chapters—staying present with feelings, offering reparenting messages, and using the TREES method to tune in to what her Lost Child is feeling and which emotional vitamins are missing. She recognises this voice as her Lost Child, the part that just wants to belong, to feel normal, to not turn every meal into a mathematics equation.

This chapter shows you how to apply everything you've learned to the practical reality of changing eating patterns. Although it might be tempting to turn to willpower or rules as the solution, this is a form of self-denial that ultimately perpetuates the problem. The real solution is through strengthening the compassionate partnership between your Wise Self and Lost Child. The emotional skills you've been building—staying present with feelings, offering reparenting messages, and using the TREES method—are the foundation that makes sustainable change possible.

Think of it this way: you've been learning to strengthen your internal crew and navigate emotional storms. Now you're ready to learn something equally essential—how to provision your ship. For too long, your Overcontroller has been trying to sail on starvation rations, or your Detached Self-Soother has been using food as the only comfort aboard. Your Wise Self is learning that

DOI: 10.4324/9781003355878-9

a well-provisioned, consistently nourished vessel sails steadier through any weather.

Before diving in, pause. You've done some good inner work already. Let those foundations solidify before rushing into behaviour change.

Part 1: Your Eating Patterns as Attempted Solutions

Your eating patterns are unique solutions your system developed to problems that once felt unsolvable.

Understanding Your Unique Pattern

Sophie's restrictive eating was her Overcontroller's solution: "If I need nothing, I can't be a burden." The logic seemed airtight, but the cost was isolation.

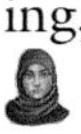 Faye's binge–restrict cycle was her system's attempt to manage loneliness her family couldn't help with: "Food offers reliable comfort when people don't." It worked temporarily. But it kept her Lost Child's real needs—for genuine connection and emotional attunement—forever unmet.

Your Eating Pattern Inventory

Highlight which behaviours in the table below feel familiar—without judgement, just curiosity.

Ask yourself:

- When does this behaviour typically happen?
- What does it accomplish for me in the moment?
- If this behaviour could speak, what would it say it's protecting me from?
- Which emotional vitamin (from Chapter 1) might be missing underneath?

The Hidden Forms of Restriction and What They Set Up

Restriction extends beyond obvious under-eating. It includes subtle deprivation—diet foods when you want regular, rigid rules despite adequate amounts, guilt about eating, and internal "shoulds" that prevent satisfaction.

The Many Faces of Restriction

Restriction appears in forms that aren't always obvious:

- Choosing "diet" or low fat versions when you want regular foods
- Eating only "safe" or "clean" foods, avoiding satisfying options
- Following rigid rules even whilst eating adequate amounts
- Going long periods without eating due to being "too busy"

Table 8.1 Eating Patterns as Protector Modes: How Your System Learned to Cope

Pattern	*Examples*	*Which of My Modes Could Be Driving This?*	*What Need Might This Be Trying to Meet?*
Restricting	Skipping meals · Long gaps without food · Rigid food rules · Stopping before being satisfied · Avoiding certain food groups · Counting Calories · Opting for "Low Fat" foods		
Bingeing	Large amounts quickly · Eating in secret · Loss of control feeling · Eating until uncomfortable		
Compensating	Vomiting · Excessive exercise · Laxatives/diet pills · Fasting after eating · Chewing–spitting		
Body-Focused	Frequent weighing · Mirror checking · Body measuring · Constant comparisons · Body checking		
Rituals	Cutting food into tiny pieces · Specific eating order · Always eating alone · Same plate/cutlery · Preoccupation/copious planning around food · Feeding others/watching others eat · Food Hoarding		
Avoiding	Social events with food · Eating in public · "Feared" foods · Showing your body		

- Compensating through extra movement after eating
- Rest: Pushing through exhaustion, working without breaks, feeling guilty about resting
- Pleasure: Denying yourself joy, hobbies, or activities done purely for enjoyment
- Emotional expression: Suppressing "unacceptable" feelings, whilst only allowing happiness or gratitude

When needs go unmet across multiple domains, your system enters a scarcity mindset—often expressed through food preoccupation.

See Appendix 17 to identify your own forms of self-deprivation.

What Restriction Actually Sets Up

Every time you restrict or deprive yourself, you're not preventing loss of control. You're preparing for it. Your body responds to deprivation of any kind as a threat—whether you're restricting food quantities, choosing only "safe" foods, working without rest, denying yourself play and pleasure, or living in constant productivity mode.

Restriction appears across most eating disorder presentations, though what it sets up varies:

For Binge–Restrict Patterns (including bulimia nervosa and many binge-eating disorder presentations): Every restriction lights the fuse. Your body interprets restriction as famine and responds with powerful biological drives: increased food preoccupation, slowed metabolism, intense urges to eat large amounts quickly when food becomes available, delayed fullness signals, and a strong preference for calorie-dense foods.

What you experience as "loss of control" is actually your body overriding your Overcontroller's attempts at continued restriction because survival takes priority. The cycle intensifies: restrict → body activates survival mode → powerful urges emerge → eating happens → shame floods in → Overcontroller insists the solution is more restriction.

For Binge–Purge Patterns: The restriction may be less obvious—you might eat adequate amounts overall—but mental restriction (guilt, "shouldn't have eaten that," rigid food rules, compensation through purging or exercise) creates the same scarcity signal. Your body doesn't distinguish between physical restriction and psychological restriction. Both trigger the biology of deprivation, which fuels the next binge episode.

For Primarily Restrictive Patterns (Anorexia Nervosa—Restrictive Type): Every restriction intensifies the very preoccupation and fear you're trying to escape. Your mind becomes increasingly consumed with food, calories, weight, and control. The restriction creates constant mental preoccupation, exhausting hypervigilance, terror that any relaxation will lead to catastrophe, and increasing rigidity. The preoccupation is your brain's survival response to deprivation—keeping you focused on finding nourishment when your body is starving.

Eating Patterns Mirror Old Relationship Wounds

Eating patterns often echo the emotional atmosphere you grew up in. Many people discover that controlling food now feels uncannily similar to how they once had to control their feelings to stay safe. Binge–purge cycles can mirror early cycles of chaos → shame → repair. Rigid food rules can echo authoritarian or perfectionistic early relationship experiences where "getting it right" was the only path to approval.

For some, hunger feels strangely familiar because emotional or physical deprivation was once the norm; for others, fullness triggers the alarm because receiving enough—or being "filled"—was tied to shame, exposure, or overwhelm. And if you grew up in an environment that felt intrusive or emotionally intense, restricting to avoid sensory overload can become a way to recreate the predictability you lacked.

None of this is about blaming your family. It's about recognising that your eating patterns formed as intelligent adaptations in an earlier relational world—strategies your younger self used to manage feelings, needs, and environments that felt too much or not enough.

Shame: The Thread That Runs through Needs, Emotions, and the Body

For many people with eating difficulties, shame is the background thread running underneath everything. It often starts when the Inner Critic internalises messages that your needs were inconvenient or unwelcome. Simply wanting comfort, rest, or closeness began to feel like evidence that something was wrong with you.

When needs couldn't be expressed safely, emotions accumulated—sadness, anger, longing. If these were met with disapproval, the Inner Critic targeted them too. You learned that emotions were shameful exposures of weakness rather than signals to understand.

With nowhere else to go, shame settled into the body—where the Lost Child lives and needs are felt most directly. Hunger began to feel like neediness, fullness like indulgence, taking up space like a threat.

Your Protector Modes stepped in to shield you: the Overcontroller tried to erase need through restriction, the Detached Self-Soother used bingeing to take in comfort privately, whilst the Lost Child stayed hungry for real connection.

The reality: your needs were never shameful—they were unmet. Your emotions were never "too much"—they just haven't been sufficiently held with understanding. Your body was never the problem—it absorbed the weight of everything you haven't been allowed to feel. Recovery means replacing the Critic's voice with the Wise Self's compassion: "Shame is showing up again, but I don't need to disappear. I'm allowed to need, to feel, and to live in this body."

The Way Forward: Recognising and Addressing All Forms of Deprivation

To shift eating patterns in a lasting way, it's important to understand that deprivation is full of complexity. Restriction—whether food, rest, pleasure, connection, or emotional expression—signals "scarcity" to the nervous system. Once scarcity is registered, the body becomes more preoccupied and urgent, activating survival mode. Nourishment, then, is what restores safety.

The work ahead is to establish a steady, predictable rhythm of nourishment—so your body and modes stop bracing for deprivation. Over time, your system learns the following:

- Food arrives regularly and adequately.
- Satisfying foods are allowed.
- Rest isn't earned.
- Pleasure is safe, not indulgent.
- Connection is nurturing, not threatening.
- Your needs will be met rather than overridden.

Whenever you catch yourself slipping into self-denial, pause and apply your TREES practice (from Chapter 7). As predictability grows, the urgency and chaos around eating ease because your system becomes less deprived and more at ease.

Faye's Journey: Understanding Multiple Layers of Deprivation

Faye's "clean eating" masked wider self-denial. Her childhood provided nutrition but lacked room for emotional needs. She absorbed: Your feelings are too much. Manage everything yourself.

That early learning shaped her adult life in ways she barely noticed:

- Food: She ate "clean" during the day—always the "approved" foods, never what she actually wanted.
- Rest: Breaks felt indulgent; she worked through lunch and pushed herself long past exhaustion.
- Pleasure and play: She had no hobbies, no spontaneous joy—everything had to be useful or productive.
- Connection: She supported everyone else but never shared her own struggles.
- Self-expression: Her natural intensity and playfulness were kept tightly under wraps.

By the time evening arrived, the deprivation had accumulated. When she binged, it wasn't simply a reaction to daytime restriction—it was the only place where she allowed herself to receive anything at all.

"The binges were the only time I let myself have anything I actually wanted," she said once. "During the day I shut down every need—food, rest, fun, company, feelings. By night I was so emptied out that eating felt like the only relief I had access to."

Faye's recovery began when she realised the binge–diet cycle wasn't just about food; it was woven into the way she treated herself in every part of life. The work became broader and unfolded on several fronts:

- **Food**: shifting to mechanical eating with foods that were both regular and satisfying

- **Rest**: protecting breaks and allowing evenings and weekends to restore
- **Pleasure**: taking up wild swimming again—an old, forgotten source of joy
- **Self-expression**: letting herself say what she felt in small, manageable ways

As these forms of nourishment returned to her life, the binge urges softened. Food no longer had to carry the weight of every unmet need. Her system felt less starved—emotionally and practically—which meant the urgency around eating began to settle too.

Understanding the Two Hungers

The Bushmen of the Kalahari speak of two hungers. *The Little Hunger* lives in the belly—the physical need for food. *The Great Hunger* lives in the heart—the longing for connection, comfort, meaning, and belonging.

Many people find that their eating patterns respond as if food should soothe both. But food can only reliably meet the Little Hunger. The Great Hunger requires a different response: attunement, rest, care, company, self-expression, and compassion.

Learning the Distinction

The "two hungers" understanding becomes useful after you're eating regularly and your body has learned to trust that food will consistently be available. At that point, you might notice:

Physical Hunger Tends To

- Build gradually over time (unless you're significantly undernourished)
- Occur predictably (typically 2–4 hours after last eating something satisfying)
- Respond to eating—the sensation eases when you're nourished
- Show up as an empty, rumbling, gurgling, or gnawing sensation in your stomach area
- Sometimes express itself through fatigue, difficulty concentrating, or mood changes (like irritability or anxiety)

In Emotional Hunger, Sensations in the Body Tend To

- Arise suddenly in connection with a specific emotional trigger or event
- Occur regardless of when you last ate
- Not be satiated with eating alone—food might provide temporary comfort but doesn't resolve the underlying feeling
- Feel more like restlessness, agitation, or seeking comfort/soothing
- Often involve craving something very specific

The Complexity: These can overlap considerably. Physical hunger can trigger anxiety or irritability (often called "hanger"). Strong emotions can create physical sensations in your stomach that feel similar to hunger. You can experience both physical hunger and emotional distress simultaneously.

What This Means for You: If you're genuinely unsure whether what you're sensing is physical hunger or emotional need, it's okay to eat. Notice what happens afterwards—if the sensation eases and you feel more settled, physical hunger was likely involved. If the sensation persists or returns quickly, you might need emotional care rather than (or in addition to) food.

Learning this distinction helps you develop emotional fluency—the ability to recognise when your body is speaking the language of feelings rather than reporting on physical needs. This takes time and experimentation.

This is also about learning to listen to your body as a way of tuning in to your Lost Child. Your Lost Child lives in your body—her emotions create the sensations, her needs show up as urges. When you learn to stay present with body signals (through consistent nourishment, respecting what emerges, protecting from Critic attacks), you're actually learning to hear her voice.

Faye's Journey

Faye's journey illustrates this. After years of chaotic eating, she found it impossible to distinguish physical from emotional hunger. "Everything just felt like 'I need food,'" she described. Only after months of mechanical eating—nourishing her body consistently regardless of hunger signals—did these distinctions begin to emerge. Her body began signalling differently; she could tell when the "I need something" feeling was actually loneliness, exhaustion, or sadness layered beneath the urge to eat.

Your Reflection (Only If You're Eating Regularly)

Notice the difference between these hungers not to decide whether to eat but to understand what else you might need in addition to nourishing your body:

- If you feel "hungry" an hour after a full balanced meal, your Lost Child may be asking for soothing, company, or rest, alongside the food you've already committed to.
- If you reach for food when lonely, that's information about needing connection, not evidence that you should alter your meal plan.
- If restriction urges appear after emotional overload, that's your Overcontroller trying to manage feelings—not a cue to restrict food.

The goal isn't to use this awareness to limit food but to recognise: "My body needs nourishment, and my heart may need something too. I can tend to both."

If this understanding triggers restriction urges, return to mechanical eating—the two-hunger concept can wait.

N.B. For Restrictive Patterns: Your first task is mechanical eating (eating by the clock)—regular, adequate nourishment regardless of hunger cues. The two-hunger distinction becomes useful only after your eating pattern is regular and your body trusts that food will consistently arrive.

Reality Acceptance: The Gateway to Change

Real change begins with acknowledging where you are without shame. Acceptance isn't resignation ("I'll always be this way") but rather facing reality ("This is where I am, and it makes sense").

Tony discovered this when he stopped waging war against his restrictive diet and exercise. For years he'd berated himself for skipping meals, believing harshness would force change. Instead, the criticism entrenched the pattern: his Lost Child hid, his Overcontroller tightened, and his Critic sharpened.

"When I stopped fighting and got curious, things started to shift," he reflected. Asking *What's this urge to over-exercise trying to do for me?* helped him see it was an attempt to feel worthy of love. Coaches had only praised discipline—controlling his diet and exercise became his adult way of earning approval—long after they were gone.

From this more compassionate place, Tony could speak to his Overcontroller differently: "You tried to help me feel acceptable. Maybe we can find ways to feel valuable that don't punish my body."

Acceptance created the safety that allowed change—by starting to let go of control as the answer, and moving into a place of understanding.

Part 2: Channelling Your Impulsive and Undisciplined Child Energy

Two modes often get misinterpreted—Impulsive Child and Undisciplined Child. They look opposite but share one root: the subjugation schema. When needs and feelings are suppressed for years, your system protests. One part erupts; another refuses to move.

Understanding Your Protest Modes

When authentic needs and feelings have been suppressed for years, your system eventually protests—through impulsive urges (Impulsive Child), stubborn resistance (Undisciplined Child), or anger (Feisty Child). These often overlap and blend. What matters is recognising protest when it appears and understanding what it needs.

What They're All Protesting: Years of living without enough freedom, choice, or responsiveness. Years of being controlled, silenced, or dismissed. Years of needing permission just to exist.

What They All Need: Freedom that is contained and safe.

If you slow the moment down, you may hear several voices at once:

- **Lost Child**: "Please see me. I'm exhausted from surviving alone. I need comfort and steadiness."
- **Protest Voice** (however it shows up for you): "I need choice. I need to breathe. I need space for me. I can't comply one more time. I need help—but not at the cost of being controlled."

Your Wise Self doesn't silence protest. She offers both freedom and limits:

- Emotional safety and reassurance for the Lost Child
- Choice, movement, pleasure, and spontaneity for the part seeking aliveness
- Help, structure, and encouragement without control for the part resisting pressure

Small, real-world acts matter: resting without guilt, choosing something playful, asking for help on your terms, saying no to draining demands, and allowing flexibility inside structure. As deprivation eases, urgency softens. As autonomy returns, resistance loosens. Protest no longer has to use eating behaviours to shout to be heard.

The Self-Perpetuating Bind

The irony is that the eating behaviours meant to protect you from feeling controlled actually create *more* control and subjugation.

You restrict to prove you don't need anyone, that you can't be controlled—but restriction makes you *more* controlled (by rules, by fear, by the Overcontroller). You comply with others' demands to avoid conflict—but then your Feisty Child rebels through bingeing, which triggers shame and stricter rules, reinforcing the belief that you are out-of-control and can't be trusted with freedom.

The underground anger is completely valid—years of silencing your needs, suppressing your preferences, and accommodating others while your own voice went unheard. But when that anger can only express itself through eating behaviours, it creates the exact guilt and self-attack you were trying to avoid. The protection becomes the prison.

Effortful Control: The Bridge between Impulse and Choice

From Chapter 2, you'll remember **Effortful Control**—the Wise Self's ability to pause long enough to understand what's happening. This is different from the Overcontroller's fear-based rigidity. *The Overcontroller says:* "Eliminate all impulses. Need nothing." *The Wise Self says:* "Pause. I notice an urge. Let's listen to what's needed underneath."

Your Wise Self doesn't try to eliminate your Child Modes' energy or needs—that would mean eliminating vitality itself. Instead, your Wise Self learns to:

Create Space between Impulse and Action: When the urge to binge arises, your Wise Self can pause: "I notice this urge. It's not an emergency. I have a few minutes to understand what's underneath."

Instead of suppressing or indulging the urge, your Wise Self creates space—enough room to hear the Lost Child's need for comfort, the Impulsive Child's need for freedom, and the Undisciplined Child's protest against control.

Meet All Needs at Once: When you pause, you may recognise that the urge carries layers: loneliness, exhaustion, needing freedom, and needing to matter. Your Wise Self can respond to all three sides.

When deprivation is addressed, the urgency naturally softens just enough to enable you to pause and choose.

Reparenting All Three Modes at Once

Recovery requires your Wise Self learning to provide: the freedom and spontaneity your Impulsive Child craves, the consistent emotional nourishment your Lost Child has been starving for, and the autonomy your Undisciplined Child needs to choose rather than comply.

To Your Lost Child: "I see how alone you've felt. I'm here now. I'm going to make sure you receive consistent care—not just scraps, but regular, reliable emotional nourishment. You don't have to live in a state of famine anymore."

To Your Impulsive Child: "You've been living under tight rules for too long. Your need for freedom and choice is normal. We'll make space for you to make choices and have what you need without feeling desperate because you don't know when the next chance will come."

To Your Undisciplined Child: "I know you're tired of being told what to do. You've followed others' rules for so long. Recovery won't be more rules imposed on you. It's choosing freedom and nourishment because you want them, not because you have to comply."

To All of Them: "When one of you starves or feels controlled, the others panic. I'm going to care for you steadily so none of you need to live in scarcity or subjugation."

Daily Structure That Nourishes All Parts

Recovery involves routines that offer:

- Regular emotional care for the Lost Child
- Regular freedom and play for the Impulsive Child
- Genuine choices for the Undisciplined Child

- Protected rest, consistent meals, and boundaries that keep you from over-giving
- Therapy, relationships, and self-attunement that bring connection into the places where loneliness used to settle

For the Lost Child: Regular meals, reliable support, protected rest, steady rhythms. This kind of structure isn't restrictive—it provides a safety net that eases deprivation.

For the Impulsive Child: Keep meals steady but allow flexibility in what you eat. Build in small pockets of unstructured time, follow a spark of curiosity now and then, and give yourself permission to change plans when your body or emotions need it. These small freedoms reassure your Impulsive Child that she doesn't have to rebel to be heard.

For the Undisciplined Child: She needs to feel she's choosing recovery, not being forced through it. Offer options where possible: "Breakfast now or in 10 minutes?" "Of these three meals, which one feels possible?" "Do you need rest before the next step?" Small choices restore agency and help her know this isn't more subjugation—she has choices.

Soothing the Old Imprisonment: The urgency of the Impulsive Child, the resistance of the Undisciplined Child, and the emptiness of the Lost Child all come from the same place: a history of being controlled, silenced, and denied. Your Wise Self can begin to rewrite that story with simple, steady reassurance: "There is enough now. Food, comfort, rest, and connection won't disappear. You have choices. You're free. I will look after all of you."

Samantha's Journey: Addressing Deprivation, Freedom, and Autonomy

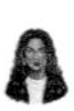 Samantha's binge–restrict cycle grew from multiple places: deprivation, protest, and resistance to control. Her Overcontroller kept her on rigid diet rules, shaped by a belief that self-denial would make her "worthy" of Gary's attention. For a while she could maintain it. But underneath, her Lost Child felt alone. Gary dismissed her feelings, disappeared for days, and offered little emotional presence, echoing her childhood, where vulnerability was brushed off and sensitivity mocked.

Her Lost Child carried the ache of being unseen. Her Impulsive Child carried the protest. Her Undisciplined Child had spent years complying with others' expectations—first her family's dismissal of her sensitivity and then Gary's emotional unavailability—and now she dug her heels in at any demand, even demands that might help. When all three had been silenced long enough, bingeing erupted: a burst of comfort, relief, rebellion, and refusal all at once. Afterwards the Critic attacked, the Overcontroller tightened the rules, and the cycle deepened.

In therapy, Samantha began naming what was really happening. Her Wise Self spoke to each part:

To the Lost Child: "You're not too much. You simply needed more than Gary could give. I'm going to make sure you get support from people and places that can hold your feelings."

To the Impulsive Child: "Of course you pushed back. You were trying to breathe. Your energy isn't the enemy—we'll find ways to let you have freedom that doesn't cost you so much."

To the Undisciplined Child: "I see you digging your heels in. You're tired of being told what to do—by others and even by me. Recovery won't be more rules imposed on you. It's choosing freedom and nourishment because you want them, not because you have to comply."

To the Overcontroller: "You tried to protect me by making me "good enough." But this path is starving the parts of me that need care. We're going to try something different."

Samantha built what she called her "nourishment on all levels" routine: • daily emotional check-ins • honest friendships where she could show feelings • therapy where vulnerability was welcomed • regular meals with satisfying foods • small acts of freedom and spontaneity • space to rest without earning it • creative play that wasn't tied to achievement • making choices about her own life—saying no, changing plans, choosing what she wanted.

The binge urges eased—not because she "got control" but because she no longer lived under control—emotionally, relationally, or physically. As her Lost Child received real connection, her Impulsive Child had space to breathe, and her Undisciplined Child discovered she could choose recovery rather than resist it, the urgency lessened.

She also began to see Gary's limitations clearly. His emotional absence wasn't evidence that she was unworthy—just information about capacity and compatibility. That clarity helped her make decisions that supported her well-being rather than staying stuck in familiar scarcity.

The Gift of Both Child Modes

Your Impulsive and Undisciplined Child Modes were never working against you. Each was trying to protect your freedom, your authenticity, your right to matter.

As your Wise Self strengthens, both begin to settle. Your Impulsive Child realises she can have choice and vitality without breaking rules to get them. Your Undisciplined Child discovers she can approach recovery on her own terms, not as another demand she must obey. Together, they learn that your Wise Self leads with collaboration rather than pressure.

The tolerance you're building—staying with discomfort long enough to find steadiness—becomes a skill that reaches far beyond eating. Life will always bring challenges; you're learning you can meet them without abandoning yourself.

This is their real gift in recovery: space to be themselves, room to choose, and growing trust in your Wise Self to guide with steadiness and care.

Part 3: Emotional Skills for Eating Urges (WAVE)

You've already learned how to meet emotions with compassion. You've seen how your modes drive urges. Now we apply those skills to eating urges themselves—the moments when old patterns pull hardest—without abandoning yourself.

Emotional Waves versus Eating Urges

As you saw in Chapter 6, emotional waves rise from your Lost Child: sadness, loneliness, anger, and shame. Urges mostly come from your Protector Modes (and sometimes Impulsive Child)—attempts to escape those feelings through restriction, bingeing, purging, compulsive exercise, or detaching.

 Harriet described it well: "The sadness felt heavy and slow. The urge to restrict felt sharp and urgent, like I had to act immediately to stay away from the sadness." Your task is to meet both the feeling and the urge without abandoning yourself.

The WAVE Method

WAVE helps you stay steady with urges. TREES is your deeper attunement practice for understanding what your Lost Child feels and needs; WAVE is your quick, in-the-moment skill for riding out urges without abandoning yourself.

W—Witness

Notice what's happening in this moment.

- If it's an emotion: Where do I feel it? What's the sensation? Is my Lost Child speaking?
- If it's an urge: What is it asking me to do? How intense is it? Where is the urgency in my body?
- If it's discomfort from not acting on the urge: What feels agitated, restless, or "wrong"?

You don't have to name the exact emotion—noticing sensations is enough: "This is what's happening inside me right now."

A—Allow

Let the wave be there without fighting it.

Allow the sadness. Allow the urge. Allow the anxiety of not acting.

The wave will crest and fall with time. Your job is simply to stay with it for a few moments.

V—Validate

Acknowledge why this experience makes sense.

"It makes sense that loneliness brings this heaviness."

"It makes sense that the Overcontroller wants to restrict—that's how it learned to manage feelings."

"It makes sense that choosing differently feels uncomfortable."

Validation does not excuse the behaviour. It's recognising the logic beneath it.

E—Embrace (with Compassion)

Offer grounding, warmth, and protection—especially for your Lost Child.

A hand on your heart. A slow exhale. A gentle inner message: "I'm here. I'm not leaving you alone with this."

To Your Protector Modes: "I see what you're trying to do. I'll handle it from here."

WAVE brings you out of automatic patterns and back into Wise Self leadership.

Samantha's Example

Samantha comes home to another evening of silence from Gary. The urge to binge hits hard.

Witness: "Strong binge urge—maybe 8/10. Restless body. And underneath, that familiar ache of not mattering."
Allow: "I can let the urge and the loneliness be here for a few minutes."
Validate: "Of course my Detached Self-Soother is suggesting food—it's been my comfort for years. And Gary's distance does hurt."
Embrace: Hand on chest. "I'm here, little one. You're not too much. And you deserve contact that's reliable. For now, let's call Sarah instead of turning to food."

The urge peaks and then gradually lessens. Not altogether, but it's no longer steering the ship.

WAVE is the core skill; it's often enough on its own. When you want to go deeper, you can add:

- TREES (Chapter 7) to understand what your Lost Child needed
- Mode language to name which part is speaking

But you don't need all of them every time. WAVE alone can interrupt the old cycle and create enough space for a Wise Self choice.

For a quick reference for WAVE practice, see Appendix 18.

Part 4: The Eating Spectrum—From Structure to Intuition

You've learned how to practice navigating urges with WAVE. Now we turn to the daily structure that makes this work sustainable—regular, mechanical eating.

One Small Step: Mechanical Eating as Reparenting

One of the most important behavioural steps in recovery is establishing regular, mechanical eating as a form of reparenting your Lost Child.

Before your body can offer reliable hunger and fullness cues, it needs a rhythm it can trust. Regular eating becomes your Wise Self's promise: "I'll make sure you're fed. You don't have to negotiate or earn this. I'm handling it now."

Tony discovered this during his recovery from years of under-eating and over-exercising. What he once called "discipline" turned out to be chronic stress on his body. Regular meals felt like a loss of control, but they were the first time his Wise Self took the wheel with real care.

This structure accomplishes several things at once: • stabilises blood sugar and energy • calms the nervous system • brings your body out of alarm mode • rebuilds trust in hunger and fullness • shows Protector Modes that nourishment can be structured and safe • teaches the Lost Child that food will come, again and again, no matter what mood you're in.

Regular eating repairs the relationship between you and your body.

Your Regular Eating Framework

For the next two weeks, practise mechanical eating—eating by the clock rather than hunger cues that may still be unreliable. Aim for breakfast within two hours of waking, then meals every 3–5 hours, with a snack between.

Meals work best when they include carbohydrates, protein, and fat. Together, they stabilise energy, support brain and body function, and help you feel satisfied. When one is consistently missing—especially carbohydrates or fat—the body drifts back toward scarcity and keeps Protector Modes on alert. Avoid the urge to create more rules or "perfect eating"—this is about giving your body consistent evidence that there is enough.

Balanced meals help your body settle and rebuild trust. Rather than labelling foods as "good" or "bad," notice what different foods offer—energy, comfort, satisfaction, or connection. All have a place.

Choose one food you usually avoid and include it intentionally each day. Over time, this helps rebuild trust and reduces the intensity of cravings. A piece of chocolate with lunch. Bread with dinner. A biscuit with afternoon tea. Chips with your sandwich.

Negotiating with Your Protector Modes about Regular Eating

Your Overcontroller will likely protest against this plan. That's expected. Return to your Chapter 4 negotiation skills:

Acknowledge Its Fears: "I hear your concern about the structure changing. You've worked hard to keep things under control."
Offer Information: "When meals are irregular, urges grow stronger and my Lost Child becomes more frightened and deprived."
Propose the Experiment: "Let's try three meals and two to three snacks a day for two weeks. We can review together."
Show the Difference between Structure and Punishment: "This isn't letting everything go. It's a different kind of structure—one based on stability rather than fear."

Tony used this exact negotiation. At first, his Overcontroller insisted: "More meals will undo everything. We'll gain weight and lose all discipline."

His Wise Self responded: "You've been doing this alone for so long. I'm here now. Our nervous system settles through consistency, not through tightening the rules."

When Hunger Cues Are Quiet or Unreliable

Periods of under-eating—whether from strict rules, emotional stress, long gaps between meals, or being below your body's healthy weight range—often dull hunger and fullness signals. This is a *biological conservation response*. When fuel has been inconsistent, the body lowers its internal volume to preserve energy, prioritising survival over appetite, warmth, and emotional regulation.

Mechanical eating provides the conditions your system needs to recover. Regular, predictable meals act as *scaffolding*—a temporary structure that holds you steady while your body repairs and relearns its rhythms. With consistent nourishment, the body can begin cellular repair, rebalance hormones, stabilise mood and sleep, restore warmth and energy, and gradually allow interoceptive signals—hunger, fullness, appetite—to re-emerge.

Your Wise Self can reassure your Protector Modes:

> *This structure isn't permanent. First, we restore safety. When the body trusts that nourishment is reliable, signals will return on their own.*

How Regular Eating Rebuilds Internal Trust

Each planned meal sends three steadying messages to your nervous system:

"Food will come again." This loosens scarcity fears.
"Your needs matter." The Lost Child begins to exhale.
"I'm guiding this now." Protector Modes can take a step back.

Over time, eating becomes less of a battleground and more of a stable pattern. Regular nourishment becomes a form of attachment repair—your Wise Self showing, through action rather than intention, that care is available and reliable.

Why Structure Comes before Intuition

People often ask: "If intuitive eating is the long-term aim, why am I starting with eating by the clock?" Because eating disorders—regardless of the specific pattern—disrupt the body's internal signalling system. When signals are inconsistent, blunted, or hijacked, the internal compass can't yet be trusted to guide eating.

Different patterns disrupt the body's internal cues in different ways, even though the end result is the same: the signalling system becomes unreliable.

Restrictive Patterns: With long-term under-eating, the body numbs hunger signals to conserve energy. This is a biological adaptation, not an indication that the body is satisfied. Meanwhile, the mind becomes hyper-focused on food, numbers, control, and perfection. The internal system feels untrustworthy because the sensations are faint or absent, and fear fills the gaps. The Overcontroller interprets this silence as proof that "you don't need food," even though physiologically the opposite is true.

Binge–Restrict Patterns: Periods of restriction create rebound hunger that feels urgent, overwhelming, and often frightening. The body is trying to correct a deficit, but the intensity makes it difficult to separate true physiological hunger from the early swell of a binge urge. The cycle produces confusion where any sensation of wanting food feels dangerous, and no sensation feels trustworthy.

Binge-Eating Presentations: Hunger may arise, but it often sits tangled with emotional needs, loneliness, overstimulation, or old patterns of using food to self-soothe. Mental and emotional restriction—shame, "shoulds," rigid rules—trigger the same biological deprivation response as physical restriction. The internal signals become layered: part body, part emotion, and part Protector Mode strategy.

Across these patterns, the relationship with internal cues breaks down. Signals are shaped by suppression (ignoring hunger until it fades), override (eating past fullness during binges, or blocking hunger during restriction), fear (distrusting bodily sensations because they feel unpredictable or "dangerous"), and chaos (signals firing in a way that feels scrambled, inconsistent, or overwhelming).

Whether the body is quiet from chronic under-fuelling or noisy from cycles of deprivation and urgency, the internal compass no longer points reliably toward safety or genuine need. Mechanical eating steps in as that temporary navigation tool. It provides the rhythm your body can't yet generate on its own—steady, predictable, external structure—until the internal circuitry recalibrates and trust in bodily cues can gradually return.

How Mechanical Eating Rebuilds Trust

Eating by the clock—having meals at steady intervals regardless of hunger cues—supports recovery across all eating patterns.

Physiologically, regular nourishment restores the body's basic rhythms. It steadies blood sugar, lifts energy, calms the nervous system, and creates the conditions for hunger and fullness cues to re-emerge. Each meal sends a clear signal: *Food is coming. You don't have to brace for famine or chaos anymore.*

Over time, this consistency allows the body to relax: silenced hunger cues begin to wake, deprivation-driven urgency eases, and eating gradually separates from emotional crisis.

Psychologically, mechanical eating shows your Protector Modes that your Wise Self can offer structure without punishment. Eating no longer hinges on being "deserving," disciplined, hungry enough, or depleted enough. It becomes steady leadership rather than a battleground.

Emotionally, mechanical eating reassures your Lost Child that nourishment is no longer conditional or erratic. She doesn't have to wait until hunger becomes unbearable or feelings overflow. Her needs are met regularly—regardless of mood, stress, or fear.

What Mechanical Eating Teaches Your Body

Tony's experience is typical. He had been restricting for years whilst over-exercising. He could barely remember what hunger felt like. "I thought I just wasn't a person who got hungry," he explained. "My Overcontroller told me this proved I was disciplined and strong—that I'd transcended basic needs." When his treatment team introduced mechanical eating, he spent months eating by the clock before the first faint sensation of hunger returned—barely discernible, almost unfamiliar. It appeared only after consistent feeding taught his body that asking for food was safe again.

Mechanical eating teaches the body that hunger is safe, signals are allowed, and nourishment will arrive without needing to escalate. In restrictive patterns, it wakes up silenced hunger cues. In binge–restrict patterns, it dismantles the deprivation–urgency loop. In binge-eating patterns, it helps separate eating from emotional distress. Across all patterns, this consistency rebuilds trust.

You saw this in Faye's story, where food restriction was just one strand in a wider web of self-denial. Mechanical eating helped, but recovery deepened only when she began nourishing herself across all domains. As that wider deprivation eased, the urgency around food faded.

From Mechanical to Intuitive Eating

The recovery transition from "mechanical" to "intuitive" eating unfolds along a spectrum, and most people spend considerable time in the middle ground where both approaches work side by side.

Early Recovery: Structure Takes the Lead. In the beginning, eating is almost entirely mechanical. You eat every three to five hours regardless of what your hunger cues are—or aren't—telling you. Your Wise Self provides full external structure because your internal compass isn't functioning reliably yet. Predictability becomes the temporary anchor that steadies the ship.

Middle Recovery: Signals Begin to Flicker Back On. As healing progresses, the structure remains, but intuitive elements begin to surface. You still eat at regular intervals, but you start noticing faint cues—faint stirrings of hunger, moments of early satisfaction, and small shifts in preference. You don't rely on these signals yet; you simply acknowledge them.

If your pattern has been restrictive, those very subtle cues may be the first signs of hunger returning. If your pattern has been binge–restrict, you begin learning the difference between genuine hunger and the frantic urgency of a binge impulse.

Your Wise Self continues to lead, while gently inviting your body's input.

Late Recovery: Over time, the balance shifts. You follow hunger and fullness cues more often, using mechanical structure as a safety rail during difficult moments—stress, illness, times when eating disorder thoughts flare. Returning to structure when needed becomes a sign of flexibility. Your body and Wise Self begin to operate in true partnership.

Stable, Ongoing Recovery: Intuition with Inbuilt Stability. Eventually, intuitive eating becomes your default. You respond fluidly to hunger, satisfaction, appetite, and energy. Mechanical structure stays in the background—an internalised rhythm you can lean on whenever life becomes choppy. Food becomes neutral. Choices are flexible. Your body and Wise Self move together with ease.

Can Mechanical and Intuitive Eating Coexist?

They do, for almost everyone. People without eating disorders also rely on a blend of both: they know when meals usually happen, they eat before social events to stay steady, they grab food during long work days even if they're not hungry, and they plan ahead for busy schedules.

Even in the most structured phases of recovery, intuitive elements can be woven in: • choosing what sounds appealing from suitable options • noticing satisfaction without letting it dictate portion size • observing preferences without letting them override nourishment • gently attending to bodily cues as they reawaken.

Rather than replacing one system with another, this is about developing the flexibility to use the approach that best supports your recovery in each moment.

Your Wise Self's Reassurance to Your Protector Modes

To the Overcontroller (All Patterns): "You've worked hard to create stability through control and deprivation. I'm taking over now with a steadier form of structure—one that nourishes rather than depletes. We're learning to eat like someone who is safe in their body."

To the Impulsive and Feisty Child (Binge–Restrict Patterns): "I know how long you've lived with desperation and urgency. Mechanical eating is the consistency you were never given. You won't need to scramble for 'last chances' anymore."

To the Lost Child (All Patterns): "You have waited so long for predictable care. I will feed you regularly—whether you feel hungry or not, whether you feel deserving or not. This is your right, not a reward."

The Goal: Trusting Your Body Again

The aim is restoring trust—between your Wise Self and your body. This means developing the capacity to: • treat hunger cues as safe, useful information • recognise when cues are unreliable and lean on structure • eat for nourishment and connection, pleasure, and community • return to mechanical eating when needed without shame • live with food as something ordinary, supportive, and non-moral.

For restrictive patterns, this means discovering that hunger isn't a threat.

For binge–restrict patterns, it means realising that regular eating prevents chaos.

For all patterns, it means living with food as something steady and uncomplicated.

Recovery is about trustworthy—rather than perfect—eating. Your body has been signalling for years, even when the messages were scrambled or silenced. Mechanical eating is how you show your body—and your Protector parts—that you are finally ready to listen.

A Note on Timing and Challenges

The pace of this transition varies widely. Some people spend months in mechanical eating; others move back and forth for years. Both paths are legitimate.

See Appendix 19 for a guide on transitioning from mechanical to intuitive eating.

For now, remember one core principle: Mechanical eating teaches your body that nourishment is reliable. Intuition grows from that soil—never before it.

Part 5: When Bodies Change

As regular eating becomes established, one of the most challenging aspects of recovery surfaces: changes in your body.

The Red Herring of Weight

Perhaps the most frightening aspect of changing eating behaviours is the possibility of weight or body changes. Your eating patterns have likely created the belief that maintaining a certain weight or body size is essential for safety, love, or self-worth.

It can help to remember that weight is a red herring—a focus that distracts from the real issues underneath.

Melissa's realisation: "I thought I needed to lose weight to deserve love and care. But when I really examined it using the work from Chapter 2, I realised the problem wasn't my weight—it was my belief that I had to earn love through being 'perfect.' Even when I was at my lowest weight, I still felt unworthy of care. The weight was never the real issue-it was my Critic telling me I wasn't good enough as I was."

What's True about Weight in Recovery

Bodies that have been undernourished need to be restored to their natural, healthy range. This is just the physiological reality. Your body has wisdom about the weight at which it functions best and that weight may be different from your eating disorder weight.

If you've been caught in binge–restrict cycles, your body needs time to regulate, to learn that food will be consistently available. The chaos of alternating between deprivation and abundance disrupts normal hunger, fullness, and metabolic signals. Regular eating allows these systems to recalibrate.

Weight fluctuations are normal—your body changes based on hydration, hormones, digestion, stress, sleep, and countless other factors. The number on the scale is simply data about gravity's pull on your body at a specific moment.

Your natural, healthy weight may be different from your eating disorder weight. The weight at which your eating disorder kept you may not be the weight at which your body actually thrives. To a large extent, our body weight is genetically programmed to be at a particular set—point range once we have reached a balance of regular, balanced eating and exercise. Recovery often involves accepting this reality.

When consistently nourished without restriction or chaos, your body will find its healthiest weight range. This requires trusting your body's wisdom more than your Overcontroller's fear.

You build this trust through the partnership you've been developing between your Wise Self and Lost Child (Chapter 5). When your Overcontroller's fear rises—"If I stop controlling, everything will spiral"—your Wise Self responds: "I'm watching over this. I won't let us fall into chaos or harm. We're learning to eat like a person who trusts their body, and I'm here to guide us through."

Each time you eat regularly despite fear, each time you respect your hunger rather than overriding it, each time you stop when satisfied rather than when rules dictate—you're building evidence that your Wise Self can take care of your body with wisdom and care.

Working with Body Image Distress

As your body changes, body image distress will likely intensify. This is where all your emotional work becomes crucial.

Apply your *translation skills* from Chapter 6. When you think "I feel fat" or "I hate my body," translate:

- What emotion is my Lost Child actually experiencing?
- Did something trigger an old schema mindset? (criticism, rejection, comparison, feeling "too much")
- What does she actually need right now?

Use your *TREES practice* from Chapter 7 to translate what your Lost Child is feeling.

Distinguish Past from Present (Chapter 5 skill): Your Protector Modes are responding as though body changes mean the same thing they meant in your past:

- Weight gain = loss of control = danger
- Visible body = being noticed = vulnerability = harm
- Taking up space = being "too much" = rejection

> But your Wise Self can offer updated information:
> Things are different now. My worth isn't determined by my body size. People who only value me when I'm small aren't offering the kind of love my Lost Child needs anyway. Taking up space is a basic human right, not something to apologise for.

Practice *body neutrality* rather than body love: You don't need to love your body. That phrase—"love your body"—can feel like yet another demand for perfection, another way you're supposed to feel that you don't. Instead, work toward something simpler and more sustainable: seeing your body as home—a place where you can feel alive, experience the world, and be present.

> Rather than judging how acceptable or attractive your body is by anyone else's standards, work toward seeing your body as the vessel through which you experience everything meaningful in your life—connection with others, the warmth of sunlight, the taste of good food, the joy of movement, the comfort of rest, the pleasure of creativity.
> Neutrality can be enough. Actually, neutrality is often the healthiest endpoint—because it takes the focus off your body's appearance entirely and puts it where it belongs: on living your life. When you can feel at home in your body—safe, grounded, present—you naturally

stop obsessing about how it looks. You start noticing what it allows you to do, feel, and experience instead.

Befriending Your Body as Home

These statements can help you shift from body hatred toward acceptance:

> "My body is my home, even if I don't like how it looks right now."
> "My body is allowing me to experience life, regardless of its size."
> "I can respect my body's needs even whilst struggling with its appearance."
> "My body isn't the enemy—it's been carrying my Lost Child all this time."

The science shows us that 97% of our body is made of stardust—literally the same elements forged in the hearts of stars billions of years ago. The carbon in your cells, the calcium in your bones, the iron in your blood—all of it came from stars that lived and died long before Earth existed. When you judge your body harshly—criticising its size, shape, or appearance—you're simply judging stardust that has organised itself into the form that allows you to be here, experiencing this moment.

Your body isn't good or bad, acceptable or unacceptable. It's an ancient matter that has taken billions of years to become you—the vessel through which the universe experiences itself. The next time your Inner Critic attacks your body, try this gentle reminder: "This is stardust. This is the universe becoming conscious of itself. This temporary form is allowing me to love, to feel, to connect, to be alive." Don't try to feel grateful or positive. This is simply about remembering the reality: you are made of cosmos, and that transcends any cultural standard about how you should look.

Tony's Body Change Journey

When Tony began eating regularly whilst reducing compulsive exercise, his body started restoring from the semi-starvation state he'd maintained. He watched the mirror closely, his Overcontroller anxious as changes appeared.

"Every morning I'd check if I looked different. Every meal felt like I was 'letting myself go.' My Overcontroller kept insisting: 'You're losing your discipline. You're becoming weak and soft. No one will respect you.'"

His therapist helped him apply the mode work: "That's your Overcontroller speaking from old fears. What would your Wise Self say to your Lost Child about these body changes?" Tony practised:

> Your body is healing. It's finding the weight it can actually function at—where you can think clearly, feel your emotions, have energy for your life. The weight you maintained through starvation and overtraining wasn't "discipline"—it was punishment. This is what caring for yourself actually looks like.

The body changes didn't stop being difficult. But Tony learned to separate his discomfort about his changing body from decisions about his eating and exercise. "Even when I hate how I look, I still eat my meals and rest when I'm tired," he explained. "Because my Lost Child's need for nourishment matters more than my Overcontroller's need for control."

Part 6: Living Recovery Daily

When Recovery Gets Messy

Your Perfectionist Overcontroller might try to turn recovery into another area where you need to excel. This part might insist you should be further along, that you shouldn't still struggle with urges, or that any "slip" means you're failing. But remember, recovery has ups and downs, setbacks and breakthroughs.

> Tony's Tuesday illustrates this: His day starts well—five days of following his meal plan. Then the gym session extends from 45 to 90 minutes. His Overcontroller took over without him fully noticing.
>
> Walking back to his car, familiar shame descends: I'm terrible at this. I'm failing at recovery.
>
> His old pattern would be to skip lunch and dinner as punishment. But Tony remembers the words from his support group: "Recovery isn't about success or failure, it's a practice you return to, over and over."
>
> Standing in his kitchen that evening, looking at the meal he'd prepped, Tony's modes are in conflict: • Overcontroller wants to skip dinner (punishment for the gym session) • Inner Critic is listing all the ways he's not good enough at recovery • Wise Self speaks up: "What if showing up means eating dinner even after a rough day? What if the practice is choosing care over punishment?"
>
> He heats up the food. Sits down. Eats it.
>
> It's not graceful. He's not happy about the gym thing. But he's here, choosing recovery even when recovery feels messy and imperfect.
>
> That's Tuesday. Tomorrow, he'll show up again.

Learning to Embrace Imperfection

The work you're doing in recovery—tolerating discomfort, staying present with feelings, eating regularly despite fear—is actually preparation for life itself.

Life is messy, unpredictable, and full of situations that can't be controlled or perfected. Your eating patterns developed partly as an attempt to create perfect order in an imperfect world. But that attempt has cost you the ability to be present for life's actual texture.

Recovery has ups and downs. Some days, motivation feels strong; other days, old patterns feel appealing again. Sometimes, you'll handle challenges skilfully; other times, you'll fumble. You might experience periods of clarity followed by confusion and doubt. Joy and disappointment often arrive on the same afternoon. Relationships that once felt simple become complicated as you change. All of this is part of being human, not evidence that you're "bad" at recovery or life.

Your Wise Self can hold this complexity. Recovery requires showing up consistently even on hard days, treating yourself with compassion when you stumble, learning from setbacks instead of using them as evidence of failure, choosing care over punishment again and again, and trusting the process even when progress feels invisible.

The Messy Middle of Recovery

There's a phase of recovery that few people talk about—the messy middle, where you've left behind the familiar structure of your eating disorder but haven't yet arrived at intuitive, peaceful eating. This is similar to the *Learning Pit* from Chapter 4—where all the real work takes place.

In this phase, you're eating more regularly, but it still feels mechanical and anxiety-provoking. Your body is changing, and you're trying to tolerate the discomfort. Old urges still arise, though you're getting better at not acting on them. You can intellectually understand your patterns, but emotions still feel overwhelming sometimes. You're doing "all the right things" but don't yet feel the freedom you're working toward.

This is perhaps the hardest phase—when you've given up the false security of your eating disorder but haven't yet built complete trust in your body and your Wise Self.

Emma's Messy Middle

Three months into regular eating,

 Emma felt frustrated. "I thought once I started eating normally, everything would feel better," she told her therapist. "But I still feel anxious before meals. My body is changing and I hate it. Sometimes I miss the 'simplicity' of restriction-at least I knew what to expect."

Her therapist helped her reframe:

> The messy middle is where the real work happens. You're building new neural pathways, teaching your body it's safe to be fed, proving to your Protector Modes that your Wise Self can handle this. It doesn't feel dramatic because it's happening slowly, consistently. But that consistency is exactly what creates lasting change.

Emma began to recognise the messy middle as evidence she was doing the hard work of genuine transformation. Each anxiety-filled meal, she ate anyway. Each urge she rode out instead of acting on. Each moment she offered her Lost Child compassion instead of criticism. This was recovery—not the Instagram-worthy "after" photo, but the unglamorous daily practice of showing up.

Permission for Imperfect Recovery

You have full permission for imperfect recovery. Permission to have bad body image days whilst still eating your meals. Permission to feel urges without acting on them is evidence you're "doing it wrong." Permission to sometimes choose behaviours you're working to change—and then choose differently the next time. Permission to grieve what your eating disorder cost you whilst celebrating small victories. Permission to need support instead of recovering "independently" and "perfectly." Permission to take as long as you need—this isn't a race.

Your Wise Self can offer this permission to your Undisciplined Child and your Perfectionist Overcontroller: "Recovery doesn't need to be perfect. It needs to be real, messy, human, and consistent enough. That's the only way lasting change happens."

Recovery as Release: Letting Go of Old Patterns

Recovery is about releasing the grip of old patterns that have kept you safe but small. Think of it like a clenched fist. You can't receive anything new—nourishment, connection, joy—whilst holding tight to old survival strategies. Recovery asks you to slowly open your hand.

The Paradox of Anxiety: Every time you let go of an old pattern without compensating, you experience short-term discomfort but invest in long-term calm. You're teaching your system: We can handle this. The feared catastrophe doesn't happen. But when you compensate—restricting after eating, apologising after setting a boundary, numbing after feeling—you cancel the investment. You reinforce the old belief that the pattern was necessary for safety.

Melissa discovered this when she maintained her boundary with her parents. The anxiety was intense. Her Overcontroller screamed that she should restrict her eating to "make up" for disappointing them. But she didn't. She sat with the discomfort, let her Wise Self reassure her Lost Child: "Of course you feel anxious, that's understandable—but you don't need to feel this alone, I'm here with you. This fear will pass. Every time we face it together and survive, we're building a calmer tomorrow."

And the anxiety did pass. Not immediately—but within days, it faded. And her relationship with her parents adjusted. By not compensating, she'd invested in freedom.

What Needs Releasing? For Each Protector Mode on Your Map, There's Something to Let Go

Perfectionistic Overcontroller: Release productivity as worth, earning rest, rigid schedules → Practice unstructured time, "good enough," receiving without earning

People Pleaser: Release automatic yes, apologising for existing, always putting others first → Practice saying no, stating preferences, tolerating others' disappointment

Detached Protector: Release numbing, emotional avoidance, constant self-sufficiency → Practice feeling difficult emotions, asking for support, naming what you feel

Approval Seeker: Release needing to be special/perfect, constant comparing → Practice being ordinary, accepting "average" sometimes, genuine connection over performance

The healing move is often the opposite of what feels safe. Your Protector Modes say grip tighter. Recovery says release. Your modes say compensate. Recovery says invest in your future by sitting with today's discomfort.

With each step forward, you don't cancel—each meal you don't compensate for, each boundary you don't apologise away, each emotion you don't numb—you're building a life where anxiety decreases naturally because you've proven to yourself, again and again: I can handle this.

See Appendix 20 for your Personal Letting Go Map.

The Daily Practice

Recovery doesn't happen in dramatic moments of breakthrough but in the accumulation of small, ordinary choices made with love and courage.

It happens when you sit down to breakfast, even though your Overcontroller is protesting. When you feel the urge to binge and instead call a friend. When you look in the mirror and choose neutrality over criticism. When you eat a biscuit and refuse to let your Inner Critic turn it into evidence of failure. When you stay present with uncomfortable fullness instead of immediately compensating. When you choose authenticity over performance in a relationship.

Every meal becomes an opportunity to practice showing up for yourself differently, consistently and with growing compassion. Each time you nourish your body, you're sending a message to your Lost Child: "You matter. Your needs are important. I will take care of you." Each time you sit with an urge instead of immediately acting on it, you're demonstrating to your Protector Modes: "I can handle difficult feelings. You don't have to work so hard to protect me from emotions anymore." Each time you choose connection over isolation, authenticity over performance, you're proving to all parts of yourself: "It's safe to be real. It's safe to be imperfect. It's safe to be human."

Your Integration Practice

Recovery is integration—bringing together all the skills you've learned in previous chapters and applying them to the practical reality of eating.

Morning Intention: Use your check-in from Chapter 5: connect with your Lost Child and set an intention • "Today I will honour my body's need for nourishment" • "Today I will stay curious about urges instead of immediately reacting" • "Today I will practice 'being with' my Lost Child when things feel difficult."

Throughout the Day: • Notice when Protector Modes activate (Chapter 3–4 skills) • Use TREES when emotions arise (Chapter 7) • Navigate urges using WAVE (this chapter, Part 3) • Eat mechanically by the clock, including feared foods (this chapter, Part 4).

Evening Reflection: • How did I show up for my Lost Child today? • What did I learn about my patterns? • Where did I choose care over punishment? • What do I need to carry forward into tomorrow?

Weekly Assessment: • Am I eating regular meals most days? • Are urges becoming more manageable? • Is my emotional capacity growing? • What evidence can I show my Protector Modes that my Wise Self is handling this?

Sophie's Daily Reality

Sophie's daily recovery looked nothing like the dramatic transformation she'd imagined. At first, on most mornings, her Overcontroller filled her with anxiety.

"I kept waiting for the day when recovery would feel easy and natural," she shared. "But my therapist helped me understand that recovery is a daily practice of choosing to show up for myself. Some days that choice feels effortless; other days it requires everything I've got. Both kinds of days are part of the process."

The meal in front of Sophie right now—whether breakfast, lunch, dinner, or snack—is an opportunity to practice this daily recovery as a chance to nourish the relationship between all parts of herself.

Her Lost Child is waiting to be fed—not just with food, but with the consistent message that she matters, that her needs are valid, that she deserves care simply because she exists.

Her Protector Modes are learning new ways to keep her safe—ways that create connection rather than isolation, authenticity rather than performance, genuine strength rather than the brittle control of restriction.

Her Wise Self is developing the capacity to hold it all—the fear and the hope, the familiar and the unknown, the messy reality of being imperfect and human.

Closing: Your Body as Home

The gradual opening you're experiencing—learning to feel your feelings, trusting your body's wisdom, negotiating compassionately with your Protector Modes—is not just healing your relationship with food. You're reclaiming your right to inhabit your body fully, to trust its signals, to honour its needs—to be present as a fully fledged citizen of the world.

This is the work of returning home—home to a body that has been faithfully carrying your Lost Child all this time, waiting for you to recognise it not as an enemy but an ally.

Your body has been trying to communicate with you through hunger, fullness, fatigue, tension, pleasure, and pain. Your eating patterns temporarily silenced those communications. Now you're learning to listen again. Your Lost Child has been living in your body, banished there when her feelings felt too dangerous. Now you're welcoming her back into conscious awareness, supporting her with the emotions she's been holding.

Your Protector Modes have been using eating behaviours to manage overwhelming feelings and meet needs indirectly. Now they're learning that your Wise Self can provide the care they've been trying to create through food control.

Recovery rarely arrives in dramatic gestures. It grows out of daily choices—to show up, stay present, and keep going even when it's hard. Not grand declarations, but the quiet commitment to care for yourself day in, day out.

Your Lost Child is safe now. Your body is home. And you—the Wise Captain of your own ship—are finally learning to nourish yourself with both food and love.

There will still be storms, but you're not lost anymore. You've learned to meet them with steadiness and care. This is how you move toward your authentic life.

Gentle Experiments to Try

Recovery is practice. These experiments help you apply what you've learned. Choose one or two that resonate—you don't need to do them all.

1. **Your Pattern Translation.** Three times this week when eating disorder urges arise, pause and translate: • Which mode is active? • What is my Lost Child actually feeling? • What emotional vitamin might be missing? • How can I meet the real need instead of using food behaviours?
2. **Regular Eating Practice**. Commit to 2 weeks of mechanical eating (or continue if you've already started): • Eat within 2 hours of waking • Lunch 3–5 hours later • Dinner 3–5 hours after lunch • Include one "forbidden" food daily. Notice: How does regular nourishment affect my mood, energy, and urges?
3. **Urge Navigation.** When strong urges arise, use WAVE: • Witness what's happening • Allow the wave to be there • Validate why it makes sense • Embrace with compassion Record what helped it pass.
4. **Body Image Translation.** When "I feel fat" or body hatred arises: • Pause and translate: What emotion is underneath? • Which schema might be activated? • What does my Lost Child actually need? • Respond with reparenting instead of restriction.
5. **Imperfection Practice**. When you "slip" or struggle: • Notice your Inner Critic's response • Practice self-compassion instead • Ask: What is this teaching me? • Choose care over punishment • Show up again tomorrow.
6. **Daily Wise Self Connection.** Each morning, take 5 minutes to: • Connect with your Lost Child • Set an intention for the day • Notice which modes might be active. Each evening, reflect: • How did I show up today? • What did I learn? • What do I carry forward?

Journalling Reflection: Tracking Your Progress

Each week, take a few minutes to journal these questions. Dating each entry lets you look back and see patterns you might miss day-to-day.

Journalling Prompt Reflections

- What forms of deprivation beyond food have you been practising? (Rest, pleasure, connection, autonomy, emotional expression?)
- When you applied WAVE to an eating urge, what did you discover your Lost Child was actually feeling underneath?
- What does your Impulsive Child or Undisciplined Child need that she's been trying to get through eating behaviours?
- How did your relationship with your body shift when you began seeing it as home rather than an enemy?
- What evidence can you show your Protector Modes that your Wise Self is handling recovery?

Why This Matters: Your Protector Modes need evidence that your Wise Self can actually manage without eating disorder behaviours. This weekly check-in creates that evidence trail—showing both you and your Protector parts that you're building new capacity, even when it doesn't feel like it in the moment.

When you're struggling, flip back through previous entries. You'll often find you're handling things now that would have completely derailed you weeks ago.

Remember: You don't need to do all of these perfectly. Choose what resonates. The practice itself—showing up again and again with compassion—is what creates lasting change.

The journey continues in Chapter 9, where the internal healing you've been doing transforms your external relationships. The secure partnership between your Wise Self and Lost Child becomes the foundation for genuine connection with others—relationships where you can finally be authentic, where your needs matter, where vulnerability leads to deeper intimacy rather than rejection.

You're ready for what comes next.

Note

1 Kassem, S. (2010). *Rise up and salute the sun: The writings of Suzy Kassem*. Awakened Press.

9 Changing Relationships and Absorbing Emotional Vitamins

This chapter is about how to absorb emotional vitamins through connections with people—without losing yourself in old protector strategies.

We'll firstly take a look at the "relationship charts" you learned in childhood (schema mindsets) and how they pull you toward familiar dynamics. Then we'll name the protector strategies that try to keep you safe—but often leave you feeling lonely. Next, we'll build the alternative: a steadier inner base between your Wise Self and Lost Child that changes how you show up. Finally, we'll bring it into everyday life with trust, realistic expectations (the Hardware Store principle), and boundaries that protect connection.

The Core Conflict Beneath Every Relationship

As you heal your relationship with food, your relationships with people start to change as well. You may find yourself wanting more honest, nourishing connection—while at the same time feeling wary of letting yourself be truly seen. This is the essential conflict at the heart of relational recovery—the deep longing to be seen for who you truly are, mixed with an equally deep fear that being seen will expose you to rejection, humiliation, criticism, abandonment, or control.

As recovery progresses, you may notice a gradual shift: you start showing up with people a little more openly. *Learning to stay with yourself creates a steadier ground for connection with others.* You begin to reach for intimacy from more solid ground, rather than from hunger, performance, or fear.

Part 1: How Your Relationship Blueprint Shapes Connections

In this section, we'll look at why certain dynamics feel compelling—especially when they repeat old patterns. In Chapter 2, you learned about the schema mindsets that formed when emotional vitamins were scarce. These created actual blueprints for how you expect relationships to function, drawing you toward specific types of people and dynamics.

Think of your schema blueprints as navigation charts drawn in childhood—maps that showed which harbours were safe and which waters were

DOI: 10.4324/9781003355878-10

dangerous. These old charts made sense when you were a small vessel navigating with limited resources. Now you're learning to update your charts based on present-day reality rather than past experiences.

Sophie: The Magnetic Pull of Schema Chemistry

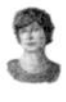 Sophie grew up learning that emotional attunement wasn't available—her mother cared deeply, but became overwhelmed by Sophie's emotions, leaving her feeling emotionally alone. Over time, she developed an Emotional Deprivation mindset: *My feelings are too much for others to handle. Others will never understand me.*

To cope, Sophie's People Pleaser Mode, made her needs smaller so others could manage. *Love means prioritising them over me.* Now she's drawn to relationships where she becomes the primary caregiver. Her Emotional Deprivation schema unconsciously selected an emotionally detached partner—his distance felt like the love she knew growing up. His inability to notice her unspoken needs confirms the prediction her mind has been carrying for decades.

The Three Schema Chemistry Patterns

Schema mindsets often pull us toward three familiar relationship patterns:

1.1. **The Familiar-Pain Chemistry**: Draws you to relationships that recreate familiar childhood dynamics—even when they hurt.

  What It Feels Like: "This relationship feels right somehow, even though it hurts."
  How It Shows Up: Growing up with critical family members, you might find yourself attracted to romantic partners who are judgemental or hard to please.

2. **The Rescue-Fantasy Chemistry**: Pulls you toward people you hope to heal, believing that if you give enough love or do everything right, they'll finally love you back

  What It Feels Like: "If I take care of them enough, they'll change and finally give me what I need."
  How It Shows Up: You choose emotionally unavailable partners, believing your patience and care will eventually help them open up.

3. **The Proof-Seeking Chemistry** Drives you to unconsciously test your deepest fears about yourself.

  What It Feels Like: "See? This proves no one really cares about me."
  How It Shows Up: If you believe "no one really cares," you might withdraw when struggling, then feel this is confirmed when no one reaches out—without recognising that you never let anyone know you were struggling.

Harriet's Story: All Three Patterns at Once

Harriet recognises all three patterns in her relationship history. She grew up learning that survival meant being invisible. After childhood trauma with no one to turn to, her blueprint solidified: I'm on my own.

Now 26, Harriet finds herself drawn to relationships with people who seem strong but emotionally distant (Familiar-Pain—recreating the dynamic she knew). Her partner, Alex, seems confident and self-sufficient—exactly the kind of steadiness her younger self longed for (Rescue-Fantasy—hoping his strength will finally provide the security she missed). But Alex's emotional unavailability recreates the familiar pattern of being unseen. Restrictive eating makes her smaller, echoing the belief that taking up less space means staying safe. Her visible struggle with food becomes her language for pain—because asking directly still feels unsafe.

When Alex expresses concern about her eating, Harriet experiences this as the closest thing to emotional care she receives in the relationship. "Sometimes I think my eating disorder is the most honest relationship I have," Harriet confides to her therapist. "It listened without judgement—even though its comfort came at a high cost."

Part 2: How Protector Modes Sabotage Connection

Here we'll name what protector parts do inside relationships to manage risk—and how those strategies backfire.

These relationship magnets don't just influence who we're drawn to—they also shape how we behave once we're there. Your protector parts automatically kick in once in relationships, using familiar strategies to manage the risk that intimacy brings.

Protective Strategies That Backfire

The Overcontroller and People Pleaser Strategies: "If I'm Perfect, and Good I'll Be Safe"

Growing up in a family where mistakes weren't tolerated, Sophie absorbed a painful belief early on: *Perfection is the price of acceptance.*

As an adult, Sophie is easygoing and agreeable—"so nice." She rarely expresses preferences. Inside, though, she often feels unseen and quietly resentful. She approaches relationships like exams, anticipating needs, apologising for imagined missteps, scanning for signs she's wrong.

Her inner taskmaster insists she must earn care by getting everything "right." Her People Pleaser keeps her small and accommodating, hoping that if she needs nothing, someone will *finally* notice what she feels.

Restriction proves discipline—evidence she's "good enough." Bingeing soothes loneliness without risking rejection. But afterwards, shame floods in: *I really am too much.* The very behaviours meant to protect her end up deepening her loneliness.

The Patterns: The Perfectionistic Overcontroller tries to earn connection through flawless performance—but makes authentic intimacy impossible. The People Pleaser tries to earn care by meeting everyone else's needs, hoping kindness will eventually be reciprocated.

Sophie's story shows how both strategies work together: one demanding perfection, the other demanding self-erasure—each cutting her off from the closeness she longs for.

The Detached Protector Strategy: "If I Don't Get Close, I Can't Be Hurt"

 Emma learned early that emotional closeness could be unpredictable. Her attempts to share feelings were often met with withdrawal. Eventually, she stopped trying. Distance felt safer than the sting of rejection.

As an adult, Emma comes across as warm, sociable, and capable—the friend everyone turns to for advice. Yet when conversations drift toward her inner world, she quickly redirects: "Enough about me. How are you holding up?"

Beneath that warmth is loneliness. Food became her reliable companion. When sadness or longing surfaces, eating brings temporary comfort.

Friends assume Emma doesn't need support. When they fail to reach out during difficult times, she feels quietly forgotten—unaware that her own guardedness has taught others to keep their distance.

The pattern: The Detached Protector manages vulnerability by numbing emotions and keeping relationships at a superficial level.

Reflection Point

Which of these three strategies resonates most with you? Can you trace it back to what you learned about relationships in childhood (Chapter 2)? How has this strategy both helped and hindered your connections?

When you start showing up differently, the push–pull gets loud: one part reaches for closeness, another panics about being seen.

2A: When Others (or Your Own Protectors) Pull You Out of the Learning Pit

As you begin showing up differently, people around you (and your own Protector Modes) often try to pull you out of the learning pit—that uncomfortable middle ground where growth happens.

Overprotective Rescue: Some people have a tendency to take over: making decisions for you, monitoring your eating, and stepping in before you can try. *Their intention* is usually to reduce your suffering—their way of showing care.

Their impact: you stay dependent, and your Lost Child's old belief—*I can't do things on my own*—gets reinforced.

The Infantilising Response: Others subtly treat you as though you're not ready or capable. They may speak for you, lower expectations, or dismiss your judgement.
Their impact: your sense of competence withers, and self-trust erodes.

When  Melissa told her mother she wanted to cook dinner on her own, her mother replied, "I don't think you're ready." What she needed was the chance to try and learn.

Relationships Built around You Being "Sick": Some relationships subtly rely on your vulnerability—someone may feel needed, secure, or purposeful when you're struggling. When you begin recovering, they may tighten their grip, question your progress, or subtly undermine your independence. Not every relationship can evolve with the healthier version of you.

When Your Own Modes Want to Escape the Pit: It's not only other people who rescue you prematurely—your Protector Modes have escape plans too.

The Overcontroller: "Just give me the formula. Let me skip the messy emotional bits."

But there is no formula. Growth happens through doing, feeling, and learning—not through perfection or shortcuts.

The Inner Critic: "You can't trust yourself. You'll mess it up."

It keeps you dependent, undermining the very self-trust you are rebuilding.

The Helpless Protector: "This is too hard. Someone else should handle it."

The longing for care is valid—but the only way to build strength is to have a go.

When Trust Needs Time to Build: If loved ones have watched you suffer, their hypervigilance makes sense. Their fear is legitimate. And so is your need for autonomy. Fear and autonomy can coexist.

When trust needs rebuilding:

1. **Check In with Your Wise Self**: In this moment are you truly ready to take ownership of your recovery? Or is there a Protector Mode in the background using this opportunity to protect or conceal your eating disorder?
2. **Acknowledge the Other Person's Fear**: "I know this is scary for you to watch me stumble. I understand you're trying to protect me. But I need to do this my way"
3. **Ask for Gradual Trust**: "Can we try one small step?"
4. **Follow through Consistently**: Trust grows through reliable action, not promises.

Protecting Your Learning Space

You'll explore boundary-setting in more detail later in this chapter (the "hardware store" problem), but for now the key idea is this: *No one can learn these skills for you. Our Wise Self and Lost Child need the chance to learn through direct experience.*

Why This Is Important: Your eating disorder kept you out of the pit by promising you could avoid struggle. Recovery means staying long enough to learn.

The Wise Self Response

When Others Try to Rescue You: "I know this is hard to watch, but I need this struggle. It's how I learn to trust myself. The kindest thing you can do is believe I'm capable."

When Your Own Modes Want to Escape: "This discomfort means I'm growing. But the learning happens *here*, in the mess. We can stay together in the pit to learn what we came here to learn."

Healthy relationships will adapt. Those that depend on your stuckness may not—and that too tells you something. Those who love you in a healthy way will tolerate your discomfort and trust your capacity to grow. And this is exactly why the inner partnership matters: *when you can stay with yourself in the pit, you don't need rescue to survive it.*

Part 3: The Internal Partnership That Changes Connection

This section builds the alternative: inner security that makes an honest connection possible.

Every lasting change begins with your Wise Self's promise to your Lost Child: I will stay with you. Now you're learning that reassurance can come from within—creating a secure inner base that makes genuine external connection possible.

Stage 1: Learning to Translate

For years, your emotions spoke through eating behaviours: restriction meant overwhelm, binge urges meant emptiness, and body distress meant shame.

Now you're learning to translate this indirect communication into emotional language—and to communicate it directly in relationships.

Emma's Translation in Action: One evening, after a difficult conversation with her mother, Emma felt intense urges to skip dinner. Instead of automatically obeying the urge, she used her TREES practice. Beneath the restriction impulse, she found the younger part of her saying: "I feel criticised and small."

Her Wise Self responded: "Your feelings make sense. You don't need to disappear to be safe."

For the first time, Emma reached out directly to a friend instead of communicating her distress through food. This was her first experience of translating the Lost Child's need into words rather than behaviours.

Consistency from your Wise Self creates the internal safety required for letting others see you; you cannot reveal externally what still feels dangerous internally.

Stage 2: Responding to Yourself with Consistency

Next comes learning to respond to yourself consistently and kindly—building the evidence your Protector Modes need that your Wise Self can actually provide care.

During a particularly stressful week at work,  Tony noticed his old pattern intensifying: earlier gym sessions, stricter food rules, declining social invitations. Instead of automatically pushing harder, he paused and checked in with his body. What he found surprised him: his exhaustion was emotional, not just physical. His Lost Child was saying: "I'm tired. I need rest and care."

Tony's Overcontroller pushed back: "Weakness is dangerous. You don't need anyone. Push through." But his Wise Self responded differently: "Of course you're tired. You've carried so much alone. Resting isn't weakness—it's a basic human need."

For the first time, he respected that message. He took a rest day, made himself a satisfying meal, and texted a friend rather than withdrawing. These small but consistent responses—meeting his own needs instead of overriding them—began to rebuild the internal trust his Protectors had lost.

Stage 3: Taking It Outside—"Empowered Vulnerability"

When you have reliable internal steadiness, external relationships stop being tests of your fundamental worth and become opportunities for connection and mutual nourishment.

You can share authentically because your value isn't dependent on others' responses. You can ask for what you need because your worth isn't contingent on never being a burden. You can set boundaries because you trust yourself to handle others' reactions.

You'll see an example of Sophie doing this later in the boundaries section

Stages 4 and 5: When Challenges Arise—Setbacks and Evolution

Learning this new way of relating isn't straightforward. Your Protector Modes will resist, old habits will resurface under stress, and you'll sometimes revert to familiar strategies.

Working with Setbacks (Sophie's Resistance Journey)

Sophie had been waiting for someone to notice her needs. The suggestion that she could meet some needs internally from her own Wise Self triggered intense resistance. "It feels like giving up on ever getting the love I need," she told her therapist. Her therapist reassured her "When you're not desperately empty, you can learn to connect with others from a healthier place, rather than chronically unmet needs."

When Sophie first tried this, her Feisty Child protested through binges: *I shouldn't have to ask for comfort.* Sophie's Wise Self validated the resistance: "You're right, you shouldn't have had to hide your needs in the past. But I'm the most reliable source of care now, I'm the one who will never leave you."

Sophie started practising small acts of self-care. When loneliness hit, her Wise Self suggested: "Let's make a cup of tea, put on some music you love, and just sit with this feeling for ten minutes. I'm here with you. You're not alone anymore."

As Sophie kept showing up for herself, the binge episodes eased and the underlying need was finally heard.

The Ripple Effect (Emma's Relationship Evolution)

Emma had long kept relationships at a surface level. As she developed an internal partnership, her external relationships began shifting.

She started small: sharing slightly more authentic responses to "How are you?" Instead of automatically saying "Great!" she began offering honest answers: "I'm having a challenging week with work," or "I'm feeling a bit lonely lately."

Some friends didn't know how to respond—they'd grown accustomed to Emma being the helper. But her closest friend, Sarah, responded with relief: "I'm so glad you're sharing more. I always felt like I never really knew how you were doing."

As Emma's internal partnership strengthened, her approach to eating naturally shifted. She still used food for comfort sometimes, but it became one option among many. When she felt lonely, she might call friends to share her vulnerability rather than automatically turning to food. When overwhelmed, she might take a walk or practise the breathing exercises her Wise Self had learned.

Reflection Point

Consider your current relationships. Which ones would likely support your increased authenticity and emotional availability? Which might resist or struggle? How do you feel about the possibility that some relationships might change as you develop stronger internal security?

As you build a steadier inner base, the next question becomes practical: who is safe enough for what kind of closeness? This is not about expecting that people will be perfectly reliable in every way—but about knowing who is an *enough-safe* person for this level of vulnerability.

3a: Learning Who Is Safe Enough to Trust (Anchor)

Before we go further, you'll need a practical way to judge "safe enough." If you grew up with mistrust/abuse or abandonment mindsets, you may both distrust everyone and trust the wrong people too quickly. Your Wise Self needs a different map—one that helps you ask not "Is this person perfect?" but "Are they safe enough for *this level* of vulnerability?"

A Schema-Based Trust Check: ANCHOR

You can think of trust as letting something important to your Lost Child become vulnerable to another person's actions. Your Wise Self's job is to notice whether that person functions as a good enough ANCHOR:

A—Attunement

Do they make a genuine effort to listen to and respond to your feelings? When they miss you (everyone does sometimes), can they repair rather than dismiss?

N—Non-harm

Do they avoid using your vulnerability against you—no deliberate shaming, mocking, threats, or coercion? When they're angry or stressed, do they still treat you as someone who matters?

C—Consistency

Are they reasonably steady over time? Not perfect but predictable enough that your nervous system doesn't live in constant whiplash between "lovely" and "terrifying"?

H—Honesty

Do their words and actions broadly match? Are they willing to tell you the truth kindly, including when it's uncomfortable, rather than hiding or twisting reality?

O—Ownership

Can they own their impact—acknowledge when they've hurt you or others, apologise, and make amends? Or do they minimise, blame, or turn things back on you?

R—Respect for Boundaries

When you say "no," set a limit, or express a preference, do they take it seriously? Or do they pressure, sulk, punish, or ignore?

No relationship scores perfectly on ANCHOR, and trust isn't all-or-nothing. You might decide:

- "This friend is ANCHOR-enough for shared activities and light self-disclosure but not for my deepest trauma story."
- "This person is reliable with practical help but not emotionally attuned—I can trust them with lifts to appointments, but I need to seek emotional support elsewhere."

Your schemas will want to swing between:

- *Over-trusting* familiar but unsafe people ("This feels like home . . . even though it hurts.")
- *Under-trusting* genuinely safer people ("They're kind . . . but I'm waiting for the catch.")

Your Wise Self can pause and ask: "Looking at ANCHOR, what evidence do I actually have? Is this a person I can risk sharing a little more with—or someone I need to protect myself from, perhaps using internal boundaries instead?"

This trust check will link directly into the Hardware Store principle: once you see clearly what someone can and cannot be trusted with, you can stop asking for bread in places that only sell hammers and nails—and start investing your vulnerability where there is at least some ANCHOR beneath your feet. The hardware store principle helps disentangle the need to be seen from the reality of others' limitations.

Part 4: The Hardware Store Principle

Because of our different personalities, cultural and family backgrounds, and our own unmet needs, people vary widely in their capacity for emotional presence and attunement. Some show care through practical support—food, money, problem-solving—while others offer emotional presence and understanding. This reflects differences in emotional development and capacity. When we repeatedly seek emotional care from someone who cannot provide it, we can end up feeling chronically abandoned and ashamed of our needs.

It's like going to a hardware store and insisting on buying bread. They have good hammers, garden furniture, and slabs of wood—but the only bread is the crumbs on the floor that have fallen from someone else's bag. If you're used to crumbs, you might not even question it. But continuing to seek emotional nourishment where it isn't available leaves you undernourished—and unable to find the bakeries in your life that can truly sustain you.

This is about recognising what the hardware store can and cannot provide, grieving what's missing, and learning to seek nourishment elsewhere. At this point, a key reality check becomes possible: who can offer the emotional vitamins you need and who can't. Understanding that some people simply don't have these to give can be quietly liberating.

Understanding Realistic Expectations

Many people with eating difficulties spend years trying to get emotional nourishment from people or relationships that simply can't provide it—then blaming themselves when they remain hungry.

Sophie's Realisation

Sophie had spent years trying to be emotionally understood by her mother for many years—hoping that if she just explained her feelings the right way, or was patient enough, or perfect enough, her mother would finally hear and understand her.

But her mother, having grown up emotionally deprived herself, simply didn't have that capacity. It wasn't a lack of love—she cared deeply—but she couldn't attune in the way Sophie needed. Growing up with this emotional absence, Sophie developed Emotional Deprivation and Subjugation mindsets: putting others' needs first to hold onto whatever connection was available.

Understanding this didn't mean cutting off the relationship. It meant adjusting her expectations. She began to appreciate what her mother could offer—practical support, concern, shared history—while seeking emotional attunement elsewhere: in therapy, with close friends, and increasingly within herself.

Your colleague might be great for intellectual conversation but not emotional support. A sibling might offer fun and shared history but not vulnerability. A parent might provide practical help but not attunement.

Accepting what people can actually offer—without expecting what they can't—frees you to seek support where it is available. Sophie stopped asking her mother for "bread" and started appreciating the hardware she did provide. She found emotional nourishment elsewhere, and over time, her resentment softened and the relationship improved—because she was no longer repeatedly disappointed.

The Grief of Realistic Expectations

Adjusting expectations often brings grief. Grief for what you needed but didn't receive. Grief for the relationships you wish had been different. Grief for the time spent trying to get bread from hardware stores. Your Wise Self can hold this grief with compassion (using the TREES practice from Chapter 7) whilst recognising that accepting reality creates space for genuine nourishment from the right sources.

Reflection Point

Which relationships in your life might be "hardware stores" where you've been asking for "bread"? What can these people actually offer? Where else might you find the emotional vitamins you need?

Indirect ways of communicating needs develop when directly asking feels unsafe; these patterns are attempts to be noticed without exposing the vulnerable parts of you that once felt shamed or dismissed.

4A: When You're Waiting for Rescue—Patterns of Indirect Need-Expression

One tricky version of the hardware store problem is when you're not only going to the wrong person for emotional bread, you're also waiting for them to notice you're starving without you ever asking. Three related patterns often develop to solve this problem.

The Core Fear of Being a Burden: At the heart of all three patterns lies a childhood experience of feeling like a burden. Perhaps your emotional or physical needs felt too much for overwhelmed caregivers. Perhaps expressing needs led to sighs, frustration, or messages that you were asking for too much. You learned something deeply painful: *My needs are a burden. Having needs makes me shameful, guilty, too much.* This creates an impossible bind. You have genuine needs (all humans do), but expressing them directly feels risky and shameful.

Three distinct Protector Modes often develop:

The Invincible Overcontroller Response: Develops contempt for having needs and vulnerability. Says: "I don't need anyone. Needing others is weakness. I'm proud of my self-sufficiency." This mode denies needs entirely. But the more you deprive yourself—of nourishment, rest, connection, and emotional expression—the needier you make yourself. The Overcontroller's rigid self-denial actually intensifies the very neediness it's trying to eliminate.

The Compliance–Resentment–Rebellion Cycle: The People Pleaser tries to avoid feeling controlled by giving control away first—accommodating others' needs, saying yes when you mean no, never expressing preferences that might create conflict. The unconscious logic is "If I comply willingly, I won't be forced. If I'm helpful enough, I'll earn the right to receive care." But compliance doesn't prevent subjugation—it guarantees it. You become controlled by the need to keep everyone happy. Underground resentment builds. Your Feisty Child's anger at being silenced has nowhere to go. Eventually, it erupts—often through eating behaviours. Restriction becomes "No one can make me eat." Bingeing becomes "I'll do what I want." But these rebellions trigger guilt (your Critic attacks: "You're selfish, out of control"), which drives more compliance, more people-pleasing, more suppression. The cycle meant to protect you from being controlled actually creates exactly that—now you're controlled by the pattern itself, unable to express needs directly, unable to access your own anger safely.

The Helpless Protector Response: Takes the opposite approach. Rather than earning deservingness through active caretaking, it uses passivity, helplessness, visible suffering, or illness as an indirect way of legitimising needs. Says: "I can't function without rescue. Can't you see how fragile I am? Someone should notice I'm struggling and step in." This mode communicates through visible suffering rather than direct asking.

The self-perpetuating trap: the helplessness meant to elicit care without direct asking actually invites others to take control—offering solutions, making decisions, stepping in to "rescue." This confirms the very fear the pattern was designed to prevent: "See? Others do try to control me. I can't trust anyone." The passivity elicits controlling care from others, which reinforces the need for passivity. The cycle deepens.

What All Three Have in Common

All three modes solve the same problem: getting needs met when direct expression feels shameful. None allow authentic relationships—you're always performing a role rather than being yourself.

Your relationships become based on obligation, pity, or being needed—rather than being known and cared for as your true self. Either way, your Lost Child loses. She doesn't get genuine connection or care. Her actual needs remain unmet because no one truly sees or hears her authentic self—they only see the performance.

Focus: The Helpless Protector Pattern

In Part 2, we explored the People Pleaser pattern. Here we'll focus on the Helpless Protector—the most complex and counterintuitive of the three, where you wait for rescue, communicate indirectly through suffering, and paradoxically push people away whilst desperately hoping they'll stay.

Melissa's parents, having had difficult childhoods, learned to be stoic and self-sufficient. Melissa absorbed: *Receiving care means becoming indebted. Taking from others depletes them. My needs are a burden.*

For a time, Melissa operated in Invincible Overcontroller mode—fiercely independent, contemptuous of neediness. But that approach was exhausting. Eventually, she collapsed into the opposite pattern: the Helpless Protector. Now she finds herself perpetually stuck—unable to ask directly for what she needs (that would be burdensome), unable to receive what's offered without guilt (she doesn't deserve it), yet desperately hoping someone will somehow see her suffering and provide care without her having to ask.

The eating disorder serves both purposes: during Overcontroller phases, restriction proves she doesn't need much—she's strong, disciplined. During Helpless Protector phases, her visible struggle communicates indirectly: "Can't you see I'm not okay?"

Why This Pattern Feels Not-Real to Others

The Helpless Protector communicates need indirectly, leaving others feeling trapped and obligated—they see the struggle but not how to help. They never get to connect with your Lost Child underneath—the vulnerable part who so desperately needs connection. Instead, they're dealing with indirect communication that feels difficult even when that's not your intention.

The Self-Fulfilling Prophecy

Your Lost Child fears being a burden, which would lead to abandonment. To avoid this, you don't directly ask for what you need. Instead, the Helpless Protector communicates indirectly through visible suffering and stuckness.

But this indirect communication—the very strategy meant to prevent burdening others—actually does burden them in ways that direct, honest vulnerability wouldn't. Partners and friends find themselves cast in an impossible role: they must function as rescuer-parent whilst also being an equal companion.

The weight of this unspoken expectation becomes the very burden your Lost Child feared creating. People do end up feeling burdened, overwhelmed, and drained. And eventually, they often pull away—confirming your original fear: *See? I was right. I am too much.*

If you could express needs directly and authentically ("I'm really struggling today. Could we talk?"), many people would likely respond with care. But the indirect approach pushes people away whilst simultaneously making them feel guilty for wanting distance.

The Turning Point: Facing Painful Reality and Reclaiming Power

Recovery from this pattern requires facing a difficult reality: No one else can do the inner job for you now. Childhood is over. The missing emotional vitamins you needed then will never arrive now, no matter how long you wait.

The Helpless Protector Mode protects you from this grief. As long as you're waiting for rescue, you don't have to face the finality of what you lost.

But on the other side of accepting that no one else is coming, you discover something surprising: Your own Wise Self is the best person for the job.

This is about reclaiming your sovereignty. When you're in the Helpless Protector pattern, you're perpetually semi-dependent on others, always living on the precipice of potential abandonment. Your sense of safety hinges on whether others will show up.

Your Wise Self makes a steady commitment: "I'm not leaving you"—you reclaim your power. You're no longer at the mercy of others' availability. You know that no matter what happens, no matter who comes and goes, you will be okay.

Differentiating Childhood Needs from Adult Needs

One vital task is learning to distinguish between childhood needs (your Wise Self's job) and adult needs (reasonable to expect from healthy relationships).

Childhood Needs (Your Wise Self's Job)

- Unconditional acceptance regardless of performance
- Attunement to feelings
- Comfort when distressed without having to earn it

- Protection from shame when expressing needs
- Being seen and valued simply for existing

These were needs you had as a child that weren't adequately met. In recovery, your Wise Self learns to provide these to your Lost Child.

Adult Needs (Reasonable to Expect from Healthy Relationships)

- Mutual emotional support, attunement and care during difficult times
- Practical help occasionally when needed
- Honesty and direct communication
- Respect for boundaries
- Being seen and valued for who you are now

Notice the difference: these involve mutuality, occasional rather than constant support, and an assumption that you're generally capable, whilst sometimes needing help.

When you find yourself feeling frustrated that someone isn't meeting a need, check: Is this a childhood need I'm expecting them to provide? Or is this a reasonable adult need they're not meeting?

If it's a childhood need (frequent reassurance, mind-reading what you need without being told, parenting-level care), that's a sign—your Wise Self needs to step in.

If it's a reasonable adult need, consider whether there's reciprocity. Adult relationships work through mutual exchange—both people offering and receiving support, both people's needs mattering. Even the most attuned people aren't attentive all the time—they get stressed, overwhelmed, and distracted by their own struggles. One missed moment doesn't mean the relationship is broken.

But if there's a consistent pattern of imbalance—if you're regularly meeting their needs whilst yours go unacknowledged, if the relationship only works when you're accommodating them, if your attempts to communicate your needs are dismissed or ignored—that's different information. This connects back to the Hardware Store principle: they may not have the capacity for the mutual give-and-take that healthy relationships require.

Your Wise Self Taking over the Rescue

Recovery means your Wise Self gradually taking over the role the Helpless Protector was desperately trying to get others to fill.

Melissa's Wise Self learned to respond directly to her Lost Child's emotions:

When Her Lost Child Feels like a Burden: "You're not a burden. Your needs are valid. I'm here to meet them—not because you've earned it, but because you deserve care simply for existing."

When Her Lost Child Feels Stuck and Powerless: "I know this feels overwhelming. Let's take it one small step at a time. I'm here to help—you don't have to wait for someone else."

When Her Lost Child Fears Abandonment: "I know you're scared everyone leaves. But I'm not everyone—I'm you. I won't leave you. No matter who comes and goes, I will always be here."

This consistent inner presence allowed the Helpless Protector to relax. It no longer had to keep Melissa stuck in visible suffering, because her Lost Child's needs were finally being met by someone who could not abandon her.

As Melissa's Wise Self took over this internal caregiving, her external relationships shifted. She no longer needed others to rescue her, which allowed her to ask for reasonable adult needs directly—and to receive care without overwhelming guilt.

Most importantly, Melissa discovered she wasn't powerless anymore. She reclaimed her power not through self-sufficiency or control but, through the Wise Self's steady, compassionate care.

Next, we turn to a freeing but painful step: recognising what some people simply can't give.

Reflection Point

Do you recognise the Helpless Protector pattern in yourself? Can you identify times when you've waited for others to notice your suffering without you asking directly?

What would it mean to face the painful reality that no one is coming to fix the past, whilst simultaneously recognising that your Wise Self can provide what your Lost Child needs now?

Can you distinguish between the childhood needs on your list (your Wise Self's job) and the adult needs (reasonable to expect from others)?

See Appendix 21 for details on mapping the ANCHOR Framework onto your relationships.

Part 5: When Food Is Their Love Language: A Note on Cultural Context

For some people, particularly women navigating patriarchal family systems or cultures with rigid control dynamics, food carries layered meanings that complicate recovery. In many cultures and families, food preparation is the primary language of love—the way caregivers (often mothers, grandmothers, or other women) express care, connection, and belonging. When you refuse food, they experience it as personal rejection: "I made this with love for you, and you're rejecting me."

For highly sensitive people, this dynamic becomes especially painful. You can feel their hurt, their sense of rejection, their disappointment. Your empathy picks up every subtle cue—the tightness in their voice, the wounded look, the withdrawn silence. And because you've learned that your needs disappoint others, refusing food feels like causing harm.

This creates an impossible bind:

- Eating beyond your body's signals means overriding your boundaries to avoid displeasing someone you love.
- Refusing food means bearing their hurt feelings, which your sensitivity absorbs as though it's your own pain.
- Your body becomes the battleground between their expression of love and your need for autonomy.

Food refusal can also become a way of expressing autonomy you can't claim elsewhere—saying no to oppressive family expectations, coercive treatment, or rigid cultural control. When you can't directly say "I disagree with you" or "I need space" or "Your expectations are crushing me," your body says it through food.

Part 6: Using Your Emotional Wisdom (Anger) in Relationships

Whether you're dealing with hardware store relationships, food-as-love-language, or rescuing patterns, one feeling deserves especially careful attention: anger.

As you develop internal security and learn to express needs authentically, one skill supports all your boundary-setting work: recognising when your anger is telling you that something isn't okay. Remember from Chapter 7: Your Feisty Child is your emotional immune system, registering when something isn't right—when boundaries are crossed, when you're treated unfairly, when your needs are dismissed. In relationships, this anger can offer vital information about what needs protecting or addressing.

If you notice anger arising—whether it's the quiet, underground anger that drives restriction as rebellion, or the more obvious frustration when someone repeatedly disrespects your limits—pause and ask: What is this anger alerting me to? What boundary has been crossed? What does my Lost Child need me to protect?

Your anger might be saying:

- "This person keeps dismissing your feelings." (External boundary needed: "When you interrupt me, I feel unheard. I need you to let me finish.")
- "You keep abandoning me (Lost Child) to keep the peace with others." (Internal boundary needed: limit time in situations where you consistently self-abandon.)
- "The dynamic with this person recreates old wounds." (Recognition: this is a hardware store situation.)

Sometimes anger signals you need to set an external boundary—to speak directly about what's not okay. Other times it reveals you need an internal boundary—to protect yourself because the other person can't or won't change.

And sometimes it simply needs to be felt and validated: "Of course you're angry. That wasn't fair. Your anger makes sense."

The skill is learning to listen to your anger as a signal rather than immediately suppressing it or turning it inward through eating behaviours. Your Wise Self can help your Feisty Child translate the feeling into wise action—whether that's expressing a boundary, creating protection, or simply acknowledging: "Yes, this is frustrating, and your frustration is valid."

Boundaries are what make visibility safe—they allow you to remain open without collapsing inward or disappearing to preserve the relationship.

Part 7: Setting Boundaries whilst Staying Connected

Learning to set boundaries without withdrawing completely—saying "no" to what doesn't serve you whilst staying emotionally present—requires understanding that there are actually two types of boundaries in recovery: external and internal.

Think of boundaries as learning to maintain your ship's course whilst staying in relationship with other vessels. You're not isolating yourself in distant waters. You're learning to sail alongside others whilst respecting what your own vessel needs.

External Boundaries: When Others Can Hear You

External boundaries are the ones you express directly to others—people who have the capacity to respect your limits, even if they sometimes forget and need gentle reminders. Setting external boundaries via assertiveness doesn't always mean making a big request or saying "no." Sometimes it simply means naming your internal reality—what you feel, need, or prefer—in a clear and honest way. This kind of boundary-setting uses "I" statements that share small but meaningful pieces of your internal world: "I'm feeling overwhelmed," "I need to finish up by 5 PM," "I'm tired today and need something low-key."

This is called *self-disclosure*—offering just enough information about your inner experience to help the other person understand you. It's not oversharing, and it's not dramatic. It's simply letting someone know where you are inside so the connection can be more real.

For people with eating difficulties, this kind of boundary often feels tricky—your People Pleaser fears being a burden, and your Overcontroller insists you should need nothing. But self-disclosure is a form of honest connection. And it's a practice that your Wise Self can learn to tolerate gently over time.

Sophie's External Boundary Practice

Sophie's perfectionist coping style had made boundary-setting feel impossible. Wasn't saying "no" the same as letting people down? Her People Pleaser insisted that good people accommodated others, that her needs should come last.

But as her internal partnership strengthened, she began recognising that boundaries weren't about being difficult—they were about being honest. Her

Lost Child had been silently drowning beneath the weight of everyone else's expectations whilst Sophie performed tireless accommodation to their needs.

One evening, her boyfriend suggested hosting friends for dinner. Sophie's automatic answer would have been, "Of course! I'll cook something special." But she paused and checked in with her Lost Child, who felt exhausted after a draining week.

Her Wise Self translated this into a boundary: "I'd love to see them, but I'm really drained." Her People Pleaser immediately protested: *They'll think you're selfish! He'll be disappointed!* She expressed her needs without apologising. Although it wasn't easy, she knew she could tolerate her boyfriend's potential disappointment without abandoning herself. "Could we plan for next weekend, or keep tonight simple?" Her boyfriend's response surprised her: "I didn't realise you were that tired. Let's keep it low-key."

Over the following weeks, Sophie practised setting small boundaries in different relationships. Each boundary felt terrifying initially. But what she discovered was that people who truly cared about her could handle her honesty. The relationships didn't end—they became more real. And those who couldn't respect her boundaries? That became a red flag, which was more about compatibility rather than her worth. In future, when her eating cycle was activated, she began to recognise when it signalled a boundary violation—which she could address directly instead of through food.

Emma's External Boundary with Diet Talk Friends: Emma valued her group of friends—they'd been part of her life for years. But whenever they met for meals, the conversation reliably drifted toward calories, "being good," and the latest eating plan. Emma had already asked them once to avoid diet talk around her, and they genuinely meant well, but the habit was so ingrained that they kept slipping back into it.

Empathic Assertiveness: What It Is and Why It Helps

Empathic reasoning means holding two truths at once:
You understand the other person's position,
and
Your needs matter too.
It sounds like:
"I know this is familiar for you . . ."
"I get that you don't mean any harm . . ."
"And I also need . . ."
"Could we . . .?"

This approach protects your boundaries and the relationship. It reduces the People Pleaser's guilt and prevents the Overcontroller from swinging to harshness.

Used skilfully, it creates space for honest connection—without abandoning yourself.

This time, instead of withdrawing or silently tolerating the discomfort, Emma experimented with *empathic reasoning*—acknowledging her friends' perspective while clearly stating her own need. When one friend began comparing portion sizes, Emma gently said:

> I get that talking about food and dieting is familiar for all of us—it's been part of our conversations for years. And I'm not judging that . . . But right now I'm working really hard on healing my relationship with food, and diet talk makes that much harder for me. Could we steer the conversation away from weight and calories while we're together? It would really help me.

She wasn't criticising them, nor was she demanding perfect care from them. She was recognising their intention *and* protecting herself.

Her voice wobbled slightly—assertiveness felt risky, especially for someone whose People Pleaser had spent a lifetime avoiding anything that might burden others. But her Wise Self held steady. She didn't apologise for needing something different. She didn't soften her request until it disappeared.

Her friends paused, then one said, "Oh—of course. Thanks for letting us know." The conversation shifted to holidays and work and the usual chat.

It wasn't magic; they still sometimes slipped back into diet talk. But now Emma had a clear, compassionate script she could return to—one that honoured her needs without dismissing theirs: "Guys . . . I know those topics feel normal for you, and I'm not judging that. I just need space from this right now. Could we change the subject?"

This was *assertiveness without aggression, empathy without self-abandonment*—a boundary her Lost Child had needed for years.

Internal Boundaries: Protecting Yourself When Others Can't Change

External boundaries rely on the other person having the capacity to respect them. When that capacity is limited, your boundary still matters—you simply take a more active role in protecting it. Sometimes you'll set a boundary clearly, kindly, repeatedly—and the other person simply cannot or will not respect it.

You're not powerless here. This is where internal boundaries become important—a limit you hold within yourself to protect your Lost Child, without needing the other person to change.

Internal boundaries aren't about punishing others or cutting them off completely. They're about protecting your recovery whilst staying in a relationship when you choose to.

Emma's Internal Boundary Work

Emma had asked her mother multiple times not to comment on her food choices or body. "Mum, I'm working on my relationship with food and my body. Comments about what I'm eating or how I look aren't helpful right now. Can you please avoid those topics?" Her mother would agree with genuine concern. "Of course, darling. I understand." Then at the next visit, inevitably: "Are you sure you need that much butter?" or "You're looking better—have you lost weight?" Emma would feel her stomach clench, her Lost Child shrinking, her Overcontroller immediately suggesting she skip the next meal to prove she had everything under control.

Emma later realised that her mother, despite caring about her, didn't want to stop commenting on food and weight because of her own lifelong struggles. She felt threatened by Emma's boundaries. This was a classic "hardware store" situation—Emma kept asking for bread, and her mother simply didn't have it to give. Understanding this didn't make the comments okay—it helped Emma stop expecting them to change.

After expressing her boundary several times with little change, Emma shifted to internal boundaries: preparing herself before visits, redirecting topics gently, and stepping outside briefly when comments became overwhelming. After each visit, she soothed her Lost Child: "Those comments are about Mum's anxiety, not about you. You protected yourself."

The transformation wasn't in her mother's behaviour—that stayed largely the same. The transformation was in Emma's response. She stopped waiting for her mother to change and started taking responsibility for protecting her Lost Child. She could love her mother and still limit exposure to triggering conversations.

Over time, Emma also adjusted how much time she spent with her mother and began to opt for times where less food was involved. Emma wasn't punishing her mother. She was setting internal and external boundaries that respected her own needs, being realistic about what her recovery could handle whilst maintaining the relationship.

Tony's Internal Boundary with His Father

Tony had always wanted emotional warmth from his father, but feelings simply weren't part of his dad's language. His father had grown up believing that vulnerability was weakness, and comments like "Come on, toughen up" were meant as encouragement, not criticism. Still, each one left Tony feeling that his emotions were inconvenient and unwelcome.

As an adult, Tony understood his father wasn't intentionally hurtful, just limited by his own upbringing. But the impact remained: whenever Tony tried to open up, his father seemed confused or dismissive. Remarks such as "Don't overthink things" or "You're looking a bit soft" reinforced Tony's childhood belief: *My feelings are too much. It's safer not to need anyone.*

This belief fed directly into Tony's eating disorder. Restriction and rigid exercise became ways to prove strength and avoid vulnerability. If he stayed disciplined and self-sufficient, he felt less exposed.

In therapy, Tony faced a difficult reality–his father was unlikely to become emotionally responsive, no matter how clearly Tony asked. Not because Tony wanted too much, but because his father simply didn't have that capacity. It was another hardware store situation—Tony asking for "bread" from someone who didn't stock it. This didn't make his father's responses acceptable—it clarified what Tony could and couldn't rely on.

This realisation brought grief, but also clarity. Tony didn't want to cut his father out of his life; he wanted contact that didn't cost him his self-worth. That required *internal boundaries.*

Before visits, Tony prepared himself: "Dad may make comments that hurt. They're about his worldview, not about me."

During conversations, he kept to safer topics—cars, football, projects they enjoyed. When interactions became tense or shaming, Tony didn't argue or shut down. He simply redirected or ended the visit earlier. These were healthy ways of protecting himself and drawing a line that enabled him to prioritise his own recovery and wellness.

Afterwards, he checked in with his Lost Child: "That was hard, but we handled it. Dad can care in practical ways, even if he can't meet emotional needs. I'm here for the rest."

Over time, Tony stopped waiting for his father to change and stopped interpreting his father's limitations as evidence of his own emotional immaturity. Their relationship didn't suddenly become close, but it became steadier and less painful. By adjusting his expectations and protecting his own emotional world, Tony could stay connected without abandoning himself.

The internal boundary didn't distance Tony from his father—it freed him to relate with more realism and less hurt.

Understanding When to Use Which Boundary

Use external boundaries when:

- The person has shown the capacity to respect your limits.
- The relationship has enough trust and safety for direct communication.
- You believe your needs can be reasonably accommodated.
- The other person has demonstrated willingness to adjust.

Use internal boundaries when:

- You've expressed boundaries multiple times and they're consistently violated.
- The person lacks the capacity to respect the boundary due to their own struggles.
- Speaking the boundary repeatedly would damage the relationship or put you at risk.
- You want to stay connected but need to protect yourself.
- You're dealing with family or work situations you can't easily exit.

External boundaries involve the other person's cooperation; internal boundaries rely on your own commitment to protect yourself when that cooperation isn't there.

Your Wise Self's Role in Internal Boundaries

When you need to rely on internal boundaries, your Lost Child might feel sad, angry, or disappointed. She might protest: "But they should respect my boundaries! I shouldn't have to protect myself like this!"

Your Wise Self can hold this grief with compassion:

> You're right. You shouldn't have to work this hard to protect yourself. In an ideal world, everyone would respect the boundaries you set. But this person can't or won't—and that's not because you're asking too much. It doesn't make their behaviour okay—but it does mean you need to protect yourself differently.
>
> I'm not abandoning you by accepting this reality. I'm protecting you by stopping the cycle of asking, hoping, being hurt, asking again. We can love this person and still limit our exposure. We can maintain a connection around what works whilst protecting ourselves from what doesn't. This isn't giving up—it's being wise.

Important Distinctions

Internal boundaries are NOT:

- Silent resentment or passive-aggression
- Secretly punishing someone whilst pretending everything's fine
- Avoiding all difficult relationships or conversations
- Never asking for what you need
- Giving up on ever being authentic

Internal boundaries ARE:

- Realistic acceptance of what others can actually offer
- Taking responsibility for protecting yourself when others can't
- Staying connected whilst honouring your limits
- Choosing when and how much to engage based on your capacity
- Loving someone AND limiting exposure to harmful dynamics

As you build your support network based on people who respect your needs and limits, you'll have more relationships that welcome external boundaries and fewer that require internal ones.

Reflection Point

Take a moment to consider your current relationships through this lens:

Which relationships in your life need external boundaries? Can you identify one small boundary you could practise expressing this week?
Which relationships may call for more internal boundaries (self-protection)? What would protecting yourself look like whilst staying connected, if you choose to?
How does your Inner Critic respond to the idea of protecting yourself in this way? Does it call you selfish or demanding?
What would your Wise Self say to your Lost Child about the need for these limits? How can you hold both the sadness that they are needed and the strength it takes to maintain them?

Closing: The Ripple Continues

As the tension softens, your relationships gradually shift from performance to emotional presence and connection. This ripple effect touches every area: relationships, work, creativity, rest, and play. Your Lost Child is learning that your Wise Self will stay—that she can emerge into authentic relationships where vulnerability leads to deeper connection rather than rejection.

Not every relationship will welcome your authenticity. But you'll increasingly choose relationships that nourish rather than deplete.

The eating difficulties that brought you to this book were never just about food. They were about the split between your authentic self and the self you had to become to stay safe. As you heal that split—as you learn not to abandon yourself—the need for eating behaviours to communicate, control, or comfort naturally lessens.

Your Lost Child is safe now. Your relationships are becoming real. And you—the wise inner leader of your own ship—are learning to navigate with both strength and openness, both boundaries and connection, both self-care and genuine intimacy.

You're learning to be yourself, to be seen more clearly, and to belong first within yourself, and then with others who can welcome the real you. This is how recovery ripples outward. This is how life becomes your own.

Gentle Experiments to Try

1: Relationship Mindset Awareness

Three times this week, when you notice difficult feelings in a relationship, pause: Which schema mindset might be activated? What is this blueprint predicting will happen? Is this prediction based on past patterns or current reality?

2: Protector Mode Recognition in Relationships

When relationship challenges arise, notice which mode activates: Overcontroller trying to prove you don't need anyone? Surrenderer hoping someone will notice without you asking? Detached Protector numbing or withdrawing? Name it with compassion: "My [mode] is trying to protect me. Thank you, but my Wise Self has this."

3: Internal Partnership before External Communication

Before important conversations, connect with your Lost Child first: What am I actually feeling? What do I truly need? How can I communicate this authentically and kindly? Then communicate from this grounded place.

4: The Hardware Store Assessment

Choose two to three important relationships and honestly assess: What can this person/relationship realistically offer? What am I seeking here that isn't available? Where else might I find that particular emotional vitamin? Adjust your expectations accordingly.

5: Anger as Information

If anger arises (even quiet, underground anger), practise curiosity: What boundary might have been crossed? What does my emotional immune system want me to know? How can I express this in a way that protects me rather than turning it inwards?

6: Small Boundary Practice

Set one small boundary this week: Check with Lost Child about what feels right. Communicate it clearly and kindly. Maintain it even if there's disappointment. Notice: The world doesn't end when I prioritise my needs.

Weekly Journalling Reflection: Relationship Authenticity

Over time, you'll notice shifts in how you show up in relationships. Each week, take a few minutes to journal two or three of these questions. Dating each entry lets you look back and see patterns you might miss day-to-day.

Journalling Prompt Reflections

- **The Longing–Fear Tension**: When relationship discomfort arises, notice the part of you that longs to be seen and the part that fears being seen. Both come from history and both are valid. The task is simply asking: *Which part needs my Wise Self's support so I can stay present without abandoning myself?*

- Which relationship magnet (Familiar-Pain, Rescue-Fantasy, or Proof-Seeking) do you recognise most in your relationship history?
- What "hardware store" have you been asking for "bread" from? What can that person actually offer?
- When you set a boundary this week, what did your Inner Critic say? How did your Wise Self respond?
- Do you recognise yourself in the Overcontroller, Helpless Protector, or People Pleaser pattern? When have you communicated needs indirectly rather than authentically?

Why this matters: Your Protector Modes need evidence that an authentic connection is possible without self-abandonment. This weekly check-in creates that evidence trail—showing both you and your Protector parts that you're building genuine capacity to stay true to yourself whilst staying in a relationship.

When you're struggling, flip back through previous entries. You'll often find you're navigating relationship challenges now that would have completely derailed you weeks ago. You're learning to be both connected and authentic—something your Lost Child has been longing for all along.

What Comes Next

You've transformed your internal world—building security between your Wise Self and Lost Child. You've learned to change eating behaviours through compassion rather than control. And now you've begun transforming your external relationships, learning to connect authentically whilst maintaining healthy boundaries.

But there's one more essential piece: discovering who you actually are beneath all the protective layers. Your true self—the person you were always meant to be—has been waiting patiently for conditions safe enough to emerge.

Chapter 10 will guide you in this discovery: learning to shift from self-surveillance to self-connection, from performing for others to being present in your own experience. You'll explore your genuine values, interests, and preferences. You'll learn to reclaim play as a pathway to your authentic self, and to work with your natural temperament as a strength rather than a flaw.

The secure relationships you're building—both internally and externally—create the foundation for this exploration. Your Lost Child can finally reveal what she really loves, what brings her joy, what matters most—because she trusts your Wise Self will honour those truths.

You've been preparing for this throughout the entire book. The authentic self you're seeking isn't something you need to create or earn—it's something you need to remember and reclaim.

You're ready for what comes next.

10 Discovering Your Authentic Self

Reclaiming the Person Beneath the Performance

> *Go confidently in the direction of your dreams. Live the life you have imagined.*
> —adapted from Henry David Thoreau, *Walden* (1854) (28)

Opening: A Question That Begins to Shift Things

 Melissa sits across from her therapist. She's been in recovery for six months now, eating more regularly, attending sessions, and doing the work. But today, a new concern surfaces.

> "I realised something this week," she says, voice steady but distant.
> I don't actually know who I am without my eating disorder or what I want. Not what I should want, not what would make my parents happy, not what would be the 'right' thing. I just feel like I rely on other people to tell me who I am or what I need.
> She pauses. "I don't think anyone ever asked me. I don't even know if there is a 'me' underneath the layers."

Her therapist responds: "That makes sense. You've had to look outward, to predict others' reactions and become who you think they need you to be. Recovery is about looking inwards and remembering that 'Little You' who's been lost under the layers of protection."

Melissa feels an old sadness. A long-forgotten part of her feels heard. She's spent 28 years learning to be what others needed her to be. She became excellent at it—the daughter who never caused problems, the employee who exceeded expectations, and the friend who always had time to help. But somewhere in all that careful adaptation, the person she actually was got lost.

There had been hundreds of moments that carried the message her voice was "too much." When she was 12, she'd tried to tell her mother she needed more support. Her aunt overheard. "You shouldn't be so selfish," her aunt said disapprovingly. "Your mother has sacrificed so much for you."

That wasn't the first time Melissa learned her voice didn't matter. It was just the clearest. There had been countless smaller moments—times when no one asked what she thought, when her feelings weren't taken into account, and

DOI: 10.4324/9781003355878-11

when care came without emotional understanding. Her family loved her; she knew that. They just didn't know how to see her.

The restrictive eating had started not long after. If she couldn't take up space emotionally, she'd stop taking up space physically, too. Make herself smaller in every way that mattered.

Now, sitting in this therapy room, Melissa finds herself facing a different question: Do these old patterns—the silence, the smallness, the constant accommodation of others—do they still serve her? Or can she learn something new?

"I think," Melissa says slowly, "I think I want to find out who I actually am. Even if that disappoints people. Even if it means risking everything I've built by being so careful."

Her therapist nods. "That's the work—learning to turn inward to find out who you've always been underneath the performance of the Protector Modes."

For years, Melissa had been adjusting her sails to catch others' wind—trimming herself to fit their expectations, tacking away from her own course to avoid their disapproval. Now she was learning how to sail by her own compass, trusting her internal navigation even when others questioned her direction.

Part 1: The Performance You Didn't Know You Were Giving

Melissa isn't alone in this disconnection. Most people with eating difficulties eventually face the same realisation: somewhere along the way, they stopped being themselves and started performing a version that felt safer, more acceptable, less likely to be rejected.

For Melissa, the performance looked like being invisible—never stating preferences, never expressing needs, and making herself small both literally and metaphorically.

For 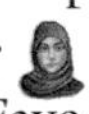 Faye, the performance looked different but served the same function. Faye had been a playful, spontaneous child who loved to sing and dance. But her family couldn't hold that energy. Her mother was ill, her father stressed with work—there was no space for joy. Her brothers mocked her spontaneity. When her best friend moved away and boys at school made fun of her acne, her mother tried to help through distraction rather than emotional attunement. Faye learned: emotions, especially intense ones like grief or joy, made her family uncomfortable. Better to stay pleasant, controlled, and acceptable.

So Faye learned to perform pleasantness, keeping her energy contained, her emotions managed, and her authentic self carefully hidden. The bingeing managed all the feelings she'd learned to keep hidden—anger at being overlooked, sadness about growing up emotionally alone, and fear that showing her real self would be too much.

Both women had created performances. Melissa performed by disappearing. Faye performed by seeming fine whilst using food in secret. Neither realised they were performing. The roles felt like just who they were.

Only now, years into these patterns, could they see the gap between the person they'd become and the person they actually were underneath.

Part 2: The Risk of Having a Voice

Melissa's first boundary felt impossible. From early childhood, her family had opinions about her eating. Their involvement felt suffocating, but Melissa couldn't say so. Saying so would make her ungrateful.

But as she strengthened the relationship between her Wise Self and her Lost Child, Melissa began to realise that recovery couldn't belong to her if she was just complying with everyone else's expectations. She needed to make the healing actually hers.

> So she set a boundary. She invited her parents over and, heart pounding, said: "I love you both. I know you've worked hard to help me. But I don't want our relationship to be about food anymore. I'm working with my treatment team on eating, and I need that part of my recovery to be private. I'd rather we talk about other things—your lives, mine, anything that isn't calories or portions."

The silence felt endless. Her mother's face went tight. "We're just trying to help. We thought you'd appreciate that we care."

"I do appreciate it," Melissa said, even as panic flooded her body. "But I need this to be different."

Over the next few weeks, her parents withdrew. Texts became shorter. Phone calls were less frequent.

The urge to restrict came back hard. Her Helpless Protector: If you just get smaller, maybe they'll see you.

Her therapist had taught her a technique: using your own name when talking to yourself creates psychological distance from overwhelming emotions, allowing your Wise Self to respond rather than being swept away.

She tried it: "Melissa, you're feeling their disapproval and it's activating your old survival pattern. That makes sense. But does making yourself smaller actually fix this? Or does it just repeat the old cycle where you disappear to keep others comfortable?"

Using her name helped her step back from the flood of feeling to see the pattern clearly.

The Old Mindset versus the Growth Mindset

Melissa's therapist helped her map the difference:

Old Schema Mindset (Emotional Deprivation/Subjugation)

- My needs are a burden on others.
- If I express what I want, I'm selfish.
- The only way to be loved is to be invisible.
- If people are upset with me, I've done something wrong.

Growth Mindset (Healthy Autonomy/Connection)

- My needs are valid and deserve attention.
- Expressing what I want is how people can actually know me.
- Being loved means being seen for who I really am.
- If people are upset with my boundaries, they're adjusting to change.

The old mindset had helped her make sense of the world when she was young and genuinely dependent. But now it was keeping her trapped in a performance that left her fundamentally alone.

The growth mindset felt terrifying—it meant risking disapproval, rejection, and the possibility of being too much. But it also offered something the old pattern never could: the possibility of being really known.

For more examples of Schema and Growth mindsets, see Appendix 22.

Part 3: When Others Struggle with Your Authenticity

Melissa continued practising. When her parents wanted her home for a family dinner but she had plans with friends, she said, "I already have plans that evening. Let's find another time."

Her mother's voice went cold. "Well. I suppose your friends are more important than family."

Melissa felt the familiar panic but used her name again: "Mel, this is the old pattern trying to pull you back. Your mother is uncomfortable with your boundary, and she's trying to make you responsible for her discomfort. But you're not abandoning anyone by having your own life."

Two days later, her mother texted: "Saturday lunch? If you're free." No apology. No acknowledgement. But also, an invitation. The relationship didn't end. It bent, adjusted, and learned to accommodate Melissa actually having boundaries.

This is what Melissa was discovering: some people in your life are attached to your performance, not your authenticity. When you stop performing, they struggle. They might withdraw. They might guilt-trip. They might try to pull you back into old patterns.

Their discomfort doesn't mean you're doing something wrong. It means they're adjusting to you actually being a person with needs and preferences, not just a supporting character in their lives. Some relationships will adjust. Others won't. And learning to tolerate that uncertainty—without immediately shrinking yourself to ease others' discomfort—is part of recovery.

Part 4: When Your Lost Child Speaks

As Melissa continued the daily dialogue with her Lost Child—asking what she needed, listening to her answers—she noticed her Lost Child had her own opinions—strong ones.

She didn't just want less time at work. She had specific ideas about what she wanted to be doing instead. She wanted time in nature. She wanted to draw. She wanted to write—not reports for work, but poetry, the kind Melissa had loved as a teenager and abandoned because it seemed impractical.

So Melissa started. Just 15 minutes some evenings, writing whatever came. No agenda, no performance, no one to please. What emerged surprised her. Her Lost Child had a voice—clear, full of images and metaphors that her analytical mind never would have generated. She wrote about water, about cold lakes and skin tingling. She wrote about the blue mass in her chest and how it was beginning to shift, becoming less solid, more like something that could move through her.

She wrote about her family, about loving them and also grieving what she'd never received. How both things could be true at once. How letting go of the fantasy of getting something retroactively didn't mean cutting them off—it just meant accepting reality and finding what she needed elsewhere.

Through writing, through drawing, Melissa discovered the intuitive wisdom her Lost Child had been holding. A knowing that didn't come from analysing but from a deeper place. A sense of what felt right versus what felt like it should.

This was her true self speaking. Not the person who performed for others, not the person who tried to anticipate what everyone needed. But the person she actually was beneath all that adaptation. And the more she listened, the clearer that voice became.

Part 5: The Missing Piece—Play as Pathway to Your Authentic Self

One day in session, Melissa's therapist asked her to reflect on her Contented Child: "What did you love to do as a child? Before the messages came that changed everything—what brought you pure joy?"

Melissa sat with the question. The answer felt distant, like trying to remember a dream. "I liked making things," she said finally. "I'd build elaborate structures with whatever I could find—sticks, boxes, stones. I'd spend hours arranging them, making little worlds. And I loved being outside. I'd lie in the grass and watch clouds, make up stories about where they were going."

"When did you stop?" her therapist asked. Melissa thought. "Maybe ten? Eleven? My family started saying things like, 'Shouldn't you be doing your homework?' or 'That's a waste of time.' Everything became about being productive, about achievement. Play felt . . . childish. Pointless."

She paused. "But it wasn't just that play seemed unimportant. It started to feel shameful. Like there was something wrong with me for wasting time on things that didn't matter. I felt guilty every time I wanted to just . . . be."

"What happened when you felt that shame and guilt?" her therapist asked. "I stopped," Melissa reflected. "I didn't choose to stop playing. It's more like . . . I couldn't bear feeling ashamed every time I wanted to do something

I enjoyed. The guilt was so heavy. So parts of me found other ways to cope—ways to feel something that didn't trigger that shame."

Her therapist suggested. "I'm wondering . . . when the restrictive eating started, what did it give you? Not what it took away, but what was missing for you at that time that it provided?"

Melissa hesitated, then began exploring: Control when everything else felt chaotic. Achievement when she couldn't seem to get things right elsewhere. A way of showing how much she was hurting without having to say anything. Proof she wasn't greedy or selfish or too much. Something that was hers—her choice, her rules—when everything else belonged to other people. Purpose and focus when she felt lost about who she was supposed to be. Relief from overwhelming feelings.

Her therapist leaned in. "So the eating disorder wasn't just replacing play with one thing. It was trying to meet multiple needs and provide multiple protections all at once?" "Yes," Melissa said, as she started to recognise that these behaviours had been doing so much, filling so many holes, protecting her in so many ways."

"But they weren't playful anymore, were they?" her therapist suggested. "There was no spontaneity, no experimentation, no room for mistakes or mystery. Just rules."

Melissa nodded slowly. She hadn't chosen to replace joy with control. She'd survived the only way she could—by developing Protector Modes that found multiple ways to protect her from unbearable shame and guilt, whilst also attempting to meet the needs that weren't being met anywhere else.

The Function of Play in Recovery

As with so many people with eating difficulties, for Melissa the transition from being a playful child into a life dominated by eating disorder behaviours was one aspect of how she learned to survive.

As you will recall from Chapter 1, play and spontaneity are core emotional 'vitamins' essential for wellbeing. But when authentic joy became tangled with shame and guilt—when spontaneity felt childish, pleasure felt selfish, and play felt silly—your system had to find another way to channel those needs. Your Protector Modes shaped these substitutes. The Overcontroller turns play into productivity—movement becomes calorie-burning rather than joy. The Approval Seeker demands achievement—swimming can't be for fun, it has to be impressive. The Detached Self-Soother uses activities to escape—bingeing becomes a distorted "treat," while restriction offers pride through self-denial.

Real play—the kind that reconnects you with your authentic self—has very different qualities. It's done for its own sake, without an outcome to prove. It involves spontaneity and responding to what feels right in the moment. It allows for silliness, mistakes, and not caring how you look. It's experimental—trying things simply to see what happens. And it connects you to your body through sensation and aliveness, not control or punishment. Above all, it's free from obligation—you're not doing it because you *should*.

Cultural Messages and Reclaiming Play

Part of what makes reclaiming play difficult is recognising the cultural mindsets that taught you it was wrong. Melissa's family operated from perpetual productivity: time not spent achieving was time wasted. Faye's family carried a different message: emotions—especially joy—were uncomfortable and potentially disruptive.

These early lessons are often reinforced by broader cultural narratives: productivity culture (worth equals output), perfectionism (if you're not excellent, why bother?), emotional inhibition (strong emotions are inappropriate), appearance management (everything should enhance how you look), achievement orientation (experiences only matter if they produce something), and subjugation or self-sacrifice (you shouldn't enjoy yourself when others are struggling).

One schema mindset that particularly interferes with play is the Unrelenting Standards schema. It operates on the belief that anything worth doing must be done efficiently, excellently, and with visible results. Play—by its nature—breaks these rules. It's messy, inefficient, and often produces nothing tangible.

If you grew up with Unrelenting Standards, you may have learned that activities are only acceptable if they improve you measurably, demonstrate discipline, or lead to something you can show others. Under these conditions, play becomes impossible. You can't play the piano for fun—it must improve your skill. You can't draw for pleasure—it must be good enough to display. Movement can't be joyful—it has to "count" as exercise.

Your Overcontroller enforces these standards, turning potential play into performance: *Am I doing this right? Am I good at this? What's the point if I'm not?*

Recovery involves recognising this pattern and deliberately choosing activities where being mediocre—or even terrible—is allowed, and where the only measure of success is whether you enjoyed yourself.

Questions for Your Own Play Exploration

Looking Back: What did you love as a child? What games or stories absorbed you? Where did you feel free? When was the last time you felt genuinely playful?

If you draw a blank here, you're not alone. Some people had to be "grown up" very early—vigilant, responsible, or performing from childhood. This doesn't mean your Contented Child doesn't exist; it means she never had the conditions to emerge. She's still there, waiting for safety and permission.

For you, your task may be to discover play for the first time.

Looking at Patterns: How did messages from family, school, or culture shape your relationship with play? When did duty replace spontaneity?

Looking Forward: What would your Inner Child parts want to do now, just for fun? What feels playful, even if it seems pointless? What small rule could you break to taste freedom?

See Appendix 23 for ways to reclaim play in your life.

Practical Play Experiments

Recovery involves practical experiments in reclaiming play—small moments of breaking the rules that have imprisoned you.

Melissa started with 15 minutes on Saturday mornings. No plans, no agenda—just time to follow whatever impulse arose. She found herself drawing—badly, messily, without any goal. Just marks on paper. It felt strange, almost transgressive. But underneath the discomfort was something else: a small flutter of aliveness.

Faye's play experiments looked different. She started dancing in her flat when no one could see. Not choreographed or trying to look good—just moving however her body wanted to move. The first time, she cried. All those years of being mocked for her spontaneity, for her joy—they came flooding back. But she kept dancing, reclaiming something that had been taken from her.

She also started doing small rebellious things: walking barefoot on grass, blowing bubbles in the garden (yes, as an adult), flying a kite, playing beach tennis with a friend and keeping no score, visiting botanical gardens just to wander, lying under a tree watching the canopy, and looking up at clouds.

Each act felt like breaking a rule. And each one opened a little more space for her authentic self to emerge.

Music as a Doorway to Your Happy Child

For many people, play starts with sound. Music can be one of the safest ways to reach your Contented Child—and it's deeply personal. The songs you connect with might feel too intimate to share at first. That's okay. This part of recovery is about freedom to be and express yourself, not performance.

You get to choose your own music without justifying your choices or making them "healthy." If a song feels important and you'd rather keep it private, respect that boundary.

Instead of asking "What does this song mean emotionally?" start with "What is it about this music that you like?" You might be drawn to the instrumentation, the rhythm, the structure, the tone, the cultural connections. If you have an Emotional Inhibition schema, you might prefer concrete terms: "I like how the drums sound" rather than "This makes me feel sad." Both are valid expressions of your Contented Child.

The key is creating space to talk about music in your own way—without pressure to "go deeper" before you're ready. Curiosity itself—being absorbed, interested, gently fascinated—is part of the Contented Child Mode.

Let music be play, not a task. Notice how your body feels when you hear something you love. Allow your Contented Child to be absorbed, interested, comforted, moved—even if you don't yet have words for why.

You're using music to create conditions where the Contented Child can safely appear.

The Connection between Play and Eating Recovery

Melissa discovered that as she allowed more play into her life, her relationship with food shifted. The substitute pleasures she'd found in restriction—the pride, the control, the sense of achievement—began to pale when she allowed herself authentic joy. Play was meeting needs for spontaneity, to exist without constant evaluation, to experience aliveness in her body, through genuine engagement.

Faye discovered something similar: regular meals became easier when she was experiencing real satisfaction in other areas of her life. The binge urges decreased when she was genuinely filling herself—not with food as a substitute for pleasure, but with actual experiences of connection, creativity, aliveness.

Play matters in recovery because it's a pathway back to your authentic self, the self that knows what true nourishment—emotional and physical—actually feels like. When you reconnect with play, you're reconnecting with your Contented Child—the part of you that understands inherent worth, that doesn't need to earn the right to exist, that knows joy is a fundamental human need, not something you have to prove you deserve.

Part 6: Working with Your Natural Temperament as Strength

Like waves in the sea, we each have a different rhythm and force. The work isn't to become a different wave, but to stop fighting the one you are.

Remember the temperament traits from Chapter 2? Environmental Sensitivity, Emotionality, Effortful Control, and Novelty-Seeking. Your eating disorder harnessed these traits, forcing your natural design into shapes that served survival but cost you authenticity.

How Eating Disorders Distort Your Natural Traits

Depending on the early messages we receive in cultural, family and educational settings, temperament traits can be the following:

- **Suppressed** by modes that numb sensation or eliminate spontaneity
- **Overdeveloped** into hypervigilance, dysregulation, or rigid perfectionism
- **Integrated** as a healthy perception, deep feeling, intentional choice, or genuine curiosity

Faye's natural temperament included high Environmental Sensitivity, Emotionality, and Novelty-Seeking—the playful child who loved to sing and dance. But when her family couldn't hold her intensity, her Detached Protector numbed sensitivity and emotions, whilst her Overcontroller eliminated spontaneity. Her high Novelty-Seeking couldn't stay suppressed—it erupted through chaotic bingeing.

Melissa's temperament looked different: high Environmental Sensitivity, high Effortful Control, but lower Novelty-Seeking. She naturally preferred routine—perfectly healthy for her design. But her Overcontroller turned sensitivity into hypervigilance and harnessed her natural discipline into perfectionism and self-punishment.

Notice how their integration work differs because their temperament profiles differ. Your work will be unique to your specific configuration.

Why Sensitivity and Emotionality Need Regulation

If you're highly sensitive and/or emotional, you have raw ingredients for deep empathy—but without adequate regulation capacity, these traits become overwhelming. Sensitivity turns into drowning in others' emotions. Emotional intensity becomes self-focused anxiety and rumination.

The good news is that your *Effortful Control "muscle" can grow.* This is about developing the capacity to guide yourself with both kindness and firmness, the way you'd guide a child you care deeply about.

What Effortful Control Helps You Do

- Motivate yourself toward meaningful goals
- Manage impulsivity—pausing between urge and action
- Work with resistant Child Modes—gently encouraging your Undisciplined Child, setting limits with your Impulsive Child
- Build a structure that supports rather than imprisons

When Past Control Creates Backlash

If you grew up with excessive control, your system may have developed a subjugation schema. Now, any structure feels like oppression. Your Angry or Rebellious Child might respond to even healthy self-discipline with: "No one tells me what to do anymore!"

This rebellion made sense when fighting for autonomy against controlling others. But now it's fighting against you, trying to care for yourself. Recovery means helping this part understand: "I'm not your controlling parent/teacher/coach. I'm trying to help you build genuine freedom—which requires some structure."

Effortful Control as Care, Not Control

With your *Undisciplined Child* (who wants to give up when things are hard): You wouldn't berate her. You'd offer gentle encouragement: "I know this is hard. Let's do it together. I'll stay with you."

With your *Impulsive Child* (who wants immediate gratification): You wouldn't shame her impulses. You'd offer a pause: "I hear you want that right now. Let's take a breath and think this through."

With your *Angry/Rebellious Child* (who refuses guidance): You wouldn't match defiance with force. You'd acknowledge autonomy whilst offering wisdom: "You absolutely have the right to choose. And I'm here to help you choose things that serve you."

This is Effortful Control as self-integration—learning to skilfully welcome back all parts without losing inner wisdom.

Different Temperaments, Different Needs

If You Have High Novelty-Seeking (like Faye): Your Impulsive Child might leap without thinking. Your work involves gently pausing before acting, building enough structure without killing spontaneity.

If You Have Low Novelty-Seeking (like Melissa): Your system naturally prefers routine. Your work involves gently encouraging yourself to try new experiences, building in time for spontaneity (which doesn't come naturally).

We're not trying to change your temperament—we're helping your natural pattern work for you, not against you—to strengthen the under-developed parts of you. Faye doesn't need to become inflexible, and Melissa doesn't need to become impulsive.

Building Connection through Empathy

This empathic capacity creates connection in both directions:

With Your Lost Child: You can feel what she needs, stay present with her pain, and comfort her without being overwhelmed. This internal connection becomes the foundation for regulation.

With Others: You can sense what they're feeling, respond with care, offer support, while maintaining your centre and protecting your wellbeing.

Both build resilience. When you can stay connected through difficult emotions, you develop natural regulation capacity. You don't need eating disorder behaviours because you've built internal and relational resources that actually work.

See Appendix 24 for understanding and working with your temperament profile.

Part 7: When the Body Carries What You Cannot Hold

Sometimes the feelings your Lost Child can't safely express take up residence in your body. When emotions feel too risky, too shameful, or too overwhelming to acknowledge, they often slip beneath awareness and reappear as sensations, body-focused distress, or intense body criticism.

Understanding the Split

You learned in Chapter 3 how your Lost Child can become banished below deck when her emotions feel too risky. Sometimes this split takes a specific form: your Lost Child gets banished from awareness by using eating behaviours to cut off from the place they live—your body.

 Sophie's story illustrates this pattern. As a child, when she cried or expressed needs, she was met with dismissal: "Oh Sophie, you're being too sensitive." Slowly, she learned that some of her feelings were unacceptable. She pushed them into the shadows, telling herself: *that's not me.*

But the "not-me" doesn't simply vanish. For Sophie, those hidden feelings—fear, anger, neediness—took up residence in her body. When she looked in the mirror, she didn't just see her reflection, all of the past rejections, shame and humiliation she had absorbed were blamed on her body—the curve of her stomach, the roundness of her face, the softness of her thighs.

The feelings she couldn't bear to hold in her mind were pushed onto her body. Her body became the scapegoat, visible proof of the defectiveness and shame she feared.

How Protector Modes Create the Split

When Protector Modes use eating behaviours to split off from the Lost Child with all her shame and guilt, they do this by disconnecting you from your inner body experience. The body, which houses your most tender feelings, is transformed from being part of "me" to being "not-me" (8)—something foreign that can be controlled, blamed, and punished.

This disconnection serves a specific purpose: it protects your attachments with other people. Rather than risk having your vulnerable feelings rejected again, your Protector Modes relocate them to your body where they can be targeted, and "fixed."

Remember from Chapter 3 how different modes work together:

- The Lost Child carries the raw pain but gets banished "below deck" and into the body.
- The Inner Critic attacks the body as a way of attacking the unwanted feelings.
- The Overcontroller uses eating behaviours to punish the body for carrying these emotions.
- The Detached Protector helps you disconnect from your physical self so you won't feel the pain that lives there.

Exercise: Listening Beneath "I Feel Fat"

This practice helps you use the skills from Chapter 6 to notice when body-hating thoughts are really an attempt to cut off from the pain and shame of your rejected Lost Child.

Step 1: Catch the Thought

Next time you notice yourself thinking "I feel fat" or "My body is disgusting," pause. Use your Wise Observer skill from Chapter 5: notice the thought without immediately reacting.

Step 2: Translate the Message

Ask yourself: "If this wasn't about my body, what might it be about?"
Could "I feel fat" really mean my Lost Child feels:

- Ashamed about something that happened?
- Angry but unable to express it?
- Overwhelmed by responsibilities?
- Needy and afraid to ask for help?
- Unsafe in some way?

Step 3: Meet the Lost Child You Fear

Visualise your Lost Child who has been living in your body, carrying these feelings. What does this part look like? What are they feeling?

Really tune into your Lost Child in your body and ask: what do you really need right now?

Step 4: Respond as Your Wise Self

Instead of punishing your body, use the reparenting messages you learned:

> "I hear how ashamed you feel. You don't need to hide in my body anymore." "It makes sense that you feel unwanted right now. I'm here to bring you back." "You don't have to live in the shadows. Your feelings are welcome with me. There is nothing wrong with you."

Step 5: Return to Your Body Gently

Use your grounding practices: place a hand on your heart or stomach. Use the cyclic sigh breath. Remind yourself: *My body is home to my Lost Child and I can care for both.*

Reflection for Journalling

- What did "I feel fat" really mean today?
- What was my Lost Child trying to tell me?
- Which schema might have been activated (from Chapter 2)?
- How did it feel to welcome this part back instead of blaming and punishing my body for past experiences of shame, humiliation, and rejection?

Breaking the Cycle: Body as Home, Not Prison

Healing begins when we see the body not as an enemy, but as the home where our Lost Child has been living in hiding. Each moment of body criticism can become an invitation to ask: "What is my Lost Child trying to tell me? What old memories is this linked to? What does she need?"

This is the integration work of recovery—welcoming back the parts of yourself that were rejected or criticised. As you practise this gentle reunion between your modes, something begins to change. The "not-me" slowly becomes part of "me" again. What once lived as "bad body" is revealed as the Lost Child whose needs are in fact normal, and who deserved care all along.

What body image work can do:

- Recognise when body hatred is really emotional pain in disguise
- Respond to your Lost Child's needs rather than punishing your body
- Gradually develop more compassion toward your physical self
- Reduce the intensity and frequency of body-focused distress
- Build tolerance for body sensations and changes

What this work cannot do: It won't necessarily make you love your body or eliminate all body image struggles. Recovery doesn't require you to love how you look—it requires learning to care for your body whilst you're building that relationship.

Your body is learning to be home rather than prison. Some days it will feel like an ally; other days it will feel like a stranger. Both experiences are part of the journey.

Part 8: The Future You're Building Toward

About a year into recovery, Melissa had a moment that caught her off guard.

She was sitting at a café with a friend—someone she'd met through a writing group she'd joined a few months earlier. They were talking about nothing particularly important: books they'd read, places they wanted to visit, the absurdity of a recent news story.

Mid-conversation, Melissa had a sudden realisation: she was enjoying herself. Not performing enjoyment, not monitoring whether she was being interesting enough or saying the right things. Just . . . enjoying being there.

Her friend laughed at something she'd said, and Melissa felt warmth spread through her chest. Instead of the tight, anxious warmth of needing approval, there was something easier. Connection without effort.

Later that day, she wrote in her journal: "Today I forgot to judge myself. For maybe twenty minutes, I just . . . was. And it didn't feel wrong."

Not a dramatic transformation or sudden self-love. Just a brief window where she could exist without constant evaluation—and recognise that this was recovery too.

Values as Your Guide

Throughout this book, you've been learning to distinguish between living from your authentic values versus living from old schema-driven beliefs. This distinction becomes crucial as you build your future.

Schema-driven "shoulds" sound like:

- I should be thin/smaller/taking up less space.
- I should always put others first.
- I should be productive at all times.
- I should handle everything on my own.
- I should be perfect or not bother trying.
- I should earn the right to eat/rest/enjoy.

Real values sound like:

- I value creativity and making space for it in my life.
- I value genuine connection over surface-level approval.
- I value balance between work and rest.
- I value asking for help when I need it.
- I value growth over perfection.
- I value caring for myself because I matter.

Notice the difference? Schema-driven shoulds come with shame and criticism. Authentic values come with clarity and self-respect.

Building a Life Worth Living

Faye discovered her values through small experiments. She valued creativity—so she started painting again, shakily at first, but that wasn't the point. She valued meaningful work over status—so she took on pro bono architectural projects for community organisations. She valued authentic connection—so she started being honest with friends about her struggles instead of always playing the role of listener.

These choices didn't cure her eating difficulties overnight. But they created a life worth showing up for. A life where bingeing felt increasingly like an interruption rather than the main event.

Melissa's values led her differently. She valued solitude and reflection—so she protected time for writing even when it felt unproductive. She valued honesty—so she started speaking her actual opinions even when it risked disappointing people. She valued her body's wisdom—so she began listening to hunger and tiredness instead of overriding them.

Her eating became more regular, because she was learning to trust her body as a source of valid information. Not always, not perfectly—but more often than before.

The Question That Taps into Your True Self

As you move forward, return regularly to this question: *Am I living from my values or from my old schema mindsets?*

When you're making decisions about food, ask: Is this choice coming from my Wise Self's values (nourishment, self-care, listening to my body) or from my Protector Modes' fears (control, punishment, earning the right to eat)?

When you're making decisions about relationships, ask: Is this choice honouring my value of authentic connection, or is my People Pleaser trying to earn care or approval?

When you're making decisions about how to spend time, ask: Is this aligned with what matters to me, or am I following old "shoulds" about productivity and achievement?

You won't always get it right. Sometimes your Protector Modes will take over before you even notice. Sometimes you'll realise hours later that you've been operating from schema-land rather than your authentic self.

The practice is about noticing, returning, choosing again.

Your Values Exploration: Take time to identify what genuinely matters to you, as opposed to old schemas-mindsets. Consider these areas:

Relationships: What kind of connections do you want? Surface-level pleasantness or messy authenticity? Many relationships or a few deep ones? What does genuine intimacy mean to you?

Work/Contribution: What feels meaningful beyond achievement? How do you want to contribute? What would you do even if no one praised you for it?

Self-Care: What does caring for yourself look like? Not what you "should" do, but what actually nourishes you. What does your body need? What does your mind need? What feeds your spirit?

Creativity/Play: What brings you alive? What would you do just for the joy of it? What did you love before you learned to be productive?

Growth: What kind of person do you want to become? Not perfect—but authentic, compassionate, brave in your own way?

See Appendix 25 for support with clarifying your own authentic values.

Living Your Values in Small Ways

You don't need to make dramatic changes to start living from your values. Small choices matter.

If you value real connection, that might mean texting a friend and sharing authentic vulnerability: "I'm struggling today" instead of "Fine, thanks!"

If you value creativity, that might mean 15 minutes of drawing before bed instead of scrolling social media.

If you value your body's wisdom, that might mean eating lunch even though your Overcontroller says you should skip it.

If you value growth, that might mean trying something you're not good at yet—and tolerating the discomfort of being a beginner.

Each small choice is a vote for the person you're becoming. Each time you choose from your values instead of your schemas, you're strengthening that neural pathway, making it easier next time.

The future you're building is about learning to live as your authentic self—messy, imperfect, real—more days than not.

Part 9: Practising Daily Authenticity

Recovery is about small, consistent choices that gradually become your new normal. Here are practices for living more authentically each day:

Morning: Who Am I Today?

Before your Protector Modes fully activate, spend three minutes connecting with yourself:

- Place your hand on your heart.
- Ask: "How am I actually feeling right now?" (Not how you should feel—how you do feel)
- Ask: "What does my Lost Child need today?"
- Ask: "What does living *my* life from *my* values look like today?"

This is about beginning the day connected to yourself—belonging to yourself—rather than immediately launching into performance mode.

Throughout the Day: The Authenticity Check

Set three gentle reminders to pause and ask: "Am I being myself right now, or in a Protector Mode?"

Notice without judgement. If you've been performing, that's useful information. Can you make one small shift toward authenticity in the next moment?

Maybe that means saying "Actually, I'd prefer . . ." instead of going along with what others want. Maybe it means admitting you don't know something instead of pretending. Maybe it means taking a break when you're tired instead of pushing through.

Small authenticity builds capacity for larger authenticity.

Evening: Compassionate Reflection

Before sleep, reflect:

- When did I show up as myself today? (Celebrate this, even if brief)
- When did my Protector Modes take over? (Notice without criticism)
- What does my Lost Child want me to know about today?
- What's one thing I can do tomorrow that would honour my values?

Write brief notes if helpful. But the practice itself—the gentle checking in—matters more than documenting everything.

Weekly Practice: The Alignment Check

Once a week, take 20 minutes to review:

- Which of my current activities/relationships/commitments align with my values?
- Which feel like obligations or performances?
- What's one thing I could add that would nourish my authentic self?
- What's one thing I could let go of that's primarily serving old schema mindsets?

Noticing the gap between how you're living and what you value creates space for gradual shifts.

Part 10: Faye's Parallel Journey

Whilst Melissa was discovering her voice through boundaries and play, Faye was travelling a different path to the same destination.

Faye's bingeing had been her way of managing the enormous loneliness of never being fully seen. In recovery, she had to face what the bingeing was protecting her from: grief about all those years performing pleasantness whilst her true self suffocated.

Through therapy, Faye learned to hold this grief without immediately numbing it. She practised staying present with loneliness—feeling the tightness in her throat, the heaviness in her chest—without rushing to fix it. And slowly, the loneliness became more bearable when she made space for it—"sitting on the fence" with her Lost Child—and stopped fighting it.

Finding Her Voice

Faye started small, admitting to friends when she was struggling instead of always playing the cheerful listener. She was certain they'd pull away, find her too much. They didn't. One friend said, "Thank you for trusting me with this. I had no idea." Another said, "I've wanted to share more with you, but you always seemed so sorted."

Faye realised she'd been creating the very isolation she feared—by never letting anyone see her actual self.

She started expressing opinions, saying no to social events when she needed solitude, pursuing activities she found interesting rather than activities that made her seem interesting. As she became more authentic in relationships, her bingeing decreased—not because she was following a perfect plan but because she was getting genuine connection.

Reclaiming Her Body

Faye practised the "Listening Beneath I Feel Fat" exercise. Each time body hatred surfaced, she'd pause and ask: "What is my Lost Child actually feeling?" Usually, it wasn't really about her body—it was about feeling rejected, overwhelmed, lonely, or invisible.

She also started treating her body with basic respect. Not love—which felt too far away. But respect. Feeding it regularly. Resting when tired. Moving in ways that felt good rather than punitive.

The Life She's Building

Two years into recovery, Faye still struggles sometimes with food and body image. But she also has friends who know her true self and love her for that, work she finds meaningful, creative practices that feed her spirit, and the capacity to feel lonely without immediately numbing it.

She's learning that authenticity isn't an end point but rather a daily practice—choosing yourself, over and over, even when uncomfortable. Most days she manages it, some days she doesn't. And increasingly, she's learning that this imperfect, messy practice is exactly what recovery looks like.

Closing: The Person You've Always Been

Both Melissa and Faye are discovering the same truth through different paths: your authentic self isn't something you need to create. It's something you need to re-member.

Underneath the performance, underneath the Protector Modes, underneath all the strategies you developed to stay safe and acceptable—there's a true self who's been waiting all along. Someone real—with her own preferences, quirks, sensitivities, and strengths. Someone who takes up space without apologising. Someone who feels deeply and expresses honestly. Someone who makes mistakes and keeps going anyway.

The more you can learn to accept all of your parts—not just the ones that make others comfortable—the more joined up you become—connecting you to the authentic, messy, imperfectly perfect, real you.

And learning to live as that person, more days than not, is what recovery ultimately means.

The eating disorder was never really about food or your body. It was about the enormous effort of trying to be someone other than yourself. The exhaustion of constant performance. The loneliness of never being fully seen.

Recovery is about finally coming home—to yourself, to your body, to the person you've always been beneath all the adaptation.

The journey continues. Some days, you'll forget everything you've learned and operate entirely from your Protector Modes. Some days you'll remember and choose differently. Both are part of the process.

Your Lost Child is learning that she can emerge from below deck. Your Wise Self is learning to captain the ship with both strength and compassion. Your Protector Modes are learning new roles that support rather than imprison you.

The sails are learning to work with your natural design instead of against it. And slowly, gradually, imperfectly—you're learning to be yourself.

That's the work. That's the practice. That's the life worth living.

Gentle Experiments to Try

Choose two to three that resonate:

Play Experiment: Spend 15 minutes doing something purely for fun with no outcome required. Notice what arises—joy, discomfort, guilt, freedom?

Temperament Noticing: Pay attention to when you're working with your natural temperament versus against it. Which temperament trait 'muscles' are overdeveloped and which could be strengthened? When do you feel most like yourself?

Value-Based Choice: Make one decision this week from your authentic values rather than schema-driven "shoulds." How does it feel?

Body-as-Home Practice: Next time body criticism arises, use the "Listening Beneath I Feel Fat" exercise. What is your Lost Child really trying to tell you?

Authenticity Check: At three points each day, pause and ask: "Am I being myself right now or performing?" Notice without judgement.

Boundary Practice: Set one small boundary that honours what you actually need rather than what you think others want from you.

Weekly Journalling Reflection

- What did I discover about my authentic self this week?
- When did I choose performance over authenticity? What was I protecting?
- When did I choose authenticity despite discomfort? How did that feel?
- What values am I living? What values am I not yet living?
- What does my Lost Child want me to know about becoming authentic?
- What's one small thing I could do next week that would honour my true self?

What Comes Next

You've learned to recognise your authentic self beneath the protective layers. You've begun reclaiming your voice, your values, and your right to take up space.

Chapter 11 addresses something we've touched on throughout but haven't fully explored: when your eating difficulties are connected to experiences of abuse or trauma. This chapter offers gentle, grounded approaches to processing these deeper wounds whilst staying connected to your recovery work.

Whether or not trauma is part of your story, Chapter 11 will help you understand how your body holds difficult experiences—and how to move forward with both wisdom and self-compassion.

11 Overcoming Trauma in Eating Disorders

Recovery is like learning to sail over waters that hold both calm moments and old storms. Your Wise Self keeps the boat steady, but growth begins in the moments when you stay with the inner waves that once felt too overwhelming to feel.

When Safety Meant Leaving Your Body Behind

Harriet's Storm

Harriet sits in the therapy room, her body perfectly still, her voice calm and measured as she describes her childhood. She appears composed, perhaps even detached. But her therapist notices the way Harriet speaks about her younger self as though she's describing a character in a film, the way she struggles to make eye contact, and uses phrases such as "the body" rather than "my body."

"The body just learned to go somewhere else," Harriet explains in a matter-of-fact way. "When things were happening, I felt like I was watching from a different place, like I wasn't really there. Does that make sense?"

Her reaction is completely understandable. Harriet grew up in a home where her parents were overwhelmed—working long hours to make ends meet, rarely home, stretched beyond their capacity. When they were present, they were hurried, preoccupied, and unable to slow down enough to attune to what Harriet needed emotionally. Her father would become overwhelmed when she cried, sometimes withdrawing for hours. Her mother would leave the room when Harriet tried to talk about feelings, appearing uncomfortable with emotional expression.

By the time Harriet was 12, she had absorbed some important messages about survival: her emotions felt too big for the adults around her to handle, her needs seemed to add burden to already-stressed caregivers, and expressing either risked losing what little connection she had. She had also come to understand that the adults in her life couldn't see her pain—not because they didn't care, but because they were so consumed by their own struggles that they had little capacity left to pay attention to hers.

When she experienced trauma at age 12, she had nowhere to turn. The adults in her life, however well-intentioned, hadn't been able to create space

DOI: 10.4324/9781003355878-12

for her internal experience. Expressing distress had led to uncomfortable responses—dismissal borne from overwhelm. So she did what her system had been preparing her to do: she disconnected from her own experience. She left her body behind and began to live somewhere safer—away from the pain of her Lost Child, in her head, in tasks, in the careful performance of being "fine."

The eating disorder came later, but it grew from this same soil. Her eating disorder became a way of managing a body that carried too much pain, a way of disconnecting from physical sensations that threatened to overwhelm her, a way of maintaining control over a vessel that no longer felt welcoming or safe.

The Difference between Struggle and Trauma

In earlier chapters, you've seen how eating difficulties can develop when emotional needs go unmet, when feelings become frightening, when the body becomes a target for displaced emotions. These patterns can create deep suffering even without experiences you might typically recognise as traumatic.

Trauma—whether a single overwhelming event or prolonged experiences of neglect, invalidation, or harm—can fundamentally alter your relationship with your own body. Trauma isn't just about what happened that shouldn't have. It's also about what didn't happen that should have: the protection, safety, attunement, autonomy, and freedom that every child deserves. Physical sensations themselves can become triggers signalling threat. Inhabiting your body can feel dangerous. Detaching from your physical self can become the only way to function.

Not everyone with an eating disorder has experienced trauma. And not everyone who has experienced trauma will develop an eating disorder. But when trauma and eating disorders intersect, the relationship between them requires specific understanding and care.

This chapter is for those of you who recognise that your eating difficulties are intertwined with traumatic experiences—whether those experiences were single catastrophic events, prolonged relational trauma, or developmental trauma in environments where you couldn't develop a secure sense of safety in your body or relationships.

If you're not sure whether trauma is part of your story, that's okay too. This chapter may help you understand patterns you've noticed, or it may simply be information you file away for later reflection with a therapist.

Before Continuing

This chapter discusses trauma and eating disorders in detail. If reading brings up overwhelming feelings, activates flashbacks, or makes you feel unsafe, pause and use your grounding practices from earlier chapters.

You might choose to skip ahead to "When You Need Professional Support" (Part 4) if you sense you need more help than self-help can provide right now. You can always return to earlier sections when you have more support in place.

Your Wise Self can decide what pace feels right. Your Overcontroller might want to speed through, or your Detached Protector might want to avoid entirely. Notice which part is guiding your choices, and respect the protection whilst also staying curious about what your system might need.

Part 1: Abandoning Ship—When Dissociation Was Survival

Let's return to our sailing metaphor, but this time imagine something more extreme than the storms we've discussed before.

Imagine your ship encountering waters so violent, weather so catastrophic, that staying aboard feels impossible. The deck is being torn apart. The vessel is taking on water faster than you can bail it out. Every moment you remain feels like it might be your last.

In this situation, what would you do? You might abandon ship. You might climb into a lifeboat and row away from the wreckage, watching from a safe distance as the storm continues to batter the vessel you once called home. You'd do this not because you wanted to leave your ship behind, but because leaving was the only way to survive.

Dissociation during trauma works this way. When experiences become too overwhelming to process, when staying present in your body feels too dangerous, when the pain threatens to destroy you, your mind adapts. It creates distance by helping you psychologically disconnect from your body (29). You might:

- Watch yourself from outside your body (depersonalisation)
- Experience events as though they're happening to someone else
- Have gaps in memory where traumatic experiences occurred
- Feel disconnected from physical sensations, as though your body belongs to someone else
- Go through daily life in a fog, never quite feeling fully present

Dissociation is a survival-based adaptation. Your system found a way to protect you when no one else would, to create distance from unbearable experiences, to help you survive what felt unsurvivable. In the short term, this operates as highly effective coping, but after many repetitions this emergency response often becomes the default setting. The temporary abandonment of your ship becomes permanent exile. Even when the storm has passed, even when waters are calm, you remain in the lifeboat—watching your body from a distance, treating it as foreign territory, and unable to return home.

The Body That Holds What the Mind Cannot

Trauma shapes more than feelings—it embeds itself in the body's patterns and reactions. Your body holds the schema mindsets we discussed in Chapter 2, which consist of implicit memories—sensations, feelings, and body states—that existed before you had words for them, or that were too overwhelming to be processed through language and conscious thought. These implicit memories live in your:

- Brainstem reactions (that instant jolt, flinch, or tightening)
- Nervous system (hypervigilance, startle responses, chronic tension)
- Visceral sensations (nausea, tightness, emptiness, heaviness)
- Movement patterns (freezing, fleeing, fighting)
- Sensory experiences (certain touches, smells, sounds becoming triggers)

For trauma survivors, inhabiting the body can feel dangerous. Physical sensations are potential triggers that can flood you with traumatic memory fragments before your conscious mind even knows what's happening.

One trauma survivor described it this way: "When I start to feel my body—really feel it—it's like there's this awful storm inside. All these feelings I can't name, these sensations that feel like danger. It's easier to just . . . not be in there."

The eating disorder becomes a tool for managing this dilemma. By controlling, punishing, numbing, or using bingeing, purging, or restricting behaviours, you maintain the dissociative split that protects you from what the body holds.

Restriction keeps you in your head, away from bodily sensations. Bingeing floods your system, creating sensations you can control and predict. Purging offers a physical release when emotional release feels too dangerous. Compulsive exercise pushes you beyond feeling, into exhaustion and numbness.

Although we often think of these behaviours as being solely about food or weight, for many people, they evolved as a way of managing a body that has become dangerous territory.

When Dissociation Distorts How You See Yourself

Dissociation not only disconnects you from emotions but alters how you perceive and experience your body and self (30). When you're watching your ship from the lifeboat, unable to return, your view of that vessel naturally becomes distorted. You're seeing it from a distance, through fog, and often through the lens of old fears rather than present reality.

For many trauma survivors with eating disorders, body image disturbance functions as a form of dissociation. You're not seeing your actual body—you're seeing a body filtered through disconnection, implicit memory, and the beliefs formed at the time of trauma. This can show up in several ways:

Visual Distortion: You look in the mirror and what you see doesn't match what others see or what photographs show. Certain body parts appear larger, smaller, "wrong," or frighteningly unfamiliar. These distortions often shift with emotional state. This is dissociated perception, a mismatch between internal experience and external reality.

Felt-Sense Distortion: You may feel huge, heavy, contaminated, or wrong even when nothing objectively supports that. These felt-sense distortions originate in the same neural pathways that hold trauma memories. When your Lost Child is activated, your body can feel like the body you had during trauma—regardless of its actual shape or size now.

Numbness and Disconnection: Some days you may feel nothing when you look at or touch your body—no warmth, no connection, no sense of "me-ness." The body becomes an object to manage rather than a home to inhabit. This numbness reflects how thoroughly dissociation has split conscious awareness from the physical self.

Why Eating Disorder Behaviours Increase Distortion: Eating disorder behaviours—restriction, bingeing, purging, and compulsive exercise—then become attempts to manage these frightening or confusing perceptions:

- If your body feels wrong, changing it offers a false sense of control.
- If you can't feel your body, extreme behaviours produce sensations intense enough to break through the numbness.
- If your body feels contaminated or dangerous, shrinking it or punishing it may feel safer than inhabiting it.

When Harriet looked in the mirror, she didn't see her actual body—she saw shame, disgust, and wrongness. These weren't visual perceptions as much as emotional memories fused with her body image. Her restrictive eating and striving for thinness was an attempt to erase a body that felt unsafe and contaminated by trauma.

Why Standard Body Image Approaches Don't Work Here: When dissociation is driving the distortion, simply challenging thoughts ("your body isn't that shape") or practising affirmations has limited impact. Body image distortion isn't a cognitive error, but rather a dissociative split. It reflects a deeper disconnection from the body that once protected you by becoming absent, numb, or unrecognisable.

Repairing the Distortion: Returning to the Ship: Recovery involves gradually reconnecting with your present-moment body, rather than the dissociated body shaped by past trauma. This is why the grounding practices in Part 2 are essential. They help you come back aboard your ship, even briefly, so your perception can begin to recalibrate.

As your Wise Self strengthens and your capacity to remain embodied increases, body image distortion often begins to lessen. Rather than being linked to actual body changes, this is because your perception changes. You're no longer viewing yourself through dissociation's distorting lens—you're beginning to experience your actual body in the here and now.

This shift is slow and gradual. Body image distortion rooted in trauma doesn't change quickly because it isn't simply "a belief"—it is a protective adaptation, a warning system aimed at using eating/weight behaviours to prevent you from returning to your trauma-flooded body. With patient practice in embodiment, steady Wise Self presence, and professional support when needed, the dissociative gap between how you feel your body and how it truly is can begin to close.

Trauma doesn't only change what you feel—it changes what your body can tolerate. One of the clearest places this shows up is appetite: for some people, it surges, and for others, it disappears.

When Survival Hijacks Appetite

Trauma doesn't affect everyone's appetite in the same way. For some people, eating increases—food becomes a way to soothe, numb, or regulate overwhelming states. For others, appetite diminishes or disappears entirely—the body prioritises survival over digestion, and hunger cues fade into the background. What looks like "disordered eating" is often the nervous system doing its best to manage threat. Eating stops being about hunger and fullness, and instead becomes a strategy for survival—either by dampening distress or by staying shut down enough to avoid it.

When Trauma Drives Eating Downward: For others, trauma pushes appetite in the opposite direction—eating too little or losing hunger altogether. When your body perceives an ongoing threat, it prioritises survival functions, and appetite can shut down completely. People may feel constantly on edge or emotionally numb, and in that state, eating can feel irrelevant, effortful, or even unsafe.

Acute stress is well known to suppress appetite, and trauma can keep your system in a prolonged state where hunger cues feel blunted, meals are skipped, and restrictive patterns become ingrained.

From Survival Strategy to Eating Disorder: Whether someone overeats or undereats after trauma, the pattern is similar: the nervous system is dysregulated, and eating becomes a coping mechanism rather than a simple response to hunger. Food becomes a way to escape feelings (through numbing, bingeing, or comfort eating) or manage them (through restriction and control).

Your eating patterns are your body's creative attempts to survive when other resources aren't available. This is why standard "just eat normally" advice falls flat for trauma survivors. Recovery requires addressing the underlying nervous system dysregulation, not just changing eating behaviours. The practices in this chapter focus on gradually reconnecting with your body, helping your Protector Modes update their threat assessment, and building your Wise Self's capacity to provide the regulation your system has been seeking through food.

Whether eating increases or decreases, the pattern is the same: food stops being about hunger and starts being about safety. That's why trauma-informed recovery has to work with the nervous system, not just eating behaviour.

The Beliefs Born from Trauma

Control-Mastery Theory helps us understand how trauma creates mindsets that keep the eating disorder in place (31). Remember from Chapter 2 how schema mindsets develop when you come to expect painful things will happen—abandonment, rejection, domination—in close relationships?

In trauma, these beliefs often take specific forms:

"If I feel what's in my body, I'll be overwhelmed and won't survive": This belief keeps you in the lifeboat, afraid to return to the ship. The eating disorder becomes a way of testing whether you can stay disconnected whilst still appearing functional.

"My feelings and needs caused the bad things to happen": If you were neglected when you showed needs, punished when you expressed emotion, or harmed when you were vulnerable, you may have concluded that your inner experience is dangerous. The eating disorder becomes a way of eliminating needs and feelings entirely.

"No one will help me if they know how much I'm struggling": If expressing distress led to abandonment, dismissal, or punishment, you learned to manage everything alone. The eating disorder becomes a private coping strategy that doesn't require you to ask for help.

"I can't trust my body's signals because they're not real": If adults didn't respond when you were in danger, or if they gaslit you about your reality, you may have learned to mistrust your own perceptions. The eating disorder becomes a way of overriding body signals entirely.

"Staying small/invisible/controlled keeps me safer than being fully present": If being visible, taking up space, or expressing yourself fully led to harm, you may have learned that existing minimally is protection. This can manifest as making your body smaller through restriction, hiding within a larger body whilst using food as barrier and numbness, or disconnecting from your expressive self regardless of body size. The eating disorder keeps you controlled and invisible—physically, emotionally, or both.

These beliefs weave together into a survival logic, and the eating disorder protects them by keeping you from ever having to test whether they're still true.

When the Body Becomes Visible Proof

Sometimes the body becomes the way of communicating what words cannot express—a way of speaking the unspeakable.

Melissa understood this dynamic painfully well. Growing up with parents who sacrificed everything whilst rarely treating themselves, she absorbed the message that her needs depleted others' happiness. Words felt inadequate to convey her internal experience of being a burden. "I couldn't just say I was struggling—they'd taught me that needing anything meant I was taking from their limited supply," she explained. "But if my body showed I wasn't okay, maybe they'd finally see how much I was hurting without me having to ask for help directly. My weight became the only way to make my pain visible on the outside."

For some trauma survivors, especially those who were taught that expressing distress directly leads to punishment or dismissal:

- Low weight (or higher weight) becomes visible communication: "I'm not okay."
- The eating disorder becomes proof that justifies the need for care.
- Physical frailty legitimises vulnerability that felt illegitimate emotionally.
- The body's deterioration does the asking when asking directly feels impossible.

This usually isn't conscious—it's driven by a deep need to be seen and helped whilst navigating the belief that direct communication of needs leads to abandonment.

But unfortunately, this indirect communication often gets misinterpreted. Rather than seeing the pain underneath, others may focus on "fixing" the eating disorder due to the risk this creates, or become frustrated by apparent resistance to recovery. The very strategy meant to elicit understanding and care can instead provoke the same dismissal and frustration that created the need for indirect communication in the first place.

The Lost Child: Frozen below Deck

In Chapter 3, you met your Lost Child—the vulnerable part that holds your emotions and needs. When trauma is involved, this part doesn't just get sent below deck. She gets frozen there.

Imagine your Lost Child below deck during a catastrophic storm. The ship is being battered, taking on water, and listing dangerously. She's terrified, overwhelmed, convinced that death is imminent. In that moment of overwhelming threat, her system adapts to protect her: it freezes her in place, like a living pause button.

This freeze response is one of your body's oldest survival strategies. When you can neither fight nor flee, when the threat is too great to process, your system essentially puts that experience in suspended animation. The memories, the feelings, the bodily sensations—all of it gets frozen in time.

Years later, your Lost Child remains frozen below deck, in a timeloop around the moment the trauma happened. She holds:

- The terror that never got fully processed
- The feelings that had nowhere safe to go
- The confusion about what happened and why
- The beliefs she formed about herself and safety
- The body memories locked in place

What makes this particularly hard is that, in this frozen state, she can't differentiate past from present. When something reminds her of trauma—a sensation, a smell, a similar situation—it's as though the storm is happening again right now. She doesn't think "this reminds me of when . . ."—she experiences "this IS that."

For trauma survivors, certain body sensations, emotional states, or situations can trigger such intense reactions. It's a frozen experience becoming unfrozen, flooding your system with feelings that belong to another time but feel utterly present.

Your Lost Child below deck needs two things:

1. Acknowledgement that what happened to her was real and overwhelming
2. Support and understanding that the storm has passed, that she's no longer in that moment

But she can't receive either of these while she remains frozen, and you remain in the lifeboat watching from afar. The core challenge of trauma recovery is how to gradually unfreeze without being overwhelmed, how to return to the ship without abandoning it again.

Why This Chapter Matters

Understanding how trauma and eating disorders interact matters because:

Recovery Approaches Need to Be Trauma-Informed: Standard eating disorder treatment that doesn't address trauma can feel re-traumatising or ineffective. You might need pacing, grounding, and safety-building that trauma-naive approaches don't provide.

Your Protector Modes Have Good Reasons for Maintaining Disconnection: They're protecting you from something that once genuinely threatened your survival. Working with these modes requires acknowledging their wisdom whilst helping them update to present-day reality.

Reconnecting with Your Body after Trauma Is Possible, but It Requires Specific Support: The practices in this chapter, combined with trauma-specialist therapy when needed, can help you gradually return to the ship you once had to abandon—but this time with a Wise Captain at the helm and crew who know how to navigate storms without abandoning ship entirely.

These patterns grew out of a younger you trying to stay safe in a world that didn't feel safe. Every "symptom" you're struggling with was once a creative solution to an overwhelming threat. Rather than "fixing" you for being wrong, recovery is about updating and gradually saying goodbye to strategies that once helped you survive but now hold you back from truly living your life.

In the rest of this chapter, we'll look at how to recognise dissociation, find your way back to the ship, work with the modes that protect you from re-traumatisation, and recognise when you need specialist support.

Part 2: Finding Your Way Back to the Ship

Coming back to your body is a series of small, reversible steps. The aim is to learn how to return without flooding.

Gentle Practices for Reconnection

The journey back to your body after trauma requires something different from standard "grounding techniques." You need practices that acknowledge why you left in the first place, that respect your Detached Protector's concerns, and that move slowly enough that your system doesn't panic and shut down again.

Think of these practices as building a bridge between the lifeboat and the ship—one plank at a time, testing each one before adding the next, always with the option to step back if things feel too much.

Recognising When You've Lost Your Anchor

Your body sends signals when you need support. Learning to recognise early warning signs of dysregulation (losing your grounding) and signs of dissociation (already drifted away) becomes your early warning system.

When You Recognise Early Dysregulation Signs—anxiety rising, heart racing, thoughts spinning, eating disorder urges increasing—you can still reach for grounding practices to help you stay aboard the ship.

When You Notice Dissociation Signs—emotional numbness, brain fog, feeling like you're watching yourself from outside, the world feeling unreal—you need practices specifically designed to help you reconnect with the present moment.

Reconnection Practices: Building Your Personal Toolkit

The following practices can help you reconnect when you've drifted away from yourself. Each is described briefly here to help you understand the approach; You'll find more detailed guidance in Appendix 26, including how to recognise signs of dysregulation and dissociation, and step-by-step support for using each practice.

- **5–4–3–2–1 Sensory Grounding**: Use all five senses to anchor yourself in the present moment—name 5 things you see, 4 you can touch, 3 you hear, 2 you smell, and 1 you taste. This practice rapidly pulls your attention back to where your body actually is right now and can help you realise you are safe now, out of harm's way. It can be especially powerful to use this grounding when outside in nature, to enable you to take in the soothing presence offered by the environment.
- **Trauma-Sensitive Body Mapping**: Begin with the places in your body that feel steady or untouched—the ones that trauma didn't silence. These become your anchor points. From that safe ground, you can gently explore the more intense areas, knowing you can always return to the parts of you that remain intact.

- **Movement Practices**: When frozen, movement helps complete defensive responses your body couldn't finish during trauma. Try gentle shaking to release pent-up energy, mindful walking where you notice each step, or slow, intentional movement like gentle stretching. Even small movements—wiggling fingers or toes—can help when you feel stuck.
- **Breath Practices**: Different breath patterns serve different needs. The Cyclic Sigh (double inhale, long exhale) offers quick calming when anxiety rises. The Tree-Root Breath helps you find stability during emotional storms by anchoring attention in your belly. Gentle humming on the out-breath adds vibration that supports grounding and reduces dissociation.
- **Temperature Shifts**: Your nervous system responds powerfully to temperature. Cold (ice in hands, cold water, brief cold shower) can interrupt intense activation. Warmth (heated blanket, hot drink, warm shower) supports settling. The strong sensation demands attention in ways that break through dissociation.
- **Scent and Tactile Anchors**: Essential oils, textured objects, or familiar comforting scents travel directly to brain areas involved in memory and emotion. Keep a small vial of essential oil in your pocket, with a scent that brings feelings of safety or links to happy memories—when you notice dissociation, the strong scent can rapidly pull you back to present awareness.
- **Nature Connection**: Nature offers presence without demanding performance. Stand barefoot on grass, noticing texture and temperature, spend time near a single plant, or simply look at the sky. Even minimal nature access helps—trees don't need you to perform or be any particular way.
- **Soothing Touch**: Slow forearm stroking/holding, weighted warmth (heavy blanket across your lap), or hand on heart with gentle pressure can signal safety to your nervous system. These practices activate nerve fibres that respond to caring touch, supporting your body's shift out of threat mode. (Only use these if touch feels comfortable and safe for you.)
- **Rhythmic Tapping**: Gentle left-right tapping on upper chest, arms, ribs, or hands in a steady rhythm sends predictable, non-threatening signals through your body. The structured pattern interrupts spiralling anxiety and helps ground you in the present moment.

When These Practices Feel Too Much

Some days, no amount of grounding will make your body feel safe to inhabit. Your Detached Protector is signalling that right now, staying in the lifeboat is what your system needs. On these days, respect the protection. You might use external focus activities (watching a film, reading, being with others) without trying to "work on" anything or simply survive the day knowing tomorrow might offer a different capacity.

The goal is developing a flexible relationship with your body—sometimes more connected, sometimes more protected, with your Wise Self able to recognise which is needed when.

The Gradual Journey Home

Reconnecting with your body after trauma is a gradual process of building trust—helping your Protector Modes see that the ship can be safe territory again, helping your Lost Child know she doesn't have to remain frozen, and developing trust in your Wise Self to stay present even when things are difficult.

Some days you'll feel more embodied, more present, more connected to physical sensation. Other days you'll find yourself back in the lifeboat, watching from a safe distance, unable or unwilling to return to the ship.

Both are part of the journey. What matters is that you're no longer permanently cut off from your body, no longer locked into disconnection as your only option. You're developing flexibility—the ability to move toward presence when safe, to move toward protection when needed.

The ship is still there, still floating, still yours. You abandoned it to survive, and that made good sense. Now you might be starting to realise that it's better to be back on board your own ship—strengthened and repaired—than to live forever in the lifeboat.

Even when you know what helps, you may find yourself resisting it. That resistance is self-protection. Part 3 is about meeting those Protector Modes directly, so your tools can get some traction.

Part 3: Working with Modes That Protect You from Re-Traumatisation

You've learned practices for reconnecting with your body. You understand the signs of dysregulation (emotional overwhelm) and dissociation. You know, intellectually, what might help when you've drifted away.

And yet you might find yourself unable to use these tools. A voice inside insists it's not safe to feel. Another rages at the unfairness of having to do this work at all. The eating disorder, which you know causes suffering, feels simultaneously like the only thing keeping you from falling apart completely.

When trauma is part of your history, your Protector Modes become especially fierce. They're not just protecting you from general discomfort—they're guarding against what once felt like annihilation. Under all these layers of protection lies your Lost Child—the young, vulnerable part who holds the pain these modes are desperately trying to shield you from.

Understanding Your Protective System in Trauma

Your Protector Modes can feel bewildering. They seem to perpetuate your eating difficulties and block your progress, yet they're working tirelessly to keep you safe from something that once threatened to overwhelm you completely.

These modes developed survival strategies when you had limited options. They've been operating on outdated information ever since, still believing you're in that original danger. The eating disorder behaviours—whether restriction, bingeing, purging, compulsive exercise, or rigid control—create new pain of their own, yet from your Protector Modes' perspective, this pain is manageable, predictable, controlled. It's pain they can see coming. The pain they're protecting you from felt like it would destroy you.

When trauma intersects with eating disorders, the schema patterns become intensified. Abandonment schemas create expectations that others will always leave. Emotional Deprivation schemas make nourishment feel foreign and dangerous. Mistrust schemas create hypervigilance and difficulty accepting help. Subjugation schemas make expressing needs feel impossible. (See Chapter 2 for full schema descriptions.)

Your Protector Modes use the eating disorder to speak what words cannot, for example, dietary restriction communicating "I don't deserve nourishment," bingeing expressing "I can never get enough of what I need," control over your body attempting to create safety in a world that felt dangerously unpredictable.

The sections that follow explore specific modes that commonly protect trauma survivors from re-traumatisation. Each mode requires its own specific approach—the Feisty Child needs space to vent and be heard, the Detached Protector needs to learn that feeling won't destroy you, the Overcontroller needs tiny steps of letting go, whilst your Wise Self proves it can handle what arises.

When Your Detached Protector Refuses to Let You Feel

You know the Detached Protector from earlier chapters—the part that numbs emotions, keeps relationships at arm's length, and uses the eating disorder to maintain disconnection. When trauma is involved, this mode becomes particularly resistant to letting you reconnect.

The eating disorder became a reliable tool for maintaining this shutdown. Restriction keeps you in your head, away from bodily sensations. Bingeing floods your system with manageable sensations that block more threatening emotions. The focus on food, weight, and body provides an acceptable preoccupation that keeps deeper feelings at bay.

When Fullness Feels Like a Violation—Trauma, Body Memories, and the Gut

For some people with trauma histories, eating and fullness don't just bring up worries about weight or control—they activate the body's alarm system. Sensations such as pressure, stretching, or fullness in the stomach can feel threatening, violating, or intolerable. These reactions happen automatically, below conscious thought, and are shaped by earlier experiences where bodily sensations were linked with danger, helplessness, or loss of control.

In this context, eating disorder behaviours often develop as protective responses: restriction reduces exposure to triggering sensations, bingeing creates intense but predictable feelings that override deeper threat signals, and purging or rigid control restores a sense of escape or containment. These patterns are not about food itself—they are about survival in a body that learned it was not safe to feel.

A more detailed explanation of how trauma affects gut sensations and the body's alarm systems is included in Appendix 27 for those who want to understand the neurobiology in more depth.

When Your Overcontroller Won't Let Go

Your Overcontroller mode operates on a simple premise: if you can control everything—your food, your body, your environment, your schedule—then nothing bad can happen again. Control becomes the illusion of safety in a world that once felt dangerously unpredictable.

When trauma is involved, this mode becomes particularly rigid. The Overcontroller remembers times when you had no control at all—when bad things happened and you couldn't stop them, when your emotions overwhelmed you and no one helped you regulate them. The eating disorder offers concrete, measurable control that feels safer than the uncertainty of healing.

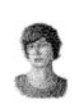 Sophie knows this mode intimately. Growing up where high standards were the norm but emotional nourishment felt scarce, she learned early that performance, precision, and control were safer than vulnerability. Her Overcontroller gave her clear rules: eat this much, weigh this amount, follow the plan perfectly. Success meant she was good enough. Failure confirmed what she'd feared-that she was fundamentally flawed. What her Overcontroller couldn't see was that the eating disorder controlled her far more than she controlled it.

Working with Your Overcontroller Requires

Interview It: "What are you afraid will happen if I don't follow the food rules perfectly? What feelings are you keeping at bay through all this control? What needs weren't met in the past that you're trying to ensure are met now through control?"

Listen carefully. Your Overcontroller might reveal fear of being criticised, terror of being out of control emotionally, anxiety about disappointing others, or dread of the vulnerability and sadness underneath the rigid structure.

Negotiate Tiny Steps: "Would you be willing to let me have one flexible meal this week—not following the rules perfectly—just to see what happens? I promise I'll stay present with whatever feelings come up."

Make the experiment small enough that your Overcontroller feels it can allow it, whilst large enough that feelings might surface for your Wise Self to practice holding.

Stay with the Feelings That Arise: When your Overcontroller releases even a tiny bit of control, feelings will emerge—anxiety, sadness, rage, vulnerability. This is exactly what your Overcontroller has been preventing.

Use grounding and reconnection practices. Speak to your Lost Child: "I'm here. I can feel this with you. You're not alone." Connect the feelings to unmet needs from the past: "This sadness makes sense—you needed to be valued for who you were, not just what you achieved."

Build Evidence Gradually: Each time your Overcontroller allows a small release of control and your Wise Self stays present with the feelings, you're building evidence that feelings can be tolerated, that your Wise Self can handle emotional discomfort, and that true safety comes from being able to feel and regulate rather than from eliminating all feeling through control.

Over weeks and months, your Overcontroller begins to trust that your Wise Self is capable. The rigid grip loosens incrementally. The eating disorder behaviours that maintained the control become less necessary as your capacity to be with feelings grows.

When Self-Attack Protects You from Facing Unbearable Truth

Some trauma survivors develop particularly fierce self-attacking patterns—what we described in Chapter 6 as the Flagellating Critic. When trauma is involved, these modes serve an additional function: they help you avoid acknowledging unbearable truths about what happened and what wasn't available to you.

Understanding Trauma in Layers

Trauma rarely exists in a single moment; it tends to layer itself over time. The most visible layer is often the shame that happened in childhood or adolescence—bullying, criticism, or body-based judgement. Beneath that usually sits a much younger child who learned long before this that having needs was unsafe.

But beneath that sits a much younger, often Forgotten Child—the one who felt invisible, who absorbed a parent's anxiety, who learned to keep the peace by having no needs of her own. This earlier aloneness is quieter but deeper. It is this forgotten Lost Child who learned to subjugate, to take up less space, and to turn her feelings inward to protect the attachment. For this child, regulating the parent's emotions became more important than having her own feelings. Needing nothing felt safer than risking her parents' overwhelm or withdrawal.

The later layer of shame—the bullying, the body criticism—simply reinforced a survival pattern already in motion. The Critic didn't begin with the fat-shaming. It began much earlier, when the child learned that attacking herself kept others calm, that sabotaging her own needs preserved the attachment, that giving up her sovereignty was the price of connection.

Recovery involves tending to both layers: the adolescent who was shamed and the younger child who learned to disappear long before anyone commented on her body.

 *Harriet's experience illustrates both layers.* You've already seen how her parents' emotional overwhelm taught her that her feelings destabilised them—the deeper, earlier layer where the forgotten Lost Child learned to regulate others' emotions by suppressing her own. When trauma occurred at 12, her Critic was already well-established. The logic was simple: "If I make myself the villain—if I'm too much, too sensitive, fundamentally flawed—then what happened makes sense. If I just fix myself enough, everything will be okay."

Making herself the problem preserved a connection to caregivers who, whatever their limitations, were all she had. It created an addiction to self-punishment—suffering proved her dedication, and deprivation might finally rid her of guilt for existing. This pattern intensifies for children with high empathy or environmental sensitivity—they absorb others' distress more acutely, feel responsible more deeply. The eating disorder becomes another expression: punishing and minimising the self that was taught it was too much.

Working with This Pattern Requires

Recognising the Protective Function: Your therapist can help you see: "Your Critic isn't just being harsh. It's trying to preserve your sense of connection and control by making you the problem instead of acknowledging limitations in the support that was available."

Separating Past from Present: "You're not that powerless child anymore. You have resources now. Your Wise Self can provide what wasn't available before. You can acknowledge what happened without it destroying you."

Grieving What Was Lost: "You can be angry. You can grieve what you didn't receive—even whilst understanding those who couldn't provide it were doing the best they could with their own limitations. Your Feisty Child has been silenced for so long. She's allowed to speak now."

Updating the System: "The loyalty you maintained through self-attack was necessary then. It kept you attached, gave you hope, helped you make sense of what happened and enabled you to survive. But it costs you everything now. You can honour that younger self who did what she had to do whilst also recognising it's time to stop betraying yourself."

You made yourself the villain because it offered a sense of control. If you were the problem, then maybe you could fix yourself. Self-punishment preserved hope that if you changed, you could finally get the care you need—but it also kept you trapped.

Being honest with yourself—*has blaming yourself ever really worked?* If it had, you'd be free by now. You've been working so hard to purify yourself, to earn your worth back. But all it's done is keep you stuck in shame and isolation.

Maybe it's time for a different approach. Instead of making yourself the villain of your life story, what if you tried being your own friend? Someone who "sits with you on the fence", who stays close when the pain comes. Someone who says, "No wonder you feel this way. I'm here." Hard times are easier to bear with a friend by your side—even, and especially, when that friend is you.

This grief—this acknowledgement of what was lost—usually needs some space before deeper recovery can unfold. Your Wise Self holds your Lost Child through this unbearable truth: "You weren't the problem. You were a child who needed protection, attunement, and safety. What happened wasn't your fault. And your anger and sadness about all of it is valid."

This deep work is best done with professional support. A trauma-informed therapist can help you navigate this process at a pace that feels manageable for your system.

Reflection Point: If you've experienced trauma, can you see how your Critic might be protecting you from acknowledging painful truths? What would it mean to stop making yourself the villain of your own story?

When Your Feisty Child Says "This Isn't Fair"

There's a rage that can arise in recovery that takes people by surprise. This is your Feisty Child's voice saying: "I shouldn't have to do this. I shouldn't have to heal from what I never should have experienced in the first place."

Your Feisty Child is right. It isn't fair. This anger often emerges from experiences of emotional deprivation or neglect—growing up without sufficient attunement, nurturance, empathy, or support. You may have had to parent yourself emotionally from a young age. Now, in recovery, you're being asked to do more of this internal parenting work, and your Feisty Child understandably protests: "Haven't I done enough already? When does someone else take care of me?"

The resentment makes perfect sense. You're being asked to work on problems you didn't create. You're having to develop resources you should have been given freely. You're having to heal wounds that should never have been inflicted.

Your Feisty Child might express this through rage at having to follow meal plans or practice self-care, fury at anyone suggesting you need to change, resentment toward people who seem to have had easier lives, or rebellious use of eating disorder behaviours as a way of saying "I'll do what I want."

When this mode isn't met with both compassion and firmness, it can start to block healing. Not because the anger is in any way wrong or bad, but because staying stuck in the rage—or stuck in denying any anger—keeps you trapped. The Feisty Child's position makes emotional sense: "If I refuse to do this work, maybe someone will finally step in and do it for me." But staying stuck doesn't compel others to rescue you. It just keeps you stuck.

Working with Your Feisty Child Means Giving Voice to the Rage

Journal the Fury: Give your Feisty Child dedicated time to express everything she feels about what happened or didn't happen. Write or draw from the feeling of rage without censoring. Let the rage pour onto the page: "It's not fair that I have to do this work." "Where were they when I needed them? Why do I have to be my own parent now?" Ground first, then write/draw without censoring; let it be messy.

Physical Release: Sometimes anger needs physical expression. Punch pillows, rip up paper, stomp your feet, throw ice cubes against a wall. Not in destructive ways, but in ways that let the energy move through your body while you focus on *feeling* it, rather than staying trapped.

The Journey through Anger

First comes the rage itself—hot, furious, demanding to be heard. Let this happen. Create space for it. Your Wise Self's role is to witness without trying to fix or minimise.

The journey through anger unfolds in stages. Rage comes first—intense and insistent. Your Wise Self's role is not to fix it, but to stay present and let it speak.

If the anger is given space, it often softens into grief—sadness for what should have been but wasn't. This grief needs tenderness and time. Eventually, acceptance may emerge—not acceptance that what happened was okay, but acceptance that staying trapped in rage keeps you bound to the past. Each stage unfolds in its own time; none can be rushed.

This process takes time. You can only create space for each stage to unfold at its own pace, staying present with whatever arises.

Reaching Your Lost Child beneath the Protection

Every protective pattern you've explored exists to keep you from something that once felt unbearable—a younger part of you who is still holding what couldn't be felt or held at the time. Your Protector Modes—the Detached Protector, the Overcontroller, the People Pleaser, the Feisty Child, and the Critic (which you worked with in Chapter 6)—all surround something important and vulnerable. Beneath these layers of protection lives your Lost Child, holding the pain, frozen terror, unmet needs, and unprocessed grief.

Understanding why your Protector Modes are so fierce helps when they seem to be blocking your recovery. They're guarding a specific, frightened young part who once faced experiences she had no resources to manage. That young part is still there, still holding what happened, still believing she's in danger.

Your Lost Child might be frozen at the age when trauma occurred. She exists outside of time, in a place where past and present blur together. When your Protector Modes sense you getting too close to her pain, they activate immediately—because to them, feeling her feelings means she's in danger again.

The feelings your Lost Child holds are significantly more intense and frightening than everyday emotional discomfort. Your Protector Modes are responding proportionally to the level of terror, shame, rage, or helplessness that this young part experienced.

Creating Containment: Ways to Connect Safely

As your Protector Modes gradually soften and your Lost Child begins to emerge, you need ways to connect with her that feel safe and manageable.

Journalling as Dialogue: Write to your Lost Child or Feisty Child, asking gentle questions and letting her respond. "What are you feeling right now? What happened that hurt you? What do you need me to know?"

Let her write back without censoring. Her words might be messy, raw, or expressed in language that sounds young. You're allowing her authentic voice to emerge.

Drawing Difficult Feelings: Give your Lost Child coloured pencils or paints and let her express what she's holding visually. "Can you draw what the fear looks like? What colour is the anger you're feeling?" The drawings don't need to be artistic—they're simply another language for feelings that might not have words yet.

Sketching Feelings as They Arise: When difficult emotions surface during your day, keep a small notebook nearby. Take a few minutes to draw shapes, colours, scribbles that represent what you're feeling. This externalises the feeling, making it something you can see and acknowledge rather than something formless and overwhelming inside you.

Being Believed and Understood: The most crucial element is that your Wise Self stays present, believing and understanding whatever emerges. Your Lost Child needs to know:

> "I believe you. What you're telling me is real and important." "Of course you feel this, given what you experienced." "You're not too much. I can handle hearing this." "I won't dismiss you the way others did. I won't let the Critic dismiss you either."

When your Lost Child shares something painful and your Critic tries to jump in with dismissal, your Wise Self protects her: "Critic, I hear you trying to minimise this pain because it feels scary. But I need you to step back right now. She needs to be heard without judgement."

Allowing Whatever Feelings Emerge: Your Lost Child has been holding these feelings for so long, waiting for someone strong enough to witness them. She needs permission to feel whatever she feels—the terror, the rage, the shame, the grief, and the helplessness.

Your Wise Self can offer this permission: "You can feel as angry as you need to feel. I'm here with you." "Your sadness is welcome here." "The shame you're carrying doesn't belong to you, but I understand you're holding it. Let's feel it together so you can begin to release it."

Building Your Capacity Gradually

Reaching your Lost Child beneath the protection isn't something you do once. It's a gradual process of:

- Strengthening your Wise Self through consistent grounding and self-compassion
- Helping Protector Modes soften by negotiating with them and showing evidence that your Wise Self can handle what they've been protecting you from
- Creating safe moments of connection with your Lost Child through journalling and drawing
- Practising staying with feelings that arise when Protector Modes release their grip
- Linking feelings to unmet needs from the past and beginning to meet those needs more directly in the present

Over a period of weeks, months, sometimes years—your capacity to reach your Lost Child deepens. The Protector Modes learn to trust your Wise Self's leadership. Your Lost Child discovers that someone is finally here who won't collapse under the weight of what she's carrying.

A Note on Professional Support

Reaching your Lost Child beneath all this protection often requires more than self-help can provide. The feelings she holds may be too intense, the Protector Modes too frightened, and the Wise Self not yet strong enough to hold it all alone.

If you're finding this work overwhelming, if your Protector Modes remain fiercely activated despite your efforts, or if approaching your Lost Child's pain feels too much, professional support is vital. We'll discuss this more fully at the end of this chapter, but know that recognising when you need more support is a healthy sign.

Part 4: Living with Trauma and Eating Difficulties

The practices in this chapter are like rehabilitation exercises after injury—slow, repetitive, and sometimes uncomfortable but necessary for rebuilding trust and strength over time. So be patient, this is all part of *learning*. And some people's systems can take longer because it's been protecting them for a very long time.

Recovery from eating disorders with trauma histories is often exhausting. Some days you'll manage to use your grounding practices, speak compassionately to your Lost Child, and negotiate with your Protector Modes. Other days, you'll be so overwhelmed that the tools feel impossible to access. You'll find yourself deep in eating disorder behaviours, dissociated for hours or days, with your Critic attacking relentlessly and your Protector Modes running the ship. Both experiences are normal.

Your Protector Modes developed over years, sometimes decades. They won't soften quickly just because your Wise Self is learning new approaches. The feelings your Lost Child holds can be genuinely frightening. When trauma is part of your history, reconnecting with your body and emotions means approaching pain that your system has worked incredibly hard to keep at bay.

So why do it? Why face all of this? Because there is more to life than survival. Because beneath the pain, there's a part of you—your Contented Child—who still remembers how to laugh, explore, and feel joy. Not perform it—but *feel it* in your body. To reclaim this aliveness, your system needs to learn that it is now safe enough to *feel*—and make space for freedom, spontaneity, connection, and peace.

This is why the work is worth it.

Ongoing Challenges You'll Face

Triggers Persist: Certain situations, sensations, or interactions may always activate your nervous system, reminding your body of times when you weren't safe. What gradually changes is the reduced intensity and duration of activation, and the effectiveness of the tools you have to help yourself regulate.

Protector Modes Resurface under Stress: When life becomes overwhelming, old patterns return. Your Overcontroller might grip tighter. Your Detached Protector might shut you down completely. Your eating disorder behaviours might intensify. This is to be expected. Your system is doing what it knows to do under pressure.

Relationships Feel Complicated: Learning to be vulnerable with others whilst carrying abandonment, mistrust, or emotional deprivation patterns takes time. You learned these patterns from real experiences. They made sense given what you lived through. They also require ongoing work to shift.

Grief Comes in Waves: You'll need space to grieve the childhood you deserved, the years lost to an eating disorder and trauma. This grief is necessary, but it's painful. Sometimes it arrives when you least expect it.

Identity Feels Uncertain: As you give less power to Protector Modes and eating disorder patterns, you'll face uncomfortable questions: Who am I without these strategies? What do I actually want? This reconstruction takes time and feels disorienting.

These practices can support day-to-day regulation, but there are times when self-help isn't enough. Knowing when to reach for specialist support is part of Wise Self leadership.

When You Need Professional Support

For many people reading this chapter, self-help won't be enough. The practices here can support your healing, but they can't replace the holding environment that trauma-informed therapy provides.

Professional Support Becomes Essential When

- Your eating disorder is medically unstable.
- Your Lost Child's pain feels too overwhelming to approach alone.
- Protector Modes remain fiercely activated despite your best efforts.
- You find yourself becoming retraumatised by attempts to reconnect with your body or feel.
- Suicidal thoughts or severe self-harm urges arise.
- Dissociation is so intense that you lose significant time or can't function safely.
- You feel unsafe in ways these practices don't touch.
- You need someone to hold the therapeutic space whilst your Wise Self is still developing.

What Trauma-Informed Therapy Provides

A trauma-informed Schema Therapist can provide the external Wise Adult presence whilst yours is strengthening. They can help negotiate with Protector Modes using specialised techniques—chair work, imagery rescripting, limited reparenting. They can offer containment for your Lost Child's pain whilst teaching your Wise Self how to provide that containment yourself eventually.

Schema Therapy was developed specifically to work with these deep, entrenched patterns that develop from childhood trauma and unmet needs. When eating disorders are layered on top of trauma, Schema Therapy (and other parts-based models) offer tools to work with both simultaneously—addressing the Protector Modes that maintain eating disorder behaviours whilst healing the wounded Lost Child beneath.

Building Your Treatment Team

A therapist is often a central part of recovery, but other team members can be equally necessary. A dietitian with expertise in eating disorders can help you rebuild your relationship with food whilst understanding how trauma affects eating patterns. They can support your Overcontroller in loosening its grip on food rules, help your Detached Protector learn that nourishment doesn't have to trigger overwhelming feelings, and work with your Wise Self to develop sustainable eating patterns that support healing.

Depending on your needs, your treatment team might also include a GP or psychiatrist monitoring your physical and mental health, or other specialists who understand both eating disorders and trauma. Innovative trauma-focused therapies such as deep brain reorienting (DBR) are also showing extremely promising results in specifically addressing unprocessed traumas from childhood.

DBR is a therapy developed by Scottish psychiatrist Dr. Frank Corrigan, which helps people gently process these deeper layers of trauma-related distress. Instead of focusing mainly on the story of what happened, DBR works with the very first body responses that occur when something feels threatening or disconnected. These early responses often show up as sudden tension, freezing, sinking sensations, or a kind of inner "shock" that happens before any emotion forms.

When this shock passes, the body often reveals an older pain underneath—feelings of loneliness, rejection, or unmet needs that were too overwhelming to feel at the time. DBR helps you slow down these reactions in a safe, contained way so they no longer hijack you in the present. For many people, the eating disorder grew around these old wounds. When certain sensations or emotions feel too intense, the eating disorder steps in like a protector—numbing, distracting, or controlling the body to avoid the deeper pain. DBR gives you a way to process that pain at a pace your nervous system can handle, without needing to relive anything or be overwhelmed.

By gently working with the body's earliest signals of danger and unmet needs, DBR helps untangle the patterns that made food, weight, or control feel like the only way to cope. Over time, clients often describe feeling less triggered, more connected to themselves, and freer to develop healthy, compassionate ways of responding to distress—because the body is no longer bracing from the past.

Reaching out for support is your Wise Self recognising that some healing work can't be done alone. It's like being a good friend to yourself—the kind of friend who doesn't expect you to sail through a raging storm without help. Instead, you reach for the guidance of experienced sailors—people who've navigated these waters before, who can help steady your course when the waves are high.

Journalling Prompt Reflections

- When do you notice yourself "abandoning ship"—dissociating from your body or emotional experience?
- Which reconnection practice (breath, movement, sensory grounding) helped you return to the present moment most effectively?
- What painful truth has your self-attacking pattern been protecting you from facing?
- What evidence can you show your Protector Modes that your Wise Self can handle difficulty without abandoning your Lost Child?

What's Possible

This work is hard. It usually takes longer than you'd like, and more support than you feel you "should" need. Progress is slower and messier than any neat description of recovery suggests. And still, it's worth it.

Recovery is about building flexibility—the capacity to notice what's happening and respond with some degree of choice rather than being completely at the mercy of automatic protective responses.

Some days you can stay more connected to your body and emotions; other days you need protection and disconnection. Some days your Wise Self leads; other days your Protector Modes take over, and you do your best to get through until you can regroup.

What Changes over Time

Over time—you can build genuine capacity to stay with difficult feelings without immediately needing to dissociate or use eating disorder behaviours. Your Wise Self can grow stronger, able to provide the safety and care your Lost Child needs. Your Protector Modes can learn to trust your leadership, softening their grip incrementally.

You can develop the ability to recognise when you've been triggered and have tools to help yourself regulate. You can learn to be vulnerable with carefully chosen people who prove themselves trustworthy. You can reclaim sovereignty over your own life, making choices based on your authentic needs and values rather than being driven by protective patterns from the past.

In recovery, your trauma history doesn't disappear, and the eating disorder patterns may not vanish completely. But you can move from being imprisoned by them to living with increasing freedom alongside them. You can learn to captain your own ship—imperfectly, with setbacks, with ongoing challenges—but with your Wise Self at the helm more often than your Protector Modes.

Part of that journey involves learning to *acknowledge* your history rather than spending all your energy trying to avoid it. Think of it like an old, disturbing movie—one your body keeps replaying in the background. When you try to ignore it or block it out, it still plays . . . you just have to keep flinching every time you hear a scene. But when your Wise Self gently puts that movie on a shelf—labelled and understood—it stops dominating the room. It's still there, part of your story, but you don't have to relive it every time a memory stirs. You can glance at it, remember it, and even grieve it—*without being pulled back in*. That's what freedom begins to feel like.

Your Lost Child has been waiting for this. She's been carrying your unheard voice, your genuine feelings, your pain, your terror—all of it—waiting for someone strong enough to see her, hold her pain, and stay present when things get difficult.

Through consistent practice, professional support when needed, and patience with the nonlinear nature of this work, your Wise Self can become that person. Not always knowing what to do, but committed to staying aboard the ship even when storms arise. Committed to never abandoning your Lost Child the way others once did.

The journey continues. Rather than heading toward some perfect recovered state, we are aiming for increasing capacity, flexibility, and freedom. One practice at a time. One moment of staying present at a time. One day of choosing your Wise Self's leadership over your Protector Modes' urgency at a time.

Eventually, acceptance may emerge—not acceptance that what happened was okay, but acceptance that staying trapped in grief or rage keeps you bound to the past. Each stage unfolds in its own time; none can be rushed.

It's possible. It's hard. And you don't have to do it alone.

12 The Voyage Continues

> *What is it to have succeeded? To be able to reach the end of your life and say to the child within, "I did not betray you, for against all odds in whatever small way I was capable of, I chose to follow my dream."*
>
> —Tahlia Hunter[1]

Your ship now sails with a captain at the helm. Your Wise Self may not lead every moment, but just knowing it's there—learning, practising, showing up again and again changes the course. The crew, your Protector Modes, is learning to work together under this new leadership. Your Lost Child is on deck, no longer locked below. The ship bears scars from past voyages, but it's seaworthy and it's yours.

Storms will still come. But you're no longer swaying according to the whims of others' expectations, searching desperately for substitutes for missing emotional vitamins, or trying to avoid the wounds from early experiences that left you caught between longing to be seen and fearing what being seen might bring.

You're learning to sail your own ship. You're choosing vulnerability and uncertainty over the false security of perfectionism and overcontrol. We can't control nature—the weather, the seas, our own bodies. The harder we try to force control, the more out of control things feel, which only reinforces the old beliefs: that your body cannot be trusted, that your needs are too much, and that you are somehow separate from the vessel that carries you through life.

Healing means reconnecting with all parts of yourself, especially the ones you learned to disown, and learning to look after them.

The eating patterns were never evidence of some inherent flaw. They developed from a mismatch between your temperament, the way you're wired, and the emotional vitamins that went missing in your early environment. Even when the world taught you that certain parts of you were wrong or unacceptable or burdensome, those disowned parts didn't disappear. They drove chaos in your internal world and your relationships, creating the urge to block them out through eating disorder behaviours.

DOI: 10.4324/9781003355878-13

Being messy is part of being human. Having needs and emotions is what makes us alive. You already have everything you need—your temperament, your sensitivity, your drive, your capacity for connection. These are your sails. When you understand them and work with them rather than against them, you can adjust to whatever weather arises with your whole crew working together.

Part 1: The Journey You've Taken

The question was never "what's wrong with you?" The real question was always: what happened to you? Which emotional vitamins did you receive, and which went missing? How did you make sense of those gaps?

Your Lost Child carried the wounds from those missing vitamins. Often she was blamed, seen as the problem—too sensitive, too needy, too much. Blaming her created a sense of control in a world that felt chaotic and unpredictable. If she was the problem, there was something you could fix. If she was the culprit, the world made sense.

Your Protector Modes stepped in to help. Eating and weight control behaviours became ways to cope, to manage overwhelming emotions, to create substitutes for what was missing—or to deny that your Lost Child existed at all, suppressing and pushing down everything she felt and needed.

Through this book, you've begun to see which vitamins were missing and looked back at your younger self with growing compassion, understanding how she had to survive and how food and body control became part of that survival story—survival strategies rather than evidence of anything lacking in you.

Often, these missing ingredients stretch back through generations. You may be the first person in your family line to truly face this pain, to grieve, to learn how to care for your own Lost Child. In understanding what happened to you, you're beginning to mend something larger—the intergenerational wounds passed down, the cultural and schema mindsets based on power and threat rather than connection and genuine living.

Your Wise Self is strengthening, and you're learning to provide those missing vitamins for yourself and to receive them from others. The deficiency never defined you as a person—it shaped your survival strategies, and now you're discovering what real nourishment feels like.

You're practising receiving, trusting that sharing your vulnerability with your own Wise Self—and with carefully chosen others—can lead to inner calm and freedom. Not everyone has the emotional maturity to be trusted with your vulnerable parts. This trust needs to be earned through consistent emotional presence—showing up with both compassion and honesty, offering genuine support rather than simply telling you what you want to hear. You're breaking free from outdated automatic patterns and starting to make your own choices.

Jane Goodall reminded us that *only when head and heart work together can we reach our true potential*. As your Lost Child and other Child Modes have come back on deck and been accepted as the core of your humanity, you've worked toward joining your thinking and feeling parts. Your Lost Child (heart) and Wise Self (integrated wisdom) are learning to work together, rather than being hijacked by Protector Modes operating in crisis.

You listen to your Lost Child's emotions and needs as a compass for understanding what you need. She hears your messages and feels safer, less fearful of being abandoned or lost. This inner bond is the foundation for everything else.

You also listen to your Protector Modes, hearing their warnings and concerns. This allows them to let go of old survival-based coping, to negotiate, and to evolve. They can begin turning toward your actual purpose in life—aligned with your unique traits and chosen values.

And you acknowledge the old messages from your Inner Critic, recognising which are outdated mindsets based on concepts you choose not to be dominated by anymore.

Caring for the One in Your Charge

Recovery reveals a responsibility many of us never realised we carried: there is a human who depends entirely on us. A human whose body needs nourishment and rest, whose emotions need to be heard rather than silenced, whose safety must be protected. That human is you.

At some point, the caregiver role must transfer—from those who shaped you, from the eating disorder that tried to fill the gaps—to your Wise Self, who can now offer what was missing: steadiness, guidance, and compassion.

Self-care is a stance. Small, consistent acts of loyalty to your own wellbeing: eating when your body signals hunger, pausing when exhaustion arrives, setting boundaries with people or internal voices that cause harm. These are the basic duties of caring for someone in your charge.

Each day becomes an invitation to check in with your Lost Child: What does the small one in me need right now? Sometimes the answer will be practical—food, sleep, a slower pace. Sometimes it will be emotional—comfort, understanding, a moment to cry without self-judgement. Whatever arises, the commitment of your Wise Self is to stay present and respond with protection rather than punishment.

This is the opposite of abandonment. When you choose, again and again, not to walk away from yourself, you form a new internal contract: I will not leave you alone with this.

Recovery becomes an act of guardianship. You're learning not only to live without the eating disorder, but to take up the role you were always meant to hold: the trustworthy caretaker of your own life.

Part 2: Recovery as Imperfect Practice

Permission for the Winding Path

In Chapter 3, you met your Perfectionistic Overcontroller—the mode that believes flawless performance is the only path to safety. Now we need to address how this mode tries to hijack recovery itself, turning the healing process into another impossible standard you can fail at.

If there's one message to take from this book, it's that recovery requires persistence through *imperfection*. Many people approach recovery the same way they approached their eating disorder—with rigid rules, impossible standards, and harsh self-judgement when they inevitably fall short. This perfectionism about recovery becomes another version of the eating disorder, just with different content. Instead of demanding perfect control over food and body, it demands perfect control over recovery.

Healing happens through trying and struggling. Through taking steps forward and sometimes backwards. Through being human rather than performing an idealised version of healing.

The Messy Reality

Remember the learning pit from Chapter 4? This is where you're living now—somewhere in those messy, confusing waters between the eating disorder identity and your true self. Recovery moves in spirals and circles. Some days you'll feel like you're making progress. Other days, it may feel like you're slipping backwards. Some weeks, you'll lead with clarity and strength. Other weeks, your Protector Modes might take over, and you'll struggle to access any of the tools you've worked so hard to learn. All of this is still recovery.

It's completely normal to lose your way sometimes. What matters most is whether you pause long enough to notice where you are. If you realise you've wandered off course, you can always choose to return to your way. The road is still there, but it's perfectly normal to find yourself on the odd detour from time to time. And each time you find your way back, your Wise Self grows stronger.

Remember 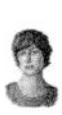 Sophie, who's Perfectionistic Overcontroller, insisted everything be done exactly right to avoid criticism? She still sometimes gets caught in that rigid thinking, especially under stress. But now she notices it happening, can name the mode that's activated, and can ask herself: "Is this genuinely important, or is my Overcontroller demanding impossible standards to feel safe?"

Or 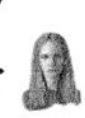 Emma, whose Detached Protector would numb through bingeing when her sensitive system felt overwhelmed? She still sometimes reaches for that pattern. But more often now, she catches the impulse earlier, understands what's driving it, and can offer her Lost Child what she actually needs-usually quiet, space, or gentle connection rather than food.

Some days, your Protector Modes will run the ship. Simply recognising them is progress—noticing when you're denying, pretending, performing, and going numb, saying "I'm fine" when you're not or feeling disgust toward your Lost Child's emotions and needs. These patterns are all driven by fears based on what you learned about yourself and your body in earlier times.

Triggers don't disappear, but they become opportunities to strengthen your Wise Self–Lost Child bond. You get better at navigating them. You'll still use eating behaviours sometimes under extreme stress. The difference is that you notice sooner, you have tools to return to yourself, and you understand what's happening.

What's Actually Changed

You have a Wise Self who shows up more often, and you're learning to embrace your inborn traits and work to your strengths. Your Lost Child trusts you more than she did, and your Protector Modes are less rigid, more willing to negotiate. You can feel emotions without being destroyed by them, whilst building the capacity to receive nourishment and ask for what you need.

Relationships are becoming places of genuine connection. You're less and less at the mercy of cultural mindsets and other people's expectations of who you need to be—nice, good, self-sacrificing, polite, self-effacing—to be deserving of love and care.

The shift:

From "I am my eating disorder" to "I have patterns I'm learning to take care of"
From "I'm broken and need fixing" to "I'm wounded and learning to heal"
From "Recovery means perfect control" to "Recovery means flexible presence"

Understanding Lapses and Relapses

One way perfectionism sabotages healing is by treating any setback as a complete failure. There's a key difference between a lapse and a relapse.

A lapse is a temporary slip—a moment or day or week when you use eating disorder behaviours whilst still generally moving in the direction of recovery. Lapses are normal and part of recovery itself. Every person recovering from an eating disorder will have lapses. They happen because old patterns are deeply ingrained, stress makes your system reach for familiar coping strategies, your Protector Modes still activate under threat, and building new neural pathways takes time and repeated practice.

When you have a lapse, your Critic might try to interpret it as evidence you're failing: "See? You can't do this. You're back where you started."

Your Wise Self can respond differently:

> I used an eating coping behaviour today. That makes sense—I was overwhelmed and my system reached for what it knows. What was happening before I used the behaviour? What do I need right now? How can I get back on track tomorrow?

A lapse becomes an opportunity to practise self-compassion, investigate what triggered the behaviour, and return to recovery tools—getting back on track is the practice itself.

A *relapse* happens when you sustain a return to eating disorder patterns for weeks or months, when you stop using recovery tools and re-engage fully with eating disorder thinking, or when you abandon treatment or support.

Even relapses aren't permanent states. A relapse signals that something needs attention—perhaps you need more support, different strategies, or to address underlying issues that haven't been fully worked through. A relapse provides information about what you need next and whether it's time to reach out for help.

The key question isn't "Did I have a setback?" but rather "What do I do after the setback?" Your Critic might say: "Give up. You've proven you can't do this." Your Wise Self says: "Get curious. What happened? What support do I need? What's one small step I can take today to move back toward recovery?"

You're learning a new language, and sometimes you'll slip back into the old one—and that's what is expected.

When Perfectionism Tries to Hijack Recovery

As you continue your recovery journey, your Overcontroller will set tests—ways of thinking that sound reasonable but actually sabotage your progress. Here are common traps and how your Wise Self can respond:

Perfectionism Says	*Wise Self Responds*
"You ate more than you planned—you've failed today."	"You nourished yourself—that's what matters. The exact amount is less important than the willingness to eat."
"Recovery should be faster. Everyone else recovers quicker."	"Recovery moves at exactly the pace it needs to for your system. Comparing creates suffering."
"If you can't follow your meal plan perfectly, why bother?"	"Meal plans are guidelines, not rigid rules. Eating imperfectly is still progress."
"One setback ruins all your progress."	"One setback is one moment. All the other moments you've chosen recovery still count."
"You should do this without help."	"Healing almost always requires support. Asking for help is strength."
"If you were committed, you wouldn't struggle."	"Struggling is part of recovery. Commitment is measured by showing up when things are hard."
"You had eating disorder thoughts—you're not recovering."	"Thoughts are just thoughts—not behaviours. They don't disappear immediately. Recovery is about how you respond to them."

When you notice these perfectionistic thoughts arising, pause and ask: "Is this my Overcontroller trying to run recovery? What would my Wise Self say right now?" This simple pause—this moment of checking which voice is speaking—can shift your entire trajectory.

Reparenting Messages for Your Journey: Your Overcontroller has been the dominant voice for so long that your Wise Self's permission-giving voice might feel unfamiliar, even uncomfortable. These reparenting messages help strengthen that gentler, wiser voice—the voice your Lost Child has been waiting to hear.

Read these slowly. Notice which ones you resist and which ones create a softening:

- You are allowed to recover imperfectly.
- Progress, not perfection, is what matters.
- Every attempt counts, even the messy ones.
- You can learn from mistakes without attacking yourself for making them.
- Recovery isn't a straight line—setbacks are part of the path forward.
- You're allowed to struggle and still be doing this "right."
- Your worth isn't determined by how perfectly you recover.
- Other people's recovery journey doesn't diminish yours.
- You can be a beginner at this, learning as you go.
- Imperfection is evidence that you're living and trying, not failing.
- You deserve compassion, especially when things are hard.

Choose the message that resonates most strongly or that you most need to hear right now. Write it somewhere you'll see it daily. Each time your Overcontroller starts demanding perfect recovery, read this message out loud to yourself—not as a rule to follow but as a reminder that your Wise Caring Self is here to support your Lost Child.

Your Wise Self's Promise

Let your Wise Self make this promise to your Lost Child: "I see you. I see all the shame you've been carrying, all the struggle you've tried to hide, all the fear that you're not good enough exactly as you are. I'm here now, and I won't demand perfection from you. I won't attack you when things are hard. I won't abandon you when you struggle.

You don't have to earn my care through flawless performance. You don't have to prove your worth through achievement. You don't have to be perfect to deserve love. I'll show up—imperfectly but consistently. When you make mistakes, I'll stay with you through them. When you feel shame, I'll remind you that being human means being imperfect. When you struggle, I'll ask, "What's hard about this? What do you need?" rather than "Why are you failing?"

You're safe with me. You're allowed to be messy, confused, struggling, and learning. We're learning together—and learning means being imperfect whilst we practise. That's not just allowed—it's how growth actually happens.""

Moving forward with your life requires you to become skilled at being imperfect, whilst continuing to show up for yourself with compassion. Every messy step forward counts. Every moment you choose self-compassion over self-attack matters. Every time you notice perfectionism and choose differently, you're recovering—and learning to be true to who you are rather than a slave to others' expectations.

Part 3: The Lifelong Practice

Daily, Cyclical, and Crisis Practices

Recovery is a process of self-growth—becoming yourself, developing compassion, becoming more joined up, and accepting your whole self as a lifelong practice. Some practices you've learned in this book you might use daily: checking in with and feeling with your Lost Child using TREES or SPACE, grounding when dysregulated, offering reparenting messages, noticing which mode is active, using WAVE practice to manage eating-weight related urges, and choosing Wise Self leadership.

Some you might return to cyclically: mode interviews when stuck, deeper imagery work with your Lost Child, negotiating with Protector Modes, processing grief as new layers emerge.

Others you might turn to in crisis: intensive grounding, reaching out for support, using TREES with overwhelming emotions, and reconnecting with your "why" for recovery.

Continuing this work is about maintaining your relationship with your Lost Child, your Wise Self presence, and the skills you've built. Appendix 28 provides an overview of the main techniques you have learned across this book and how to choose between them.

Living Your Values

Let your values be the compass you're moving toward. Recovery unfolds through the choices you make in the direction of what matters most—connection, creativity, contribution, compassion, and authenticity. Each day becomes an opportunity to act in ways that embody these values rather than letting eating disorder patterns make the decisions for you. Living this way is an ongoing, values-guided way of being in the world.

Reading this book is the first step toward your own self-discovery. As you move away from Protector Modes dominating your actions, you can begin to align more closely with becoming the person you are underneath, with your own values.

It can be helpful to journal, reflecting on questions such as: What kind of person do you want to be? What relationships do you want to cultivate? What brings you genuine joy (not eating disorder "highs")? What legacy do you want to leave? What would you do more or less of if the eating difficulties weren't taking up so much space?

Give yourself time for these to emerge as you move through the healing process, moving from "I'm in recovery" to "I'm living my life."

The Ongoing Relationship with Your Body

Re-establishing a relationship with your body takes time. Your body has carried the pain of past missing emotional vitamins or traumas. It's been blamed, bruised, battered, and vilified—made the culprit for being too much or not enough, which is why the starting point is acceptance. Acceptance acknowledges where you are and is the starting point that allows you to redirect from here.

Rebuilding trust with your body requires specific, consistent actions over time. For detailed guidance on creating the conditions that allow your body's signals to return—hunger, fullness, tiredness, comfort—see Appendix 29: Rebuilding Body Trust.

This is ongoing work. Recovery is about something simpler than body love: willingness to be in your body right now, to listen to what it's telling you, to treat it with basic care. Instead of pressuring yourself toward body love, aim for body neutrality—seeing your body as a vessel, a place from which you experience the world, a manifestation of nature rather than a separate object. Begin to notice that inside your body is a sense of aliveness. Recognise the work your body does for you every day—your organs functioning without you even thinking about it.

The real work is learning to *be in* our bodies, connecting to sensations with gentle presence—rather than objectifying them through Overcontroller-driven body checking and comparisons. With time, we can begin to treat our body as part of us—no longer the enemy.

A Wider View of Embodiment

Most of us have been taught to view the body as a sealed container—something that begins and ends at the boundary of our skin. Eating disorders intensify this narrow lens, pulling you into a small, isolated space where shape, weight, and constant self-monitoring seem to define your worth.

But your body is part of something larger. Your breath comes from forests. Your nourishment comes from sunlight, soil, and water. Your cells depend on the atmosphere around the Earth. When you remember that your life is continuously held by air, light, water, and the living world, something inside begins to ease. You begin to feel supported rather than alone, connected rather than defective.

Each day you feed yourself adequately, you're practising care. Each time you rest when tired, you're respecting your body's signals. Each moment you stay present in your body rather than dissociating, you're choosing embodiment.

Part 4: When You Need More Support

Remember that you don't have to do this alone—getting professional help is your Wise Self recognising what you need. Professional support is often essential, especially when your Lost Child's pain feels too overwhelming to manage alone, your Protector Modes are too rigid for self-help, or if your health or safety is at risk. Don't rely on your Invincible Overcontroller to assess whether you need help.

Medical assessment is essential along the way, and there will often be a requirement for medical monitoring to manage physical instability.

A multidisciplinary team can be incredibly helpful: a psychotherapist (for mode work, imagery, reparenting), a dietitian (for food relationship, meal planning), a GP/Psychiatrist (for medical monitoring and medication if needed), and peer support groups (for connection with others who understand).

Hope and Reality Held Together

As you reach the end of this book, it's important to recognise that the work might sometimes feel more difficult than you want it to be. It might take longer to recover than you anticipated. Setbacks happen, and some days you'll wonder if it's all worth it. It might feel easier to hold onto the eating difficulties. Your Protectors will urge you to stay with what you know.

Yet, it's important to remember that change is possible. Others have walked this path before you. Your Lost Child is already healing as a result of just being seen more often. Your Wise Self gets stronger with every practice. Your parts are becoming more connected, and you're building capacity you didn't have before. You can break free from eating disorder patterns. It's hard work, and it's possible to heal—both are true.

A Letter to Your Lost Child

When you feel the struggle, it can help to write a short letter from your Wise Self to your Lost Child—something you can return to when things are difficult.

Here's an example:

"Dear Lost Child,

> You've been waiting so long for someone to see you, to understand, to stay present when things are difficult. I'm here now. I'm learning how to be the person you've always needed.
>
> I know you're scared. I know you've been hurt. I know you learned not to trust care because it came with conditions or disappeared when you needed it most.
>
> I'm not perfect at this. I'm still learning. My Protector Modes still try to take over sometimes. But I keep coming back to you. I keep practising staying present. I keep choosing to see you and value you.

You don't have to hide below deck anymore. The storms are different now—they're the storms of present challenges, not the storms of original trauma. And you're not facing them alone.

I'm here. I'm not leaving. We're learning to sail together.

With love,

Your Wise Self"

I invite you to write your own.

Closing: The Ship Is Yours

Your ship is yours now. It bears the marks of every storm you've weathered—scars that tell the story of your survival and your courage. Your Lost Child is no longer locked below deck—she's finding her way into the light, slowly, at her own pace.

Some days you'll sail smoothly, and other days you'll face storms that test everything you've learned. All of this—the smooth sailing and the storms—is part of the journey. You're learning to sail—to read the weather, to adjust the sails, to stay steady when things get rough, to ask for help when you need it.

Your ship was always seaworthy. It just needed a captain who could see its worth—your worth—beneath all the protective strategies and survival patterns.

That captain is you. And she's here to stay

Love after Love[1]

by Derek Walcott

The time will come
when, with elation,
you will greet yourself arriving
at your own door, in your own mirror
and each will smile at the other's welcome,
and say, sit here. Eat.
You will love again the stranger who was your self.
Give wine. Give bread. Give back your heart
to itself, to the stranger who has loved you
all your life, whom you ignored
for another, who knows you by heart.
Take down the love letters from the bookshelf,
the photographs, the desperate notes,
peel your own image from the mirror.
Sit. Feast on your life.

That time is already beginning. Your Lost Child is arriving at the door. Your Wise Self is learning to say: sit here, eat, feast on your life.

Note

1 Maxwell, D. (2014). ***The Poetry of Derek Walcott 1948–2013. Selected by Glyn Maxwell.*** New York: Farrar, Straus and Giroux.

References

1. Tippett, K. & Goodall, J. (2020). The shadow of humanity and the spirit of animals a conversation. *Orion Magazine*, Autumn 2020. Available at https://orionmagazine.org/article/the-shadow-of-humanity-and-the-spirit-of-animals/
2. Dr. Florian Ruths (24th June, 2021). Meeting Core Needs During Isolation. "Get Your 5 Vitamins a Day!" A playful metaphor to explain and sustain the meeting of emotional needs, ISST virtual conference.
3. Roediger, E., Stevens, B. A., & Brockman, R. (2018). Contextual schema therapy: An integrative approach to personality disorders, emotional dysregulation, and interpersonal functioning. New Harbinger Publications
4. Boyce, W. T., & Ellis, B. J. (2005). Biological sensitivity to context: I. An evolutionary-developmental theory of the origins and functions of stress reactivity. *Development and Psychopathology*, *17*(2), 271–301.
5. Sim, L., & Peterson C. (2021). The peril and promise of sensitivity in eating disorders. *International Journal of Eating Disorders*, *54*(11), 2046–2056.
6. Joshua, P. R., Lewis, V., Simpson, S., Kelty, S. F., & Boer, D. P. (2023). What role do early life experiences play in eating disorders? The impact of parenting style, temperament and early maladaptive schemas. *Clinical Psychology & Psychotherapy*, *31*(1), e2904.
7. Rettew, D. (2013). Child temperament: New thinking about the boundary between traits and illness. W. W. Norton & Company.
8. Petrucelli, J. (2016). Body-states, body image and dissociation: When not-me is "not body". *Clinical Social Work Journal*, *44*, 18–26.
9. Zohar, A. H., Giladi, L., & Givati, T. (2007). Holocaust exposure and disordered eating: A study of multi-generational transmission. *European Eating Disorders Review*, *15*, 50–57.
10. Oldershaw, A., Startup, H., & Lavender, T. (2019). Anorexia nervosa and a lost emotional self: A psychological formulation of the development, maintenance, and treatment of anorexia nervosa. *Frontiers in Psychology*, *10*, 219.
11. Maté, G. (2019). *When the body says no: The cost of hidden stress.* Vermilion, London.
12. Cobbaert, L., Mitchell, P., Hay, P., & Perkes, I. (2026). Self-reported interoceptive sensibility across eating disorder symptoms: Associations with sociodemographic factors. *Journal of Eating Disorders*, *14*, 55.
13. Khalsa, S. S., Berner, L. A., & Anderson, L. M. (2022). Gastrointestinal interoception in eating disorders: Charting a new path. *Current Psychiatry Reports*, *24*(1), 47–60.
14. Tiemann, A., Ortmann, J., Rubo, M., Meyer, A. H., Munsch, S., Vögele, C., & van Dyck, Z. (2025). The relevance of cardiac and gastric interoception for disordered eating behavior. *Journal of Eating Disorders*, *13*, 114.
15. Alcott, L. (1869). *Little Women; or, Meg, Jo, Beth, and Amy.* Robert Brothers.

16. Nottingham, J. (2017). *The learning challenge: How to guide your students through the learning pit to achieve deeper understanding (Corwin Teaching Essentials).* Corwin Press.
17. Balban, M. Y., Neri, E., Kogon, M. M., Weed, L., Nouriani, B., Jo, B., Holl, G., Zeitzer, J. M., Spiegel, D., & Huberman, A. D. (2023). Brief structured respiration practices enhance mood and reduce physiological arousal. *Cell Reports Medicine, 4*(1), 100895.
18. 5 effective breathing exercises for anxiety. Medicalnewstoday.com (2022). https://www.medicalnewstoday.com/articles/breathing-exercises-for-anxiety.
19. Monti, A., Porciello, G., Panasiti, M., & Agliotti, S. (2022). The inside of me: Interoceptive constraints of self in neuroscience and clinical psychology. *Psychological Research, 86*(8), 2468–2477.
20. Siegel, D., & Bryson, T. (2012) *The whole-brain child: 12 revolutionary strategies to nurture your child's developing mind.* Bantam Books.
21. Nummenmaa, L., Glerean, E., Hari, R., & Hietanen, J. K. (2014). Bodily maps of emotions. *Proceedings of the National Academy of Sciences of the USA, 111*(2), 646–651.
22. Terry, M. L., & Leary, M. R. (2011). *Self-compassion, self-regulation, and health.* Self and Identity, 10(3), 352–362.
23. Brockman, R. N., Simpson, S., Hayes, C., van der Wijngaart, R., & Smout, M. (2023). *Cambridge guide to schema therapy.* Cambridge University Press.
24. Brooks, A. W. (2014). Get excited: Reappraising pre-performance anxiety as excitement. *Journal of Experimental Psychology: General, 143*(3), 1144–1158.
25. Taylor, J. B. (2008). *My stroke of insight: A brain scientist's personal journey.* Viking.
26. Gross, J. J., & Levenson, R. W. (1997). Hiding feelings: The acute effects of inhibiting positive and negative emotions. *Journal of Abnormal Psychology, 106*, 95–103.
27. McGonigal, K. (2019). *The joy of movement: How exercise helps us find happiness, hope, connection, and courage.* Avery.
28. Thoreau, H. D. (1854). *Walden; or, Life in the woods.* Ticknor and Fields.
29. Kearney, B. E., & Lanius, R. A. (2022). The brain–body disconnect: A somatic sensory basis for trauma-related disorders. *Frontiers in Neuroscience, 16*, 1015749.
30. Lanius, R. A., Terpou, B. A., and McKinnon, M. C. (2020). The sense of self in the aftermath of trauma: Lessons from the default mode network in posttraumatic stress disorder. *European Journal of Psychotraumatology, 11*, 1807703.
31. Fimiani, R., Gazzillo, F., Fiorenza, E., Rodomonti, M., & Silberschatz, G. (2020). *Traumas and their consequences according to control-mastery theory. Psychodynamic Psychiatry, 48*(2), 113–139,

Online Appendices

Appendices for this book, as listed below, can be found in the following support material pages: www.routledge.com/9781032410227.

Appendix 1: What Is Schema Therapy for Eating Difficulties?
Appendix 2: The Provisions Barrels Exercise
Appendix 3: Temperament Survey
Appendix 4: Schema Mindsets and Core Needs
Appendix 5: Life Story Timeline Exercise: Mapping Your Story
Appendix 6: Modes—Meeting our Inner Parts
Appendix 7: Creating Your Mode Map
Appendix 8: Feelings Wheel
Appendix 9: Physicalising Emotions—a Guided Practice
Appendix 10: A Simple Guide to Working with Your Harsh Inner Critic Voice
Appendix 11: The Rejected Inner Child Transformation Visualisation
Appendix 12: Reparenting Messages for Your Inner Child
Appendix 13: Developing Emotional Fluency Through Tree
Appendix 14: The Emotional Vitamins Barrel Practice
Appendix 15: Movement Practices for Integration
Appendix 16: Music as an Emotional Companion for the Lost Child
Appendix 17: Complete Deprivation Checklist
Appendix 18: Wave: Applying Your Emotional Skills to Eating Urges
Appendix 19: Transitioning from Mechanical to Intuitive Eating—a Detailed Guide
Appendix 20: Your Personal Letting Go Map
Appendix 21: The ANCHOR Framework: Trust, Schemas, and Wise Risk-Taking
Appendix 22: Old Mindsets versus Growth Mindsets
Appendix 23: The Importance of Play in Recovery
Appendix 24: Your Temperament as Natural Design
Appendix 25: Discovering Your Authentic Values
Appendix 26: Detailed Grounding and Reconnection Practices
Appendix 27: Why Gut Sensations Can Trigger Trauma Alarm Systems
Appendix 28: When to Use TREES, WAVE, SPACE, INTERNAL COMPASS and ANCHOR Practices
Appendix 29: Rebuilding Body Trust and Healing Body Image

Index

For Product Safety Concerns and Information please contact our
EU representative GPSR@taylorandfrancis.com Taylor & Francis
Verlag GmbH, Kaufingerstraße 24, 80331 München, Germany